Thieme Almanac 2007

Acupuncture and Chinese Medicine

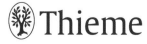 Thieme

Library of Congress Cataloging-in-Publication Data
is available from the publisher.

Calligraphies by Helmut Magel, Heilpraktiker,
Wuppertal, Germany: tcm@helmut-magel.de

We wish to thank 3B Scientific for the kind support

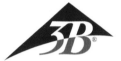

Distributor of Seirin acupuncture needles in Europe
(www.3b-akupunktur.de)

© 2007 Georg Thieme Verlag,
Rüdigerstrasse 14, 70469 Stuttgart, Germany
http://www.thieme.de
Thieme New York,
333 Seventh Avenue, New York, NY 10001, USA
http://www.thieme.com

Cover design: Original artwork by Peng Shi-qing,
Chengdu, Sichuan, China (courtesy of Paradigm
Publications, Brookline, MA, USA)
Typesetting by Druckerei Sommer, Feuchtwangen
Printed in Germany by Grafisches Centrum Cuno, Calbe

10-ISBN 3-13-142611-X (GTV)
13-ISBN 978-3-13-142611-6 (GTV)
10-ISBN 1-58890-425-3 (TNY)
13-ISBN 978-1-58890-425-6 (TNY)   1 2 3 4 5 6

Overview

Our Mission

Our mission is to bring into existence and widespread use a tool for those working in, or joining the field of acupuncture and traditional Eastern medicine, which will help them to successfully navigate the many and often-complex passageways. We aspire to create and maintain a level playing field environment that encourages diversity in approaches, recognizing that the field thrives in this diversity.

The Editors Wish to Thank:

Belgium
François Beyens

China
Dai Lin

France
Dee Braig
Patrick Shan

Germany
Gaby Balling
Helmut Magel
Oskar Mastalier
Gerd Ohmstede
Gabriel Stux
Jürgen Voigt
Velia Wortman-Chow

Israel
Yair Maimon

Italy
Roberto Gatto

The Netherlands
Junko Ida
Holly Tops
Albert de Vos

Sweden
Peter Torssell

Switzerland
Simon Becker
Marian R. Nielsen Joos

UK
Selina MacNair
Daniel Maxwell

USA
Ronald M. Bloom
Sean Donovan
Marnae Ergil
Bob Felt
Bryan Frank
Diana Fried
Bonnie Thomas
Ken Rose
Sylvia Seroussi Chartoux

Editorial Board

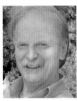
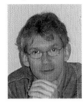

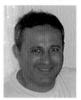

Isaac Cohen is a Guest Scientist at the University of California, San Francisco, and has been involved with the UCSF Cancer Research Center and UCSF Center for Reproductive Endocrinology for the past 10 years. He is one of the founding members of the University of California, San Francisco Carol Franc Buck Breast Care Center Complementary and Alternative Medicine Research Program. He is a co-investigator on numerous basic and clinical grants and has assembled teams of scientists from four different universities to work on his projects.

Isaac is an international leader in the study and application of natural products for cancer and women's health. He graduated from the Pacific College of Oriental Medicine in San Diego and completed his doctorate at the Postgraduate Institute of Oriental Medicine in Hong Kong, China. His expertise is in translational science and, working from the bench to the clinic, he has developed a number of products for clinical testing that have been awarded an FDA IND, as well as a pipeline of over 50 candidate drugs. Isaac is a co-founder and the President of Bionovo, Inc.

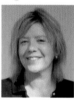

Angelika-M. Findgott started her career as a commercial apprentice in the publishing business and later concentrated on marketing and advertising. She has been with Thieme International since 1998, where she is editor in charge of the complementary medicine book program.

Table of Contents

List of Abbreviations and Acronyms

AACMA Australian Acupuncture and Chinese Medicine Association
AACP Acupuncture Association of Chartered Physiotherapists, UK
AAMA American Academy of Medical Acupuncture
AAOM American Association of Oriental Medicine
ABMA American Board of Medical Acupuncture
ACAOM Accreditation Commission for Acupuncture and Oriental Medicine, USA
ACCME Australian Council for Chinese Medicine Education
ACHI Association of Chinese Herbalists in Ireland
ACMP Association of Chinese Medicine Practitioners
ACRWG Acupuncture Regulatory Working Group, UK
ACUMEN Acupuncture for Menorrhagia, UK
ADS acupuncture detoxification specialist
AFA Association Française d'Acupuncture (French Association of Acupuncture)
AGTCM Arbeitsgemeinschaft für Klassische Akupunktur und Traditionelle Chinesische Medizin e.V. (Association for Classical Acupuncture and TCM), Germany
AHMAC Australian Health Ministers' Advisory Council
AHPA American Herbal Products Association
AIAM Associazione Italiana di Agopuntura-moxibustion e Medicina Tradizionale Cinese (Italian Association of Acupuncture-moxibustion and TCM)
AMED ancillary medicine database
AMIA Associazione Medica Italiana Agopuntura (Italian Medical Association of Acupuncture)
AOM acupuncture and Oriental medicine
ARRC Acupuncture Research Resource Centre, UK

ARRCBASE Acupuncture Research Resource Centre's bibliographic database
ART Acupuncture Randomized Trials
ARTG Australian Register of Therapeutic Goods
AWB Acupuncturists Without Borders, USA
BAAB British Acupuncture Accreditation Board
BAcC British Acupuncture Council
BMA British Medical Association
BMAS British Medical Acupuncture Society
CAM complementary and alternative medicine
CaPSURE Cancer of the Prostate Strategic Urologic Research Endeavor
CCAOM Council of Colleges of Acupuncture and Oriental Medicine, USA
CCCPH Centre for Community Care and Primary Health, UK
CE continuing education
CEDRE Centre d'Études et de Recherches en Ethnomédecine (Center for the Development and Research in Ethnomedicine), France
CF chronic fatigue
CMR Chinese Medicine Registration (Act 2000), Australia
CMRB Chinese Medicine Registration Board, Australia
CNT clean needle technique
COPA Council on Post Secondary Accreditation, USA
COPD chronic obstructive pulmonary disease
CPD Continuing Professional Development
CRREW Community Relief and Rebuilding through Education and Wellness, Pakistan
CTCMA College of Traditional Chinese Medicine Practitioners and Acupuncturists of British Columbia, Canada

DAAAM Deutsche Akademie für Akupunktur und Aurikulomedizin (German Academy for Acupuncture and Auriculomedicine)

DÄGfA Deutsche Ärztegesellschaft für Akupunktur (German Medical Association of Acupuncture)

DAGD Deutsche Akupunktur Gesellschaft Düsseldorf (German Acupuncture Society Düsseldorf)

DGfAN Deutsche Gesellschaft für Akupunktur und Neuraltherapie (German Society for Acupuncture and Neural Therapy)

DH Department of Health, UK

DPCS Drugs Poisons and Controlled Substances Act, Australia (Victoria)

DSHEA Dietary Supplement and Health Education Act, USA

EAM East Asian medicine

ECTS European Credit Transfer and Accumulation System

EHEA European Higher Education Area

EHPA European Herbal Practitioners Association

EIOM European Institute of Oriental Medicine

EMBASE Excerpta Medica Database

EMT emergency medical technician

ETCMA European Traditional Chinese Medicine Association

EUFOM Beroepsorganisatie Acupunctur (Federation for Acupuncturists), Belgium

EuroTCM European Register of Organizations of Traditional Chinese Medicine

FDA Food and Drug Administration, USA

FEMA Federal Emergency Management Agency, USA

FISA Federazione Italiana delle Società di Agopuntura (Italian Federation of the Acupuncture Society)

GERAC German Acupuncture Trials

GRICMED German Research Institute of Chinese Medicine

GST Goods and Services Tax, Australia

HCC hepatocellular carcinoma cancer

HIV human immunodeficiency virus

ICMART International Council of Medical Acupuncture and Related Techniques

IRCHM Irish Register of Chinese Herbal Medicine

JCCMA Joint Consultative Committee for Medical Acupuncture, Australia

KSAs knowledge, skills, and attitudes

MYMOP Measure Yourself Medical Outcome Profile

NAAV Nederlandse Artsen Acupunctuur Verenigung (Dutch Medical Acupuncture Association)

NADA National Acupuncture Detoxification Association, USA

NAFO Norsk akupunkturforening (Norwegian Acupuncture Association)

NASC National Academic Standards Committee, Australia

NCCAM National Center for Complementary and Alternative Medicine, USA

NCCAOM National Commission for the Certification of Acupuncture and Oriental Medicine, USA

NGO non-governmental organization

NHC National Herbal Council, Ireland

NHMRC National Health and Medical Research Centre, Australia

NHS National Health Service, UK

NIH National Institutes of Health, USA

NK natural killer

NOKUT Nasjonalt organ for kvalitet i utdanninga (Norwegian Agency for Quality Assurance in Education)

NSAIDs Non-steroidal anti-inflammatory drugs

NVA Nederlandse Verenigung voor Acupunctuur (Dutch Association for Acupuncture)

NWG National Working Group

OS over-training syndrome

OTC over-the-counter

PA Praktiserende Akupunktører (Association of Acupuncture Practitioners), Denmark

PRC People's Republic of China

PTSD post-traumatic stress disorder

RCT randomized controlled trial

RECIST response evaluation criteria in solid tumors

RMIT Royal Melbourne Institute of Technology, Australia

SAATCM	Svenska Akupunkturförbundet Traditionell Kinesik Medicin (Swedish Acupuncture Association for TCM)
SfH	Skills for Health, UK
SIA	Société Internationale d'Acupuncture (International Acupuncture Society), France
SIA	Società Italiana Agopuntura (Italian Acupuncture Society)
SPO-TCM	Swiss Professional Organization for Traditional Chinese Medicine
SMART	Self Management and Recovery Training
SR	Statutory Regulation
STRICTA	STandards for Reporting Interventions in Controlled Trials of Acupuncture, UK
SUSDP	Standard for the Uniform Prescribing of Drugs and Poisons, Australia
TCM	Traditional Chinese Medicine
TCMCI	Traditional Chinese Medicine Council of Ireland
TEAM	traditional East Asian medicine
TGA	Therapeutic Goods Administration, Australia
THMPD	Traditional Herbal Medicinal Products Directive
TIM	traditional Iranian medicine
VEGF	vascular endothelial growth factor
WFAS	World Federation of Acupuncture–moxibustion Societies, China
WFCMS	World Federation of Chinese Medicine Societies, USA
WHO	World Health Organization

For more abbreviations of US organizations please see "Organizations and Associations in the USA," p. 163, Professional Developments, Legislation, and Regulation.

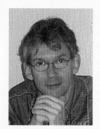

Stephen Birch

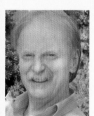

Michael McCarthy

Introduction to the Thieme Almanac

Acupuncture and Chinese herbal medicine, including the various forms of both of these therapies in many countries, and the numerous different massage therapies with their internally cultivated traditions that have come to us from Asia, are some of the therapies in the field known as traditional East Asian medicine (TEAM). This is a very large and broad area, with a great diversity of ideas and methods, which have been adapted in many different ways in the various countries where they now exist. This Almanac attempts to cover this wide range of therapies, methods, theories, and practices.

Over the years, many of us in the field of acupuncture and Chinese medicine have come to recognize both the power and weaknesses of these practices as they have developed within the twentieth and twenty-first centuries. The processes of development that have occurred in the more than one hundred countries where practitioners currently practice are extremely complex. The study, teaching, practice, and development of these systems are different in each country. Describing these alone provides work for many doctoral theses.

The therapies have developed not only because they are clinically effective but also for many other reasons. Among these are the following:

- *The therapies provide readily accessible and practical solutions to massive public health problems.*
- *They are alternative and natural, and, as such, attractive to both patients and practitioners.*
- *Because scientific research has been undertaken on them, they have become more acceptable to people living today.*
- *The therapies are less expensive.*
- *They offer hope when sometimes none is available.*
- *They allow us to marry cultures and histories in our global development.*
- *They offer us useful tools and techniques for not only maintaining our health but also developing ourselves as individuals.*
- *Some people are satisfied with the intellectual solutions the therapies offer; some with the practical solutions that they provide.*

A number of people in the field who have looked at TEAM's complex picture have traveled the world and have seen the various manifestations, developments, solutions, and problems it faces globally. Gradually an idea developed. In 2004 at the inspirational Rothenburg conference, one of these travelers, Ken Rose, first articulated this idea, and many of us jumped at what he articulated. This was that the field has no clear voice or space of its own; there is nowhere that TEAM can turn to, to find out about itself in all its complexity, diversity, and splendor.

The average practitioner in Kalamazoo, Michigan, knows as little about what a practitioner in Tokyo, Sydney, Kuala Lumpur, Dublin, Rome, Rio de Janeiro, Johannesburg, or Guang Dong is doing, any more than does the average practitioner from these places about the work being practiced in Kalamazoo. Because it is such a huge and diverse discipline, it is very difficult to find out about what is going on within the whole field. Not only that—many places have the same problems and challenges, and when solutions are found in one place, others elsewhere know nothing about them. Reinventing the wheel has a value in so far as one understands something better if one does it oneself, but on the other hand it can be a huge waste of time and resources. The field faces many challenges in many quarters, and these challenges can become smaller if a larger, more international, communication network is established. Also, if the field can find its voice through greater collaboration and communication among its diverse parts, that voice will become all the more effective and productive. In a nutshell, these are the reasons for producing this Almanac, which aims to help the field find its voice, and give wings, as it were, to our experiences, ideas, understanding, and methods. The idea is very simple, and yet very grand.

Ken's original idea was followed up by Thieme Medical Publishers through the support of Angelika Findgott and Malik Lechelt. They managed to capture the rest of us to work on his hypothesis. Stephen Birch and Isaac Cohen first came on board, followed by Felicity Moir, Michael McCarthy, Jane Lyttleton, Elisabeth Rochat de la Vallée, Mary Tagliaferri, Chris Dhaenens, and Yuhuan Zhang. Then many others came afterwards to work on this project. There have been a number of focus and editorial meetings, with many emails and conversations. Many people have offered support for the idea, which is now about to take its first flight.

It will not be possible to satisfy everyone the first time round. As yet, we are only a small group working on the Almanac, but the intention is to offer TEAM a place to find its voice. Thieme Publishing Group stands behind the idea and this publication to help to achieve that goal.

We encourage readers to contribute to future Almanac publications. In this current edition, we have put together a broad range of information from diverse sources on a wide selection of topics. Of course, not all the possibilities are covered, and equally, of course, many resources and contacts have not yet been mentioned. So please send your articles, together with your resource and contact details, to the Almanac. If you feel, for example, that your organization should be listed under the section listing groups that organize trips to poor, traumatized regions of the world, that's great. If you consider that a particular educational approach has not been properly addressed, please let us know; we all need to look at what is going on as regards the training of future practitioners. If you feel that your organization makes important contributions to, for example, research in the field, then write in and tell us about your group so that we can introduce you in the next edition of the Almanac. It is most important that you send us your contact information, so that we can expand the list of resources in the next issue.

We hope you enjoy and find value in this first edition.

Stephen Birch, Amsterdam, the Netherlands
Michael McCarthy, Dublin, Ireland

Thieme Almanac 2008 – Publishing Autumn 2007

*Personal subscription order details

USA, Mexico, Canada, Central and South America

Please add US$ 7.50 for shipping and handling. Additional shipping charges will be applied to orders from Alaska, Hawaii, Puerto Rico, and outside the USA. NY and PA residents add applicable sales tax. All prices quoted are payable in US currency or its equivalent sum in other currencies.

Europe, Africa, Asia, and Australia

For subscribers in Germany only: Order can be cancelled by giving written notice to the publisher (Georg Thieme Verlag, PF 30 11 20, 70451 Stuttgart) within 30 days of subscribing. Cancellation must be mailed within this period (date of mailing verified by postal stamp). Cancellation after this period must be received by 30th of September of the year prior to publication.

For subscribers outside of Germany: Invoices will be dispatched in each year, 4 weeks prior to publication. Cancellations must be received by 30th of September each year.

Shipping: Additional shipping and handling charges will be applied to all orders.

Written notification is required for all cancellations.

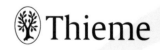

Easy ways to order:

 Visit our homepage and **order online** at **www.thieme.com**

The Americas:	customerservice @thieme.com	Thieme Publishers 333 Seventh Avenue New York, NY 10001 USA	Fax: +1 212 947 1112	Order Toll-Free 1 800 782 3488 Information: +1 212 760 0888
Rest of world:	custserv @thieme.de	Thieme International P. O. Box 30 11 20 70451 Stuttgart Germany	Fax: +49 711 8931 410	Information: +49 711 8931 421

Personal Subscription Order Form

Thieme Almanac 2008 – Publishing Autumn 2007

☐ Please enter my **personal subscription order*** for the annual **Thieme Almanac**

USA, Mexico, Canada, Central and South America US$ 49.95
Europe, Africa, Asia, and Australia € 39.95

I will be billed upon publication.

☐ **Bill me!** Please send me a proforma invoice (Bank charges extra).
☐ **Please charge my credit card:** ☐ Visa ☐ Euro-/MasterCard ☐ AMEX ☐ Access ☐ Discover

Card # ___ ___ ___ ___ - ___ ___ ___ ___ - ___ ___ ___ ___ - ___ ___ ___ Exp. Date _____

Important! Card Verification/Security code (3- or 4-digit code
found after the card number on the back of your credit card): _____

Date/Signature _____

USA only: ☐ **Check enclosed** for US$ _____ (U.S. funds, payable to Thieme)

First Name _____

Last Name _____

E-mail _____

Address _____

City/State/Postal Code _____

Country _____

Phone _____

Fax _____

EU countries only: If you are registered for VAT, please quote your VAT number: _____
For non-registered customers, applicable German VAT will be added to your invoice (excluding Germany and Austria).

☐ I want to order _____ additional copy/ies of the **Thieme Almanac 2007.** My contact details are listed above.

☐ Yes, I want to receive **Thieme Acupuncture and Oriental Medicine eNews,** an e-mail newsletter alerting me on new
publications in the field. My e-mail address is listed above.

*Please see reverse side for details.   **T538** cs X/2006   Printed in Germany. Prices subject to change.

History, Language, and Culture

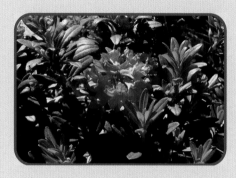

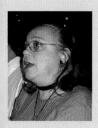

Elisabeth Rochat
de la Vallée

Introduction

This section, as indicated by its name, presents three main parts: history, language, and culture. History covers the recent as well as ancient history of Chinese medicine, within and outside of China.

The history of acupuncture and Chinese medicine in the non-Asian countries allows us to become aware of the differences existing in the origin and transmission of the practice of Chinese medicine in countries sometimes very closed, geographically and culturally. It also gives us an insight into the expansion of Chinese medicine all over the world and the tremendous change that occurred during the second half of the twentieth century.

We begin with the history of acupuncture in Italy; articles on the history of acupuncture in other countries (e.g., France, Sweden, Australia) will follow in future issues.

Some articles also relate to international achievements, such as the already long history of the Rothenburg Congress in this issue.

Concerning the history of medicine in China, the articles cover either a major evolving development or focus on a precise theme, such as the article on trepanation.

Some specific presentations are given to help readers who are not familiar with the chronology of Chinese history. A simple and general outline of the dynasties is a valuable, time-saving aid.

In future issues, we also intend to present studies on the cultural framework within which Chinese medicine was born and developed. We will have articles on the theory of acupuncture and Chinese medicine, discussions on key concepts (such as qi or shen) or on translation. Furthermore, we will have studies on the Chinese classical vision of life and the way of thinking surrounding the evolution of Chinese medicine, otherwise known as Chinese philosophy.

We wish to have in this section a variety of approaches and to provide an open platform for exchanges about these exciting topics that are not only history but also the very root of medicine and of our own understanding.

Elisabeth Rochat de la Vallée, PhD
Paris, France

Acupuncture or Trepanation?
A Study of Qin Minghe, a Skilled Physician of Tang China

Fan Ka Wai, PhD, Kowloon, Hong Kong

Abstract

In the early Tang dynasty, Emperor Gaozong summoned Qin Minghe to treat his *feng xuan* disease. Qin quickly diagnosed the emperor's malady, and was able to cure him by combining acupuncture with bloodletting. Many scholars considered that Qin's medical technique was trepanation or bloodletting. In this paper, the author will examine the studies undertaken by previous scholars, and point out that Qin Minghe relied on Chinese medicine in treating Emperor Gaozong. Qin's medical skill can be explained by Chinese medical theories and practices. The author sees no evidence for the use of trepanation or bloodletting.

Keywords

Acupuncture, bloodletting, Chinese medicine, Qin Minghe, Tang China, trepanation.

Introduction

The temptation to find evidence for foreign medical practices in pre-modern China is very great when cures are described as unexpected and extraordinary. After all, medical innovations travel readily along trade and pilgrimage routes, crossing national boundaries as readily as do bacteria. But while the history of Chinese medicine is in part the history of intercultural borrowings, in the absence of compelling evidence it is best to look first at local traditions. In this essay I will consider the evidence both for the use of indigenous medical techniques and foreign techniques in the context of Qin Minghe's (秦鳴鶴) treatment of Emperor Gaozong (唐高宗).

The illness of Emperor Gaozong (649–683 CE) allowed for a turning point in the history of the Tang Dynasty (618–907 CE). For a brief moment, Empress Wu (武則天) took advantage of the emperor's condition to seize power and establish her own dynasty, called the Zhou dynasty (690–705 CE).

From the Xianqing (顯慶) period (656–661 CE), the emperor suffered from *feng xuan* (風眩), literally "wind dizziness," which caused temporary blindness and obliged him to give up all official duties.

In the second year of Yongchun (682–683 CE) (永隆), Gaozong summoned Qin Minghe to the palace to treat his disease. Qin quickly diagnosed the emperor's malady and was able to cure him by combining acupuncture with bloodletting. Little is known about Qin, but his medical accomplishments have attracted scholarly attention, and in particular the work of the Japanese scholar Kuwabara Jitsuzo (桑原隲藏) (1870–1931) has shed a great deal of light on Tang medical practices. Kuwabara posited two related hypotheses:

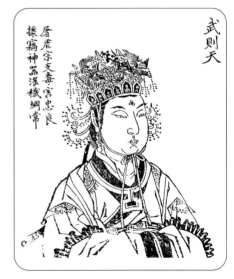

Fig. 1 Empress Wu

History, Language, and Culture

Acupuncture or Trepanation? A Study of Qin Minghe, a Skilled Physician of Tang China

first, that Qin was a foreigner, possibly from Rome, and second, that he relied heavily on trepanation. Kuwabara's article was translated into Chinese and had a great impact on many Chinese scholars.

In the present paper, I offer an alternative explanation of the treatment. In my opinion, Qin Minghe relied on Chinese medicine in treating Emperor Gaozong. I see no evidence for the use of trepanation.

Qin Minghe's Medical Technique

When he summoned Qin Minghe, the 30-year-old emperor could no longer see. The story is told in five historical works prepared in the Tang dynasty: *Jiu Tang shu* (舊唐書—Old History of the Tang Dynasty), *Xin Tang shu* (新唐書—New history of the Tang Dynasty), *Zi zhi tong jian* (資治通鑑—Comprehensive Mirror for Aid in Government), *Da Tang xin yu* (大唐新語 —A New Account of Tales from the Tang Dynasty), and *Tan bin lu* (譚賓錄—Record of Dialogues with Guests). The record of the five books may have some difference, but on the whole the story is the same. The story comprehensively states that the Emperor Gaozong had *feng xuan* disease and could not see. He summoned two court doctors, Zhang Wenzhong and Qin Minghe, to treat his disease. Doctor Qin told him that the disease was caused by an upward attack of toxic wind in his body. He also said, "Inserting a needle in your head and drawing a small amount of blood could cure the disease." At that moment, Empress Wu was standing behind a curtain. She did not want Gaozong to recover. She said, "He who proposes to cause blood to flow from the emperor's head should be killed." Qin was terrified. Gaozong said, "It is unreasonable to treat the doctor as a criminal simply because he discussed the disease with me. Since I can no longer bear the disease, let him try. Bloodletting may not yield bad results." Qin inserted a needle into two acupoints, *bai hui* (百會) and *nao hu* (腦戶). Suddenly Gaozong said, "I can see!" Empress Wu also thanked Qin and said, "Heaven brought you here to serve as our master."

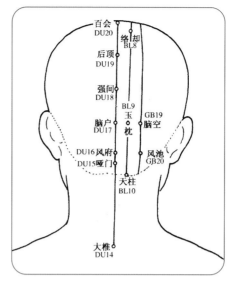

Fig. **2** *Bai hui (DU-20) and nao hu (DU-17).*

In the end, the empress bestowed great treasures upon him [1].

This is a remarkable story, and not entirely believable. The present author suspects, for example, that Qin was not entirely successful, since the emperor died the following month. And one cannot help noticing that the other court doctor, Zhang Wenzhong (張文仲), did not say anything. Why?

According to *Jiu Tang shu*, Zhang had earned great renown for curing those afflicted with *feng* diseases, of which *feng xuan* is one example, and his prescriptions were reproduced by Wang Tao (王燾—670–755 CE) in *Wai tai mi yao fang* (外台秘要方—The Secret Pharmacy of the Imperial Library) [2]. During the reign of Empress Wu, Zhang was appointed to the position of *shi yu yi* (侍御醫), or junior court doctor, and ultimately served as *shang yao feng yu* (尚藥奉御), or director of the court medical department. It is tempting to imagine that Zhang's brilliant career was as much the result of his faithful service to the empress as that of his medical expertise, and that service could well have begun before the empress took the throne. The histories indicate that she did not wish to see her husband recover from his illness. *Zi zhi tong jian* states specifically that, because Gaozong suffered from *feng xuan* disease, the empress was able

History, Language, and Culture

Acupuncture or Trepanation? A Study of Qin Minghe, a Skilled Physician of Tang China

to take control of the government [3]. In sum, anyone who obstructed the empress's ambitions by healing the emperor would not be likely to last very long.

Trepanation and Bloodletting

When writing the history of Sino-foreign medical exchange, scholars such as Kuwabara Jitsuzo, Fan Xingchun (范行準,) Jin Xianlin (季羨林), and Ma Boying (馬伯英) devoted a great deal of energy to Qin Minghe. They concluded that his skills were adapted from the medical practices of Central Asia.

In the early Tang, Du Huan (杜環), China's ambassador to the states lying to the west, wrote an account of his travels entitled *Jing xing ji* (經行錄—The Record of Du Huan's Journey). He wrote, "The people of Da Qin (Rome, 大秦) were good at curing eye diseases and dysentery. They identify the disease without seeing any symptoms and open the brain to sweep out parasites (開腦出蟲)" [4]. *Xin Tang shu* also recorded, "In Persia there are some excellent doctors able to cure diseases of the eye, to open the brain and sweep out parasites" [5].

Physicians in both Rome and Persia developed techniques for drilling holes in the skull to remove parasites. In fact, trepanation was practiced in many areas of the ancient world, including not only Europe and Asia, but also both North and South America [6]. Kuwabara Jitsuzo concluded that trepanation was fairly common in western Asia by the seventh century. He connected foreign medicine and trepanation to the Emperor Gaozong through Qin Minghe's name, pointing out that Da Qin (Romans—大秦) were often given the surname "Qin (秦)" in Chinese records [7]. While Fan Xingchun rejected this thesis as unsubstantiated speculation, other Chinese scholars followed Kuwabara's lead in trying to identify the source of Qin's medical skill [8].

Jin Xianlin rejected the notion that Qin had performed a true trepanation ("opening the brain"), and proposed that what was a simple bloodletting had been misrepresented as something far more complex and danger-

ous. As for "sweeping out parasites," that was clearly pure fantasy [9].

Ma Boying speculated that Qin may have been a Nestorian doctor. Physicians associated with this branch of Christianity based in Persia were noted for their expertise and their familiarity with Greek medicine. In the medical books of Hippocrates, which Nestorians translated into Arabic, one treatment for blindness is trepanation. Hippocrates wrote that allowing liquid to flow from the pierced head could restore the patient's vision. Ma also pointed out the widespread use of bloodletting in ancient Europe. It is possible that Nestorians brought the technique to China. Ma emphasized that the technique ascribed to Qin in historical texts is not described in any ancient Chinese medical treatise [10].

I find the hypotheses offered by these scholars to be unconvincing, largely for lack of compelling evidence. To move the discussion on a bit further, I propose that we pay more attention to two issues. First, Qin inserted a needle into two acupoints: *bai hui* and *nao hu*. Is there any evidence to show that this could cure *feng xuan* disease? Second, did Tang acupuncture practices sometimes cause blood to flow? By answering these questions I hope to address the larger question—a crucial one: is it possible to understand Qin Minghe's medical technique within the confines of Chinese medicine?

Feng Xuan and Acupuncture

In Chinese medical theory, *feng xuan* disease was typically associated with eye problems. According to *Zhu bing yuan hou lun* (諸病源候論—Treatise on the Causes and Symptoms of Diseases), a medical treatise written by a court doctor in the Sui Dynasty (581–618 CE), and the *Ling shu* (靈樞—The Spiritual Pivot), probably compiled in the era of the Warring States and Han Dynasty, (453 BCE–220 CE), *feng xuan* disease was caused by wind invading the body and the brain, which seriously impeded the production and circulation of *qi* and blood. From the viscera, the invasive wind traveled via channels (the

History, Language, and Culture

Acupuncture or Trepanation? A Study of Qin Minghe, a Skilled Physician of Tang China

main function of the channels is to transport *qi* and blood and to connect the internal viscera with other organs) to the brain and thence to the eyes, producing dizziness and blurred vision [11].

The following passage appears in the *Ling shu*: "The ascending *qi* then reaches the brain. In the rear, it emerges at the center of the nape of the neck. Therefore, when evil attacks at the nape of the neck, it meets the hollow of the body and enters deeply, penetrating the brain via the connections to the eyes. On reaching the brain, it makes it spin. This spinning leads the eyes to relate anxiously" [12]. This text draws a clear connection between *feng xuan* disease and blindness.

The *Zhu bing yuan hou lun* also states that an invasive wind would tend to go to the brain and cause blurred vision [13]. Given the widespread belief that *feng xuan* precipitated blindness, it is not surprising that Qin Minghe expected the invasive wind to travel upward in the emperor's body.

The Tang medical literature suggests a range of different methods for treating *feng*

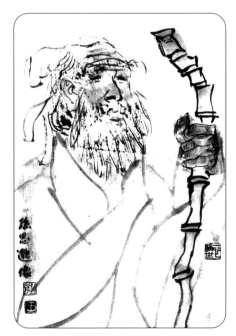

Fig. 3 Sun Simiao

xuan disease. Among the leading treatments were decoctions, acupuncture, and moxibustion. Sun Simiao (孫思邈—581–682 CE), a celebrated colleague of Qin, wrote a pair of important medical classics, *Bei ji qian jin yao fang* (備急千金要方—Invaluable Prescriptions for Ready Reference) and *Qian jin yi fang* (金翼方—Supplement to Invaluable Prescriptions for Ready Reference), which can provide insights into Qin's medical technique.

Sun identified wind (*feng*) as the origin of all diseases and recommended the use of decoctions, acupuncture, and moxibustion as treatments. Sun was partial to the use of moxibustion, and he recommended that cases of *feng xuan* disease be treated by heating the *bai hui* acupoint, as well as by giving the patient *xu ming* (續命) decoctions. In emergencies, he recommended acupuncture using heated needles [14].

In *Zhen jiu jia yi jing* (針灸甲乙經—The Systematic Classic of Acupuncture and Moxibustion), Huangfu Mi (皇甫謐—215–282 CE) identified the acupuncture points said to have been used to treat Emperor Gaozong as falling along the *du* channel (督脈). He located the *bai hui* point at the midpoint of the front of the head, one-and-a-half *cun*s above the posterior forehead and at the center of the brainpan. The needle was to be inserted three *fen*s into the acupoint. He located the *nao hu* on the back of the head, close to the upper border of the occipital bone. The *nao hu* acupoint could be used to treat serious headaches, dizziness, wind invading the brain, and other ailments [15].

An early medical classic, *Su wen* (素問—Plain Questions), was probably compiled in the era of the Warring States and Han dynasty, and stated, "If the physician inserts the acupuncture needle too deeply at the head's *nao hu* point, the brain will be injured and death will be immediate" [16].

In *Bei ji qian jin yao fang,* Sun Simiao described the function of the *bai hui* acupoint, noting that it could be used to treat *xie feng* (邪風—evil wind), blurred vision, and dizziness. He also pointed out that while the effects of invasive wind on the body and internal organs could lead to death, inserting a

History, Language, and Culture

Acupuncture or Trepanation? A Study of Qin Minghe, a Skilled Physician of Tang China

needle three *fens* into the *bai hui* acupoint could strengthen the body [17].

Qin Minghe and Zhang Wenzhong, both of whom served as court doctors, would have appreciated that *bai hui* and *nao hu* were very important acupoints, and that they had to be punctured very carefully, never deeply. My brief survey of the extant literature on Chinese medicine has revealed that it was acceptable for Qin to prick the two acupoints in order to treat a case of *feng xuan* disease that exhibited symptoms of headache and dizziness. Clearly, he did not make a hole in Emperor Gaozong's skull. In addition, Qin was not the first to treat *feng xuan* disease with acupuncture. It is recounted in *San Guo zhi* (三國志—History of the Three Kingdoms] that Hua Tao (華佗) used acupuncture to treat Cao Cao (曹操), whose case of *feng xuan* disease affected his head [18].

It was upon hearing that Qin Minghe intended to draw blood from the emperor's head that Empress Wu spoke of executing Qin. According to the *Ling shu,* there were nine kinds of acupuncture needles in ancient times. One was called the lance needle; it had three sharp cutting edges and was used in cases of chronic illness [19]. Furthermore, some physicians intentionally let the acupoints bleed slightly [20]. Sun Simiao indicated that if too much blood was drawn from acupoints on the head, the result could be blindness [21]. Although there is no way to know whether Qin used a lance needle or not, it was an acceptable acupuncture tool, as long as little blood flowed. As to Ma Boying's suggestion that Qin's medical skill was bloodletting technique, the records are clear in their evocation of acupuncture points, and there is no evidence of the existence of bloodletting proper in pre-modern China.

Conclusion

Scholars who have investigated Qin Minghe's treatment of Emperor Gaozong's *feng xuan* disease have set forth unnecessary and unconvincing hypotheses to explain a miraculous cure. Obsessed by the idea that strange practi-

ces must have been involved, they have failed to see that Chinese medical theories and practices can explain Qin's medical skill. The *bai hui* and *nao hu* acupoints that were said to have been used by Qin were recognized by contemporaneous and earlier specialists as efficacious in treating *feng xuan* disease, especially in cases that involved blindness. In my opinion, there was no connection between Qin's medical repertoire and trepanation. Finally, the suggestion that Qin's cure went beyond what could be expected of seventh-century Chinese science is invalidated by one indisputable fact: Emperor Gaozong died in the month following the treatment.

References

1. Liu Xu. *Jiu Tang shu* [Old history of the Tang Dynasty]. Beijing: Zhonghua shu ju; 1975:111; Ouyang Xiu. *Xin Tang shu* [New History of the Tang Dynasty]. Beijing: Zhonghua shu ju; 1975: 3477; Sima Guang. *Zi zhi tong jian* [Comprehensive Mirror for Aid in Government]. Shanghai: Shanghai guji chubanshe; 1997:1864; Liu Su. *Da Tang xin yu* [A New Account of Tales from the Tang Dynasty]. Beijing: Zhonghua shu ju; 1984:141–42; Hu Qu. *Tan bin lu* [Record of Dialogues with Guests]. In: Li Fang, *Taiping guang ji* [Extensive Records of the Reign of the Grand Tranquility]. Beijing: Zhonghua shu ju; 1961:1671.
2. Wang Tao. *Wai tai mi yao fang* [The Secret Pharmacy of the Imperial Library]. Beijing: Hua xia chubanshe; 1993:268–69.
3. See ref 1, Sima Guang, *Zi zhi tong jian,* p. 1864.
4. Du Huan. *Jing xing ji* [The Record of Du Huan's Journey]. In: Du You, *Tong Dian* [Encyclopedic History of Institutions]. Beijing: Zhonghua shu ju; 1988:5266.
5. See ref 1, Ouyang Xiu, *Xin Tang shu,* p. 6261.
6. Harold Ellis. *A History of Surgery.* London: Greenwich Medical Media; 2001:5–7.
7. Kuwabara Jitsuzo. *Sui Tang shidai Xiyu ren Hua hua kao* [Sinicization of Central Asian People During the Sui and Tang Periods], He Jianmin, trans., 1939. Reprint Taibei: Xin wen feng chuban gongsi; 1979:30.
8. Fan Xingchun. Gudai Zhong Xi yiyao zhi guanxi [Medical exchange between China and the West in ancient times]. *Zhong Xi yiyao* [Medicine East and West]. 1936;2(10):26.

History, Language, and Culture

Acupuncture or Trepanation? A Study of Qin Minghe, a Skilled Physician of Tang China

9. Jin Xianlin. Yindu yanke yishu chuan ru Zhong-guo [Indian ophthalmology in China]. *Guoxue yanjiu* [Studies in Sinology]. 1994;2:555–60.

10. Ma Boying. *Yixue shi yu Zhongguo wenhua* [Chinese Culture and the History of Medicine]. Shanghai: Shanghai renmin chubanshe; 1995: 303.

11. Chao Yuanfeng. *Zhu bing yuan hou lun* [Treatise on the Causes and Symptoms of Diseases]. Bei-jing: Renmin weisheng chubanshe; 1991:55.

12. Wu Jingnuan (translator): *Ling shu.* Honolulu: University of Hawaii Press; 1993:269.

13. See ref 11, p. 52.

14. Sun Simiao. *Qian jin yi fang* [Supplement to Invaluable Prescriptions for Ready Reference]. Shanghai: Shanghai guji chubanshe; 1999:469.

15. Huangfu Mi. *Zhen jiu jia yi jing* [Systematic Classics on Acupuncture and Moxibustion]. Beijing: Renmin weisheng chubanshe; 1996:470, 1688.

16. Ni Maoshing. *The Yellow Emperor's Classic of Internal Medicine*: *A New Translation of the "Neijing Suwen" with Commentary.* Boston and London: Shambhala; 1995:187.

17. Sun Simiao. *Bei ji qian jin yao fang* [Invaluable Prescriptions for Ready Reference]. Beijing: Renmin weisheng chubanshe; 1997:1071.

18. Chen Shou. *San Guo zhi* [History of the Three Kingdoms]. Beijing: Zhonghua shu ju; 1977:802.

19. See ref 12, p. 3.

20. See ref 2, p. 709.

21. See ref 17, p 199.

Further Reading

A Study of Medicine in China: Its Legacies, Inheritance and Integration during the Medieval Period. Hong Kong: Chinese University Press.

Couching for cataract and Sino-Indian medical exchange from the sixth to the twelfth century AD. *Clin Experiment Ophthalmol.* Apr 2005; 33(2):188–90.

Foot massage in Chinese medical history. *J Altern Complement Med.* 2006, Jan–Feb; 12(1):1–3.

Jiao qi disease in medieval China. *Am J Chin Med.* 2004;32(6):999–1011.

On Hua Tuo's position in the history of Chinese medicine. *Am J Chin Med.* 2004;32(4):313–320.

Online research databases and journals of Chinese medicine. *J Altern Complement Med.* 2004; 10(6):1123–1128.

Review of the national center for complementary and alternative medicine website. *JMLA.* 2005; 93(3):104–106.

The complementary and alternative medicine information source book. *Evidence-Based Complementary and Alternative Medicine.* 2005;2(2):261–262.

The guide to complementary and alternative medicine on the internet. *Complementary Therapies in Medicine.* 2006;14(2):2006:167–168.

Contact Details

Fan Ka Wai, PhD, Lecturer
Chinese Civilization Center
City University of Hong Kong
www.cityu.edu.hk
Adjunct Assistant Professor
School of Chinese Medicine
Chinese University of Hong Kong
www.cuhk.edu.hk

The History of the Rothenburg Conference for Traditional Chinese Medicine, Germany

Gerd Ohmstede, Heilpraktiker, Aachen, Germany

The Conference for Traditional Chinese Medicine (TCM) that takes place in Rothenburg, Germany, is the largest in Europe. This international conference attracts audiences and speakers from 16 countries. It is a non-commercial event and is supported by many TCM societies and professionals. It is managed by the *Arbeitsgemeinschaft* (AGTCM), but is owned and run by and for TCM practitioners and enthusiasts as a forum for education, discussion, and networking. This annual event brings together the many well-educated and trained TCM professionals who have a wonderful creative power and deep understanding of nature gained through the practice of TCM. Many schools of thought are accepted within TCM; the forum invites discussion on these different schools of thought and philosophies of both scientists and healers, who have a well-based foundation upon which they construct their ideas and beliefs.

The first congress took place in 1968, 15 years after the foundation of the AGTCM. A group of up to 30 acupuncturists met in Rothenburg to enhance their understanding of the ancient medicine.

The German term *Arbeitsgemeinschaft* expresses the idea behind the unity of this group: a companionship working hard for something. The AGTCM is a community (*Gemeinschaft*) that meets to exchange information. At the same time, there is the work (*Arbeit*) for the common cause and for the continuing training in acupuncture and Chinese medicine. Back in the 1960s, only a few good textbooks were available in Germany, which meant that those wanting to deepen their understanding of the subject were re-

The "Wildbad," Rothenburg

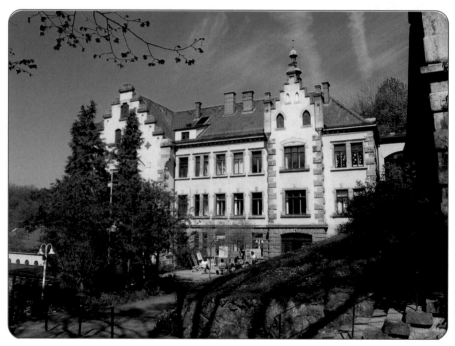

© Gaby Balling

quired to meet with like-minded people. That is how the Rothenburg conferences began.

An old medieval town forms part of Rothenburg, and this is where the conference center is situated. It is located within an art-deco-style building in an historic park near a river. This is a symbol for Chinese medicine: an ancient place for an ancient medicine.

The first-ever-documented conference was held in 1971 and lasted two and a half days. In 1989 it was a great honor for the AGTCM to organize the Global Conference for Acupuncture (in Düsseldorf) on behalf of the Société Internationale d'Acupuncture (SIA) (see also p. 12, History). The AGTCM was a member of this French-based global organization, made up of acupuncture associations. The global conference took place over a period of three days and included 33 lectures and 10 workshops. In 2006, the conference took place over five days, with 60 courses and two full mornings of plenary sessions. Eight hundred participants and 51 international speakers were registered. Approximately half the lectures were given in English.

Even in the early years of the conference, the most renowned speakers of their time lectured in Rothenburg: Jack Worsley, Dr Van Buren, and Nguyen van Nghi. From 1979–1994, Professor Porkert regularly visited Rothenburg and introduced Chinese herbal therapy to the AGTCM. He was responsible for clarifying some apparent confusion regarding terminology used in the field at that time, and decisively supported and determined the development of Chinese medicine within the AGTCM in the 1980s.

The conference's light and open atmosphere and environment, as well as direct interaction on the part of the speakers, and the open networking in which the participants engage, have always been practiced and encouraged in Rothenburg. The medieval setting of the town may have greatly contributed to this. As a result, the conference has become a living example of the Chinese medicine ideal: the free flow of *qi* and *xue* and an open space for *shen*. Both speakers and practitioners agree that we all share the same concern in trying to alleviate suffering and cure disease,

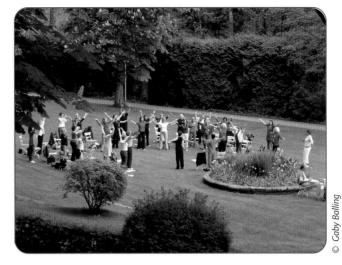

© Gaby Balling

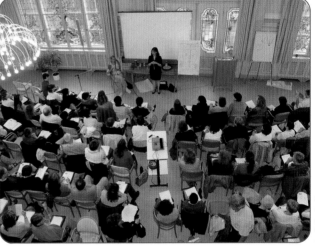

© Gaby Balling

although there are different methods of diagnostics and therapy in Chinese medicine that lead to this same goal. This point of view represents a very important step toward unity within the profession, as well as broad acceptance of Chinese medicine in Germany and across Europe.

The conference management is an independent department of the managing committee of the AGTCM.

Contact Details

www.tcm-congress.de

Chinese Medicine in Italy: Integrated into the Modern Medical System

Subhuti Dharmananda, PhD, Portland, Oregon, USA

Background

Italy has a long history of interaction with China. Two famous early Italian visitors to China were the Venetian Marco Polo (1254–1324) and the Jesuit priest from Macerata, Matteo Ricci (1552–1610). Chinese medicine made its way to Italy primarily via its development in France during the 20th century.

Acupuncture, as a medical practice rather than a curiosity, was brought to France though the efforts of George Soulié de Morant (see Appendices 1 and 2), who was engaged in the French diplomatic service in China between 1901 and 1917. Soulié de Morant published articles and French translations of Chinese and Japanese medical texts, and on his return to France taught clinical applications of acupuncture to French physicians. He also systematically introduced acupuncture theory taken from the classical texts to the physicians. A unique approach to acupuncture therapy was developed by the French proponents, which has come to be known as "French Energetic Acupuncture." Among its basic principles is the concept, common in the Chinese system, that diseases and symptoms, particularly pain, are related to blockages in the flow

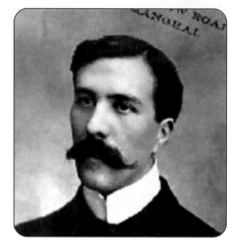

Soulié de Morant

of *qi*. With this as a point of emphasis, there is a high reliance on acupuncture points that are designated "barrier points" (see Table **1** for a brief review of the diagnostic approach and point selection; see also Appendix 3). This system developed within the medical community, so it has primarily influenced medical doctors who practice Chinese medicine, including those in Italy and the USA.

A student of Soulié de Morant, Dr Albert Chamfrault, helped to establish the Association Française d'Acupuncture (AFA—French Association of Acupuncture) in 1945. By 1966, this association had set up six teaching centers in France: in Paris, Bordeaux, Limoges, Nice, Strasbourg, and Toulouse. With the establishment of formal teaching opportunities, some doctors from Italy studied acupuncture in France during the late 1960s, and then returned to found the Società Italiana Agopuntura (SIA—Italian Society for Acupuncture) in 1968, one of the numerous professional organizations that was founded in Europe at that time. This Italian society has produced numerous workshops, congresses, and a jour-

Table 1 Barrier points in the French Energetic Acupuncture system

	Yang exiting	*Yang* entering	*Yin* exiting	*Yin* entering
Shoulder	SI-11	LI-15	LU-2	PC-2
Elbow	TB-13	TB-7	HT-6	HT-6
Wrist	LI-9	SI-6	PC-4	LU-6
Hip	BL-29	ST-31	SP-12	LV-11
Knee	GB-33	GB-36	KI-5	KI-5
Ankle	ST-37	BL-63	LV-6	SP-8

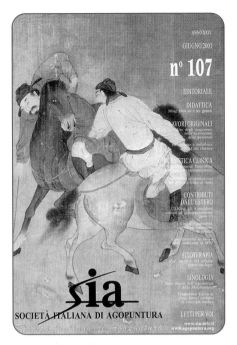

nal, now in its 25th year, with a quarterly publication. Several schools of acupuncture were developed in Italy (there are at least 16 at present), one of the largest being So-Wen, the Scuola di Medicina Naturale (School of Natural Medicine) in Milan, which opened its doors in 1973. Initially, the schools taught only the French Energetic method.

During the 1980s, when China had become more open to foreign visitors, several SIA members developed new contacts with Mainland China. This revealed the more complete system of Chinese acupuncture that existed in the country, as well as the extensive system of herbal medicine that had not previously been introduced into Italy (or France, to any extent). While French Energetic Acupuncture relies mostly on the systematic study of the channels, Chinese herbal therapies rely more on the *zang fu* theory. It took several years to introduce and develop the *zang fu* framework in Italian schools. So-Wen and a few other advanced schools quickly turned to teaching this subject; as early as 1987 Dr Grazia Rotolo and Dr Caterina Martucci (authors of *Farmacoterapia Cinese*) introduced the first herbal seminars. Even so, up to the late 1990s most

students of Chinese medicine in Italy were not able to understand and apply herbal medicine. This, however, has changed over the past five years. Presently, 80 % of the schools have adopted a Chinese program that includes both acupuncture and herbs according to the full Traditional Chinese Medicine (TCM) system. Roberto Gatto (president of the SIA), Sonia Benassi (head of Lao Dan, an herb company), and a few other doctors who have visited China and attended many international seminars, continue to develop and promote the TCM system, including herbal prescribing.

Aside from SIA, other organizations grew up. For example, the Associazione Italiana di Agopuntura-moxibustion e Medicina Tradizionale Cinese (AIAM—Italian Association of Acupuncture-Moxibustion and Traditional Chinese Medicine) was established in 1987 with three central committees: scientific, educational, and legislative. It also incorporates the Inter-University Commission for Acupuncture Research. Additionally, there is an Italian Medical Association of Acupuncture (AMIA) in Rome and the Fondazione Matteo Ricci (Matteo Ricci Foundation), which includes a school in Bologna, a journal, and several workshops. There are now a sufficient number of acupuncture organizations in Italy to enable a coordinating organization to be established: the Federazione Italiana delle Società di Agopuntura (FISA—Italian Federation of Acupuncture Societies), with 2500 members. A plethora of schools and professional organizations have arisen in other European countries as well, and a coordinating organization for Europe has been established, called EuroTCM (see also "European Register of Organizations of Traditional Chinese Medicine [EuroTCM]," p. 177, Professional Developments, Legislation, and Regulation).

The Extent and Nature of Acupuncture in Italy

According to the Italian law, only medical doctors can perform acupuncture therapy; this has also been the case in France, Belgium, Denmark, and the Scandinavian countries (see also the section Professional Developments, Legislation, and Regulation, p. 107). The So-Wen database of MD acupuncturists, the largest file available in Italy, counts more than 7000 names. The total number of Italian MDs trained in acupuncture is likely to be about 10 000. As in France, this represents one of the highest densities of Chinese medical practitioners outside East Asia. (Holland, which does not restrict acupuncture to medical doctors, has the highest density, with an estimated one practitioner for every 3200 people.) The population of Italy is about 56 million, that is, less than one-fifth that of the USA, which has a more liberal legal status for acupuncture, yet has only about 15 000 licensed acupuncturists and about 5000 medical acupuncturists. It has been reported that about 16 % of Italy's population uses various types of alternative medicine, including Chinese medicine, and that many would like to see these therapies covered by health insurance. (For further information on regulations, see also the section Professional Developments, Legislation, and Regulation, p. 107.)

The study of acupuncture in Italy involves 400–500 hours of training over a four-year period. Since the students are medical doctors already in practice, they can only attend weekend seminars, which accounts for the long total duration of the courses. The cost of the program is about € 5000 ($US 6000 in 2004). The Italian programs provide about twice the training that medical acupuncturists receive in the USA at the main training center at UCLA School of Medicine (where French acupuncture has been a major theme). Chinese herbal medicine has been treated as an independent course in Italy (about 250–300 hours of study over a two-year period), which is taken by some doctors after their graduation from acupuncture studies. Since the duration of training is so long (six years with the added herb courses), most students do not pursue herbal training (see also the section Education, p. 193).

Many of the acupuncturists are family doctors (general practitioners) who still rely on the use of modern drug therapies. They have pursued acupuncture studies because of their concerns about drug side effects, and the desire to find alternatives to the less than adequate drug therapies. A few of the doctors add Western herbs or homeopathic remedies to their prescription range; now several hundred have included prescribing Chinese herbs.

In Italy, a limited selection of herb products (and other natural supplements) are sold in stores or via the Internet as non-prescription items. These herb products do not have a good reputation among the medical doctors, who would prefer to prescribe specific remedies, including Chinese herbs, based on their diagnostic work. According to Italian law, however, medical doctors are not allowed to sell or give any prescription, either drugs or herbs, directly to the patient; they have to refer patients to a pharmacy that will carry the appropriate herbal products. Unfortunately, the quality of some of the Chinese herb products that were initially introduced into Italy was often poor, and there have been concerns about contamination of those coming from China. Because the term "herbal therapy" in Italy (and throughout Europe) means the use of plants only, some people have argued against inclusion of any of the traditional animals and minerals as commonly found in many Chinese products. The concern for high-quality products, coupled with the small number of prescribers, has resulted in expensive products. All these factors have restricted the use of Chinese herbs in Italy. As a result, many Italian acupuncturists apply acupuncture to treat pain and certain acute symptoms, but do not deal with internal medicine (that is, herbal medicine). Research has focused on acupuncture therapy.

Things are gradually changing in this regard. The introduction of Chinese herb courses (involving about 500 doctors) has stimulated greater interest in prescribing herbal remedies. A small herbal company began developing a product line in 1988 that has expanded to include over 30 traditional formulas relying solely on plant materials, with herb extraction carried out in Italy to ensure quality.

This company specifically aims to ensure the high quality of raw materials and manufacturing, correct formulation, and proper distribution. Because of low levels of demand at the present time, it is difficult for the company to develop a full range of products, partly because all sales have to go through pharmacies; it is estimated that only about 400 medical acupuncturists are routinely prescribing the relevant items. Other small product lines have also appeared in Italy during the past few years, including a line of topical and internal remedies with a focus on orthopedics and traumatology, especially sports applications. These were developed by Dr Karl Zippelius, who immigrated to Florence, Italy, from Germany, having studied acupuncture and herbs there. The products include pastes, salves, tinctures, and tablets.

Over the next three years, the new programs of herbal medicine education will have the capability to train about 500 new practitioners. Additionally, through seminars, as many as 1000 current practitioners could receive continuing education on the topics. It is unlikely, however, that these participation levels will be met; the actual attendance may be only 20–30 % of the potential audience, owing to scheduling conflicts and concerns about the ability to readily obtain and utilize the herbal remedies. Perhaps with positive response to the therapies the demand for training will increase in the coming decade.

Promise and Challenges

Background

So far, the historical development of Chinese medicine in Italy has been reviewed, and the fact that acupuncture has been entirely within the modern medical profession has been highlighted. This situation differs from that in the USA and other English-speaking countries, such as Canada, Great Britain, Australia, and New Zealand, where acupuncturists can be licensed or registered separately from any modern medical licensing. In the USA, for example, about 75 % of acupuncture practitioners are not medical doctors, and more than 90 % of the practitioners who prescribe Chinese herbs are not medical doctors. This section of the article provides further description of the promise of, and challenges to, Chinese medicine in Italy, which may be representative of trends in the future throughout all of southern Europe and, perhaps, most of Europe.

The Promise

There is a growing sense among medical doctors in Italy that their patients have a need for therapies that are not currently included within orthodox medical practices, which are dominated by drugs, surgery, and allied techniques. This is because of requests by the patients themselves for alternatives, and a significant number of situations where doctors clearly see that the modern medical therapies they can offer are either not tolerated by some patients or are not sufficiently successful for certain diseases. The area of neurological and psychological disorders, for example, has been the focus of concern in this regard.

The interest in Chinese medicine in Italy is clearly growing, and the desire for training in this field may be illustrated by the lengths that doctors will go to in order to access quality courses. For example, several doctors have been willing to travel for many hours to reach the site of weekend seminars, and travel thus repeatedly throughout a year or more to complete a course. Weekend training is undertaken, because all the students are already doctors in practice who have to spend the weekdays seeing patients. In part, the solution to this lengthy travel time is to open schools in several cities, and this is being done. Even so, there are still only a few large-scale programs, such as the ones operated by So-Wen in Milan and in Naples. It may require several years to broaden other programs for the convenience of local physicians.

With an increase in the number of medical doctors practicing Chinese medicine, there is now the opportunity to establish clinics where two or more such doctors practice. This will enable patients to access a central clinical site for this type of therapy. Also, some doctors of Chinese medicine have been able to bring their skills into a few hospitals. Until recently, in order to receive Chinese medicine treatment, it was necessary to go to the private office of a doctor practicing the therapy in isolation, and this is still the usual situation that prevails today.

The study of Chinese herbal medicine is now offered routinely, whereas in the past doctors might learn only acupuncture. As a result, it is possible for patients to gain access to both methods of therapy. With more doctors using Chinese herbs, the range of products available for them to prescribe will increase, since there needs to be a certain level of demand for an herb or formulation to enter into commerce and remain there, and especially to have the appropriate labeling for Italy.

The Challenges

The challenges to enhancing the use of Chinese medicine in Italy are great. At the present time, acupuncture is not formally recognized as a medical specialty, and so doctors are not able publicly to proclaim the fact that they provide acupuncture. Whereas in the USA anyone can put up a sign advertising, for example, acupuncture therapy or Chinese medicine, in Italy the doctor's offer of acupuncture has to be made known by word of mouth. For people who are not yet aware of this therapeutic method, therefore, they will not know that it is potentially available for them, and unless someone lets them know about Chinese medicine, they won't be able to find out how extensive the use of this technique might be.

The situation as regards herbal medicine is even more difficult. There are actually two herbal systems operating simultaneously, both at a low level. The officially sanctioned system involves herb products that are subjected to rigorous testing and quality control standards, and are sold only through pharmacists. The stringent controls on the products raise the costs and limit the number of formulations that can be offered, while the requirement of sale through a pharmacy (the routine method in Europe) complicates the task of getting the formulas to the patients. A second group of products is sold outside of this controlled situation, at some risk to those involved. Such products may come from Europe, the USA, or China; depending on their

nature, they may be sold over the counter or be prescribed directly by the doctor. Because of the tenuous position of the products, however, they are neither widely distributed nor promoted.

A bigger problem—only now becoming evident—is that the governments of Europe are putting together lists of herbs (and various dietary supplements) that are considered unacceptable for use in the products. Several entries on these lists seem to have been added without much justification, so that commonly used herbs that have no significant safety problems attached to them are, or soon will be, banned. Italy may be the most restrictive country and have the longest list at the present time, but over the next few years, what is banned in one country in Europe is bound to be banned in the others. As examples, notice was given this year in Italy that two commonly used herbs, polygala (*yuan zhi*) and ganoderma (*ling zhi*), will no longer be permitted for sale, either alone or in products. One can only speculate as to how these two herbs came to be listed. By banning even a few commonly used ingredients, dozens of standard traditional formulas will have to be reformulated without them. Already, European governments do not allow herb products to include most of the animal and mineral ingredients found in many traditional Chinese herb formulations. For some herbs, one species is permitted but another is not, without any clear explanation—for example, *Lycium chinense* (*di gu pi*) is not allowed, but *Lycium barbarum* (*gou qi zi*) is allowed, yet both herbs are used interchangeably in China.

Rules under development for the past few years aim virtually to block marketing of any new formulations, without extensive pre-market testing, and allow only those that have been used for a long time. Thus, one of the rules will require that a Chinese herb formula to be marketed in Europe must have been used in China for at least 30 years and in Europe for at least 15 years. The first requirement is relatively easy, since most of the traditional formulas of interest have been used for much longer than that in China. The second requirement is far more difficult to meet, since records from 15 years ago may well be limited and several important formulas not extensively used. Further, with the growing list of herbs not permitted in formulas, the prior use of them loses some significance, since the formula must now be changed to meet the new regulations.

Research in Italy

In the *Journal of Traditional Chinese Medicine* (2000;20(3):231–240), a group of eight Italian medical acupuncturists reported on their comparison of drug therapy versus acupuncture for migraine. They evaluated 120 patients affected by migraine treated at four public health centers. Acupuncture therapy focused on the use of five points: *tou wei* (ST-8), *xuan lu* (GB-5), *feng chi* (GB-20), *lie que* (LU-7), and *da zhui* (GV-14); all but the last mentioned point were treated bilaterally. Patients were evaluated after six and 12 months of therapy. The authors concluded that acupuncture was a cost-effective alternative to modern drug treatments.

Numerous clinical reports are published in Italian, mainly in the *SIA Journal.*

The following is a sample abstract of a report on the use of acupuncture for pain:
Title: Acupuncture Therapy for Dysmenorrhea
Authors: Stefania Bresciani, Raffaella Mezzopane, Roberto Malavasi, and Alberto Lomuscio
Institutions: Scuola di Medicina Naturale and Divisione di Ginecologia Ospedale San Paolo, Milan
Published in: *SIA Journal*, December 2003; 108:36–40

Summary: Thirty women with primary dysmenorrhea have been treated with acupuncture, following a fixed protocol. The authors have evaluated the intensity and duration of pain, the number of work days lost every month, the amount of drugs used to control the pain of menstruation, and associated symptoms. The results show a very significant reduction of all these parameters. It is suggested that acupuncture therapy should be used together with classical Western therapy in all cases of primary dysmenorrhea.

Contact Details

Subhuti Dharmananda, PhD, Director, Institute for Traditional Medicine, Portland, OR, USA
www.itmonline.org

Today, the Internet is the fastest growing method of retrieving information about Chinese medicine. Numerous articles are posted, practitioners are listed, or have their own websites, and associations present their newsletters and alert people to seminars. Italian Chinese medicine organizations have been slow to develop the benefits of an Internet presence, and increased exchange of information by Internet may be vital to help the field develop further. A few of the websites found are the following:

Associazione Medica per lo Studio dell'Agopuntura: www.agopuntura.org

Federazione Italiana delle Società di Agopuntura (Federation of Italian Societies of Acupuncture): www.agopuntura-fisa.it

Societá Italiana Agopunctura (Italian Society of Acupuncture): www.sia-mtc.it

Centro di Energia per la vita (Center for Life Energy): www.energiaperlavita.it/perimedia.asp

Fondazione Matteo Ricci (Matteo Ricci Foundation): www.fondazionericci.it

Istituto Orientale di Medicina Energetica (Institute of Oriental Energetic Medicine): www.iomeitalia.org/lascuola.htm

So-Wen (the So-Wen School of Traditional Chinese Medicine): www.sowen.it

(The first part of this article was originally published on the itm website, www.itmonline.org, in September 2004.)

Appendices

Appendix 1:

Early European Exposure to Acupuncture
Prior to the work of George Soulié de Morant, a few Westerners had described acupuncture therapy, and some had used it. They failed, however, to generate sufficient interest in the field for it to develop formally. The first records relating to Chinese medicine date back to 1671, when a French Jesuit priest named P.P. Harvieu, who had served in China, published *Les secrets de la médecine des chinois* (Secrets of Chinese Medicine). There was brief mention of acupuncture from time to time after that, but then a number of articles and books appeared in the nineteenth century, outlined in Table **2** (adapted from *Understanding Acupuncture* by Stephen Birch and Robert Felt, New York: Churchill Livingstone, 1999).

Appendix 2:

**Soulié de Morant's Introduction
of Chinese Medicine to Europe**
Peter Eckman, in his book *In the Footsteps of the Yellow Emperor* (San Francisco: Cypress Book Company, 1996), presents the results of his intensive research into the development of acupuncture therapy in Europe. The main purpose of his effort was to discover the influences on J.R. Worsley, who became a significant figure in the development of acupuncture in England and America, two countries where Eckman has lived and worked. He was able to trace significant influences from both Japan (via visiting Japanese practitioners and teachers) and from China (mainly via George Soulié de Morant), as well as some influences from Vietnam and Korea, together with the interaction with German naturopathy and homeopathy. Regarding George Soulié de Morant, he wrote the following (edited here for presentation):

I think we can say that contemporary traditional acupuncture in the West started with George Soulié de Morant (1878–1955) in 1927

in France. Prior to that date, there had been scattered accounts and even some books about acupuncture in Western languages, but no attempt to formulate a systematic understanding of acupuncture based on points, meridians, the circulation of qi and its management and reflection in pulse diagnosis. Soulié de Morant grew up in an unusual family that encouraged him to learn Chinese from the age of eight. He was originally schooled by the Jesuits and intended to study medicine, but had to give up that ambition when his father died.

At 21 (1899), based on his linguistic skills, he got a secretarial job in China, and happened to be in Beijing during a cholera epidemic. Soulié de Morant became acquainted with a Dr Yang, who was considered extraordinarily successful in treating cholera victims with acupuncture (typical formula of points: ST-25, ST-36, LI-10, and points surrounding CV-8). Soulié de Morant's curiosity was piqued to the point that he began studying with Dr Yang, who let him do some of the treatments under his guidance.

Soulié de Morant was subsequently appointed to the French Consular Corps and sent to various cities in China, in each of which he sought out acupuncture teachers, including several in Yunnan, which is contiguous with Indochina. It is likely that the initial Vietnamese influence on French acupuncture was a consequence of his studies in Yunnan [though France had ruled over Indochina since 1887, which may have allowed for other routes of influence, such as Vietnamese traditional doctors living in France.] Soulié de Morant adopted local custom as his own, and it was said that when he dressed up, his speech and manner were indistinguishable from a native Chinese, and so he earned the respect and trust of his teachers, who supplied him with the most precious texts and instruction. He became so proficient a practitioner that in 1908 the Viceroy of Yunnan certified him as a "Master Physician-Acupuncturist" [just four years after meeting Dr Yang and beginning the study of acupuncture.]

One other Oriental influence on Soulié de Morant came from Japan, where he spent a month in 1906 because of his poor state of health, and is reflected in his later citation of

Table 2 Some 19th century references to acupuncture in the West

Date	Country	Author(s)	Nature of publication
1802	UK	W. Coley	Article on the uses of acupuncture
1816	France	L. Berlioz	Book on acupuncture for chronic disorders
1820	Italy	S. Bozetti	Book on acupuncture
1821	UK	J.M. Churchill	Article on using acupuncture for treating rheumatism
1822	USA	Anonymous	Medical journal commentary favorable to acupuncture
1825	France	J.B. Sarlandiere	Article on the use of electro-acupuncture for gout
1825	Italy	A. Carraro	Article on the uses of acupuncture
1826	USA	F. Bache	Article on the uses of acupuncture
1826	UK	D. Wandsworth	Article on using acupuncture for pain relief
1826	Germany	G.E. Woorst	Review article on the status of acupuncture
1827	UK	J. Elliotson	Article on using acupuncture for rheumatism
1828	Germany	J. Bernstein	Article on using acupuncture for rheumatism
1828	Germany	L.H.A. Lohmayer	Article on using acupuncture for rheumatism
1828	France	J. Cloquet, T.M. Dantu	Book on acupuncture
1833	USA	W.M. Lee	Article on using acupuncture for rheumatism
1834	Italy	F.S. da Camin	Describing Sarlandiere's work on electro-acupuncture
1871	UK	T.P. Teale	Article on acupuncture for pain relief

Japanese works in his publications. Thus, from its inception, the European acupuncture that Soulié de Morant inaugurated reflected aspects of Chinese, Japanese, and Vietnamese traditions. In fact, Soulié de Morant also cited several classical Korean texts, so that that tradition was also represented.

Soulié de Morant returned to France in 1918, but it was not until 1927 that his career in acupuncture really began there. At that time, he brought his daughter for medical treatment to Dr Paul Ferreyrolles (1880–1955), a member of a study group of physicians investigating alternative medicine. This study group prevailed upon Soulié de Morant to abandon all his other interests and translate the classical Chinese medical texts into French and train them in acupuncture treatment. This he did, while also developing his own clinical practice, first under medical supervision in several hospitals, and later in private practice. He also experimented on himself, needling different points to see their effects, and kept careful records that he used in his subsequent publications.

Among Soulié de Morant's sources, aside from his extensive practical training, were many classical Oriental texts, the main ones being two Ming Dynasty Chinese texts: Zhen Jiu Da Cheng (Great Compendium of Acupuncture and Moxibustion, 1601) and Yi Xue Ru Men (Basics of Medical Studies, 1575). He was also influenced by the Japanese work of Sawada, as communicated by Nakayama, whose book Soulié de Morant translated into French with the assistance of the Japanese George Ohsawa (Japanese name: Sakurazawa Nyoitchi; 1893–1966, one of the originators of "macrobiotics").

His first writing about acupuncture was an article in a French homeopathic journal in 1929, in collaboration with Ferreyrolles, and his first serious book about acupuncture, Précis de la vrai acuponcture chinoise, was published in 1934. Altogether, he wrote over 20 articles and books on acupuncture, his magnum opus being L'Acuponcture Chinoise, the first part of which appeared from 1939–1941, but was only published in its entirety posthumously in 1957, and later in English translation (Chinese Acupuncture) by Paradigm Press (1994) (see above).

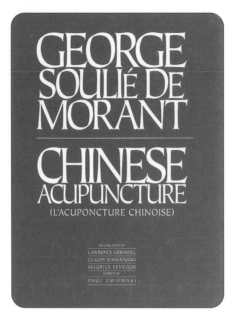

The students of Soulié de Morant, including Jean Niboyet (1913–1968, founder of the Mediteranian Acupuncture Association), Albert Chamfrault (c.1912–1971, of the French Association of Acupuncture), and Roger de la Fuÿe (1890–1961), pushed forward the field of acupuncture with translations, associations, conferences, and developing clinical practices.

Appendix 3:

French Acupuncture and the Barrier Points

During the 20th century, many of the European writings about acupuncture focused on its use for rheumatism, gout, and other pain disorders. This emphasis continues to this day; the dominant use of acupuncture in the West, especially amongst medical acupuncturists, is for "musculoskeletal" problems. The unique approach taken in France, which has been formalized and promoted in the study groups and workshops of the Association Française d'Acupuncture (AFA) [French Acupuncture Association], led to the description of two groups of points. According to the French medical acupuncturists Gérard Guillaume and Mach Chieu (as described in their book *Rheumatology in Chinese Medicine*, Vista:

Eastland Press, 1996), one type of points can have either global effects or affect an entire channel, or axis—see below. These include most of the transport points, cleft points, source points, and connecting points. The others type are specific for the area to be treated, and include mainly associated points, alarm points, and barrier points. Guillaume and Chieu point out that "barrier points are extremely important in the treatment of pain."

Dan Bensky has written about the French system (www.siom.com), and a portion of his presentation has been adopted for presentation here. Among the key concepts of the French system are the use of the eight diagnostic parameters, grouping of acupuncture channels into axes, and the above-mentioned focus on barrier points.

In the French system, the eight diagnostic categories (vacuity/repletion or deficiency/excess, cold/hot, interior/exterior, *yin/yang*) are applied to the diagnosis of local musculoskeletal pain, particularly joint pain, rather than only to the general syndromes as is commonly practiced within the TCM system. For example, pain that is lessened with pressure or support is classified as vacuous or deficient, while pain that worsens is considered to be of replete nature. Pain that is lessened by heat and increased by cold is considered to be of a cold nature, and conversely for pain that is increased by heat. The pain may come from invasion of external pathogenic factors and be lodged in a painful joint or muscle, or may come from interior disharmonies of the internal organs, and migrate from there to the affected part. A *yin*-type pain is dull, throbbing, of moderate intensity, chronic, occurring or aggravated at night, and deep. A *yang*-type pain is sharp, violent, paroxysmal, stabbing, burning, intense, acute, diurnal, and superficial.

The French place a strong emphasis on the channels, more so than on point sets as is often the case in modern TCM in China. The 12 channels are viewed as six pairs of channels: two greater *yin* channels, two lesser *yang* channels, etc., taken from the six-fold system depicted in the *Nei Jing Su Wen* (Yellow Emperor's Classic of Internal Medicine: Book of Common Questions) for acupuncture and repeated in the *Shang Han Lun* (On Cold Damage) for herbs. The functions of the two channels within each pair are understood to be related, and so are the manifestations of their disharmonies. Each of these pairs is known as an axis, or great channel.

The concept of barrier points originally came from the Chinese word *guan*, often translated as barrier or gate. Several French doctors were struck by the number of points that have this word in their name, either primary name or alternate, and they also noted the importance of the concept of barriers or gates in the discussion of joint problems in Chapter 60 of the *Nei Jing Su Wen*. Using this as a point of departure, they described each joint as a place through which physiologic energies (*qi* and blood in TCM terms) pass, as through an open gate; under certain pathological circumstances the joint space can turn into a barrier (closed gate) that obstructs the circulation. The *yin* and *yang qi* enter and exit the joints. Utilizing the eight categories and properties of channel flow in the axes, the practitioner has to determine the fundamental nature of the disorder, specifically whether the blockage involves the *yin* or *yang qi* as it is either entering or exiting the joint. The barrier points (which are originally picked on the basis of traditional descriptions of their channels, specific point indications, the point names, and other factors) are then to be selected as the main part of treatment.

A Concise Chronology of Chinese History

Period of the Five Legendary Rulers c. 2600 BCE–1600 BCE		Huang Di Zhuan Xu Di Ku Yao of Tang Shun of Yu	
Xia Dynasty		c. 2100 BCE–c.1600 BCE	
Shang Dynasty		c. 1600 BCE–c.1045 BCE	
Western Zhou Dynasty		c. 1045 BCE–c.771 BCE	
Eastern Zhou Dynasty 770 BCE–256 BCE	Spring and Autumn Period	722 BCE–481 BCE	
	Warring States Period	453 (403) BCE–222 BCE	
Qin Dynasty		221 BCE–206 BCE	
Han Dynasty 206 BCE–220 CE	Western Han	206 BCE–8 CE	
	Eastern Han	25–220 CE	
Three Kingdoms 220–280 CE	Wei	220–265 CE	
	Shu Han	221–263 CE	
	Wu	222–280 CE	
Jin Dynasty 265–420 CE	Western Jin	265–316 CE	
	Eastern Jin	317–420 CE	
Northern and Southern Dynasties 386–589 CE	Southern Dynasties	Song	420–479 CE
		Qi	479–502 CE
		Liang	502–557 CE
		Chen	557–589 CE
	Northern Dynasties	Northern Wei	386–534 CE
		Eastern Wei	534–550 CE
		Northern Qi	550–577 CE
		Western Wei	535–556 CE
		Northern Zhou	557–581 CE
Sui Dynasty		581–618 CE	
Tang Dynasty		618–907 CE	
Five Dynasties and Ten States	Five Dynasties 907–960 CE	Later Liang	907–923 CE
		Later Tang	923–936 CE
		Later Jin	936–946 CE
		Later Han	947–950 CE
		Later Zhou	951–960 CE

Five Dynasties and Ten States	Ten States 902–979 CE	Northern Han	951–979 CE
		Wu	902–937 CE
		Southern Tang	937–975 CE
		Wu Yue	907–978 CE
		Min	909–945 CE
		Southern Han	917–971 CE
		Chu	927–951 CE
		Jing Nan (Nan Ping)	924–963 CE
		Former Shu	907–925 CE
		Later Shu	934–965 CE
Song Dynasty 960–1279 CE	Northern Song	960–1127 CE	
	Southern Song	1127–1279 CE	
Liao (or Qi Dan, or Chi Tan)		916–1125 CE	
Jin		1115–1234 CE	
Xi Xia (or Tangut)		1038–1227 CE	
Yuan Dynasty		1279–1368 CE (established 1206)	
Ming Dynasty		1368–1644 CE	
Qing Dynasty		1644–1911 CE	
Republic of China		1912–1949 CE	
People's Republic of China		1949 CE–	

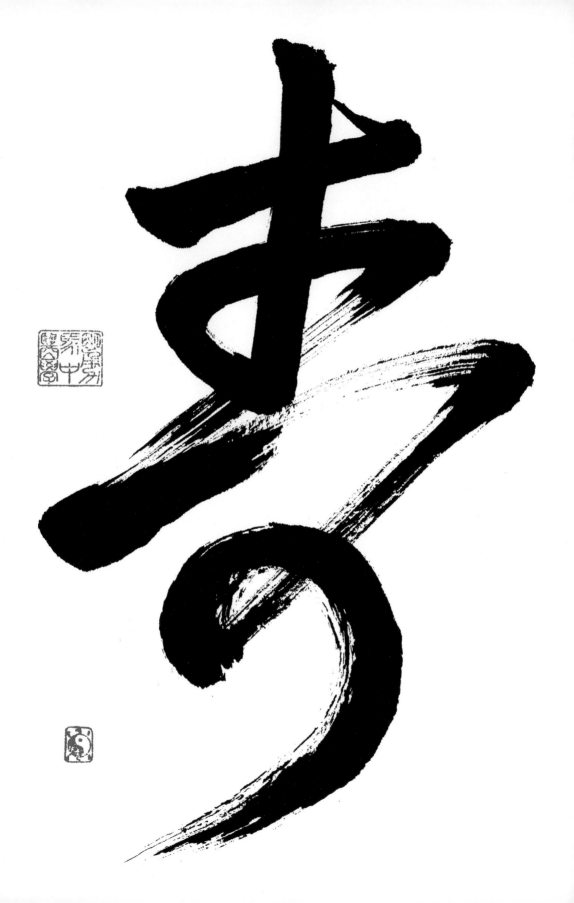

Research

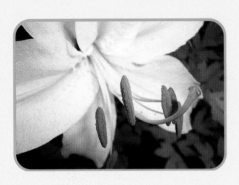

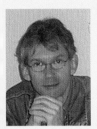

Introduction

A Voice for Research

Stephen Birch

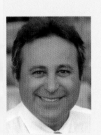

Isaac Cohen

In attempting to bridge modern and traditional, East and West, with the enormous diversity of voices in the field, the Almanac must naturally find a voice for research. In fact, given the changes in modern thinking and health care taking place everywhere, we cannot avoid approaching the topic of research. For many, research is the currency of acculturation as Traditional East Asian Medicine (TEAM), acupuncture, and Chinese medicine continue growing in the West. Both public and private medical services and institutions have come to depend on research as a way of helping sort through the masses of data and claims about therapies, therapists, and their theories. As witnessed in the pieces below, research clearly has both clinical and social ramifications. While research on TEAM does not yet seem to be a major player in public health care policy decision-making in Asia, it may end up playing that role as the traditional medicines of Asia gradually continue to lose ground.

Over the years discussing the topic of research with colleagues in the West and in Japan, I have found that many of us feel intimidated because we feel we don't understand its raison d'être. Many of us also feel inflammatory about the subject because it involves big business, it is not humanistic or philosophically satisfying, it seems unrelated to clinical practice, or it has little impact on how we help our patients. There are many reasons to turn away from research but it is there, whether we like it or not. More importantly, if we as a community can approach it more openly and try to influence its use and development more actively, we can make it do service for us. Research has been used to attempt to club us as practitioners but we don't have to be clubbed by it; we can choose a different way.

This section is therefore not, on the whole, written in a very technical format, with facts, tables, figures, and data. We have attempted to write in a way that will help you to approach research in the field. There are many places researchers can publish their data and papers; the Almanac is a perfect place for us to digest and discuss them. Hence the approach of this section is to help to understand what resources are available, to look at what is going on, to deconstruct important studies and help to interpret them. (Here it should perhaps be noted that often the conclusions of a researcher do not follow from their study and results.) We are fortunate, of course, to have some papers included that are rather more technical in their approach—that is to be expected. Nevertheless, the main aim of this section is to expose information and make the data clearer to understand. As will be shown, some of the research has clear social and clinical implications.

How have acupuncturists and acupuncture organizations come to grips with research? In the non-physician acupuncture community in the UK we have two exemplary models that can inspire us to do better. We have a very powerful voice and presence, if only we can learn to use them.

Hugh MacPherson, who has a research degree from years ago, gradually turned back to research after years of practicing and teaching acupuncture. The effects of this have been profound; he has made huge contributions to the field. His story is included in the article on the UK-based Foundation for Traditional Chinese Medicine. Hugh now runs a group ensconced within the research medical community at York University. This shows what openness and a little perseverance can achieve.

The British Acupuncture Council (BAcC) established the Acupuncture Research Resource Council (ARRC) in collaboration with academia, and hired Mark Bovey to run the organization. The purpose of the ARRC is to provide up-to-date access and summaries of research data for BAcC members, and to promote research among members and through collaboration with the research community. The success of these two groups in the UK shows what can happen when the acupuncture community comes together and collaborates on joint projects.

Isaac Cohen from California has written a piece that is a little more technical, but his topic and content is very important. The paper is fascinating, as it shows how our treatment options are opening up into new areas of clinical practice, specifically the treatment of cancer with herbal medicine. Isaac is heavily involved in research of Chinese herbal medicines and has already made huge contributions in this area. It is possible that his review only scratches the surface of this sector, and his own contributions to it, but it does expose what is fast becoming clear, namely that Chinese medicine may well have a place in the future treatment of cancer.

The next topic includes several pieces about the large new acupuncture studies recently completed in Germany. Included in this is my own overview of the studies, written to help us understand what they mean and how to cope with the contradictory results and interpretations. There is also a short piece by Velia Wortman expressing her dissatisfaction with the research and an article by Marcus Baecker and Gustav Dobos about the studies. Discussion of these studies will continue for a long time to come, so please read Gabriel Stux's piece about them in the Legislation, Regulation, and Professional Development section. His piece helps to explain not only their social ramifications but also some of their scientific aspects.

The Clinical Practice section includes a paper by Marian Fixler that presents data from a simple study she undertook. It is included in that section because it has clear clinical implications and is a great example of how practitioners can, with a little support, undertake some simple research in their own practice. It is useful to look at this paper if you are interested in getting involved in research. I have submitted a case history for the Clinical Practice section that highlights some research issues, which bring further perspective to the discussions in this section.

We hope to encourage greater cooperation among research groups, researchers, and practitioners, and more support for research among practitioners. In future issues of the Almanac we plan to publish more material and resources to further these goals.

Stephen Birch, PhD, LAc
The Stitching (Foundation) for Study of Traditional East Asian Medicine, Amsterdam, the Netherlands

Acupuncture Quo Vadis?—On the Current Discussion Around its Effectiveness and "Point Specificity"

Marcus Baecker, MD, Iven Tao, MA, and Professor Gustav J. Dobos, MD, Essen, Germany

Summary

The results of the Acupuncture Randomized Trials (ART) and German Acupuncture Trials (GERAC) illustrate the real effectiveness of acupuncture in the treatment of migraines, tension type headache, osteoarthritis of the knee, and chronic lower back pain. Acupuncture appears to be far superior to conventional standard treatment for the latter two indications. The results of the ART and GERAC studies, however, show that the relevance of "point specific" effects has been overestimated for some indications. The review discusses these results, based on an explanation of the various effect categories of acupuncture therapy. It is thereby shown that the current data does not support the postulate of a "no matter where acupuncture," nor can they justify the irrefutability of the theories of Chinese medicine. Future studies will be required to determine more accurately by which mechanisms the therapeutic effects of acupuncture are mediated. Furthermore, it will be necessary to define more clearly for which indications the location of the needle is the crucial part of the overall treatment effect, and for which indications other factors, such as needle stimulation intensity or the physician-to-patient interactions, are the dominating factors. Acupuncture research is still in its infancy. It is therefore advisable not to be tempted by the current data to make unreliable judgements.

Keywords

Acupuncture, ART, GERAC, effectiveness, effect categories

Abstract

The model projects carried out by health insurance companies in the study of the effectiveness of acupuncture have allowed a new dimension to acupuncture research and raised numerous questions. The results of the ART and GERAC trials are discussed in the review, as are their implications for acupuncture.

Introduction

The Acupuncture Randomized Trials (ART) and German Acupuncture Trials (GERAC) were conducted to study the effectiveness of acupuncture in the context of model projects, sponsored by the Geman health insurance companies, to improve the evidence base for acupuncture in pain treatment. After the initial results of the ART and GERAC studies became known, a discussion developed that was characterized more by journalistic marketing polemics than by scientific argument. In this paper, the substantial results of the ART and GERAC studies will be discussed, as well as their implications for acupuncture. There will be a discussion relating to the categories of treatment effects that occur with acupuncture therapy. We feel that understanding these categories is very important for the classification of the results of acupuncture studies. Furthermore, questions resulting from the current data are raised, and necessary research projects are addressed. Finally, possible consequences for practice and training are highlighted.

The ART and GERAC Studies

There were four randomized studies in both ART and GERAC for the indications of migraine, tension tpye headache, osteoarthritis of the knee, and chronic lower back pain. In the ART studies, respectively 300 patients were included, while the GERAC studies each had around 1000 patients per indication. These are the largest number of patients in randomized controlled trials (RCTs) of acupuncture recorded to date. They used a semi-standardized acupuncture therapy. Each used freely selectable points, combined with compulsory points. In order to examine the clinical effectiveness ("therapeutic effect," Fig. 1) the acupuncture in the GERAC study was compared with a guideline-oriented, conventional standard therapy, and in the ART study with a group of waiting listed patients. In order to investigate the effect mechanism, in particular the relevance of "point-specific effects" (Fig. 1), both sets of studies used a third group where "minimal acupuncture" was used. This consisted of some superficial needling of "non acupuncture points," without further stimulation. The essential results of ART and GERAC can be summarized as follows [1–5]:

- Acupuncture clearly showed a better therapeutic effect compared with the conventional standard therapy for osteoarthritis of the knee and chronic lower back pain (GERAC), as well as a clearly better result than "no treatment" (waiting list) with osteoarthritis of the knee, chronic lower back pain, migraine, and tension headache (ART). Acupuncture was comparably more effec-

tive than pharmacological standard treatment in migraine.

- Acupuncture showed a significantly better effect in the treatment of osteoarthritis of the knee in the ART study when compared with minimal acupuncture, while it showed no statistically significant difference between the types of acupuncture used in the treatment of migraines, tension headaches, and chronic lower back pain.

- So far, the GERAC study results do not show a significant different therapy effect for the main outcome measures between acupuncture and minimal acupuncture for chronic lower back pain, osteoarthritis of the knee, or for migraine.

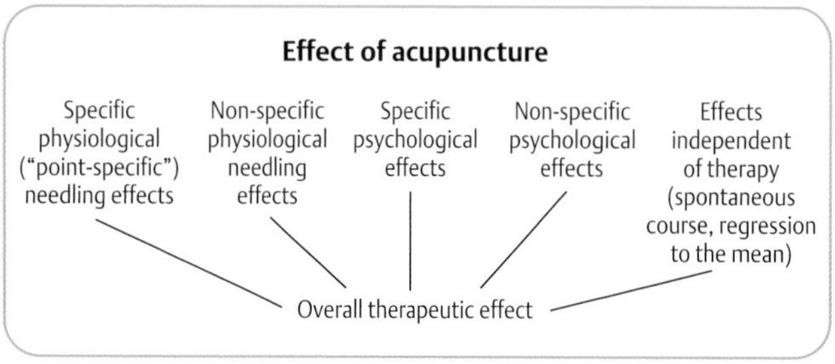

Definition: Effect Categories of Acupuncture Therapy

In order to elucidate the effectiveness and effect mechanisms of acupuncture in discussions of the ART and GERAC study results, it is helpful to clarify different effect categories resulting in acupuncture therapy.

1 Physiological needle effects are effects that derive primarily from the response of the organism to the somatosensory (mostly nociceptive) needle stimulus on the level of tissue and organ systems (nervous system, immune system, cardiovascular system).

1a Specific, physiological needle effects can be evoked only by the needling of a certain area of the body in a specific manner. Specific physiological needle effects can be triggered through treatment of points local to the problem, in painful local areas or on specific points remote to the affected region. At present, "point-specific" effects have been established only for a very limited number of points. Here the antiemetic effect of PC-6 shown in multiple randomized controlled trials can be mentioned [6]. To what extent the effect of an area can be considered as specific depends on the definition of the size of the area (point, surface, segment, dermatome, myotome, etc). In the original acupuncture texts [7], acupunc-

Effect of acupuncture

Specific physiological ("point-specific") needling effects	Non-specific physiological needling effects	Specific psychological effects	Non-specific psychological effects	Effects independent of therapy (spontaneous course, regression to the mean)

Overall therapeutic effect

Fig. 1 The overall therapeutic effect of acupuncture comprises various elements. To simplify, these can be categorized into psychological effects and physiological needling effects, with respective specific and non-specific parts. As in all other therapies, factors independent of therapy also occur, such as the natural spontaneous course of an illness or statistical regression to the mean.

Table 1 Therapeutic effects (main objective parameters) in the ART studies

	Acupuncture Group (VA)	Sham Acupuncture Group (SA)	Waiting List (WL)	Difference VA vs. SA	Difference VA vs. WL
Chronic lumbago Reduction (std) in the level of pain on visual analog scale (in week 8)	28.7 (30.3)	23.6 (31.0)	6.9 (22.0)	n.s.	P<0.001
Migraine Reduction (std) in days with severe headaches (migraine)/month (in weeks 9 to 12)	2.2 (2.7)	2.2 (2.7)	0.8 (2.2)	n.s.	P<0.001
Tension headache Reduction (std) in days/month with headaches (in weeks 9 to 12)	7.2 (6.5)	6.6 (6.0)	1.5 (3.7)	n.s.	P<0.001
Gonarthrosis OMAC score[1] (std) at the end of treatment (week 9)	26.9 (1.4)	35.8 (1.9)	49.6 (2.9)	P<0.0002	P<0.0001

[1] Complaint index that reflects restriction of movement and pain

ture points are topographically described on the basis of salient body places (bones, skin folds, etc). In this way, located points serve as reference points for others. Inevitably these distinctions tend to leave us with the picture of a "reactive area" rather than a "point." It would be conceivable that, in the course of further scientific investigations, the classical concept of "point specificity" is replaced by a concept of "reactive areas."

1b Non-specific, physiological needle effects are defined as mechanisms that can be triggered by treatment of different areas of the body to the same or comparable extent. From a psychophysiological point of view, the needle stimulus represents a stressor for the patient, initially owing to its usually painful character. This evokes a distinct increase of sympathetic nerve activity during needling and a sympathetic withdrawal after the needling [8, 9]. This "post-stimulative" decrease of sympathetic nerve activity [10] might be an explanation for the frequently reported relaxing effect patients experience directly following acupuncture. Psychophysiological investigations show that repeated stimulation leads

to a change in the reaction of the organism, which is due to an adaptation to the stimulus [11]. These findings might offer an approach for the understanding of long-term effects of acupuncture [12]. For migraine patients it can be shown that during an acupuncture treatment there is a reduction in the previously increased cerebrovascular irritability in the course of ten acupuncture sessions [13]. Furthermore, a reduction of the sympathetic tone over the course of twelve acupuncture treatments has been observed in migraine patients [14]. The intensity of stimulation used is substantial for adaptive processes [15]. The stimulation intensity (that is, strength of needle manipulation, number and thickness of the needles, frequency and duration of the treatments) may also play a role in acupuncture-induced, non-specific, physiological effects. Related psychophysiological studies on this are required.

2 Psychological effects are defined as the effects that arise on the basis of the interaction between physician and patient, and the psychological processing of the therapy situation by the patient.

Table 2 Therapeutic effects (main objective parameters) in the GERAC studies

	Acupuncture Group (VA)	Sham Acupuncture Group (SA)	Standard Therapy (ST)	Difference VA vs. SA	Difference VA vs. ST
Chronic lumbago Responder rate: improvement of at least 33 % in three items on "Van Korff Pain" questionnaire (after 6 months)	47.6 %	44.2 %	27.4 %	–[2]	+[2]
Migraine Reduction in days with migraine/ month (after 6 months)	2.3	1.5	2.1	–[2]	+[2]
Tension headache Responder rate: reduction in days with headaches by at least 50 % (after 6 months)	33 %	27 %	Study cancelled[3]	–[2]	+[2]
Gonarthrosis Responder rate: improvement of at least 36 % on WOMAC score[1] (after 6 months)	51 %	48 %	28 %	–[2]	+[2]

[1] Complaint index that reflects restriction of movement and pain
[2] Details of significance level not previously published in writing
[3] The study was concluded on 03/05 as not enough patients could be recruited for the standard therapy

2a **Specific, psychological effects** are effects that result from the specific nature of the acupuncture treatment. For this, like Paterson and Dieppe [16], we count and formulate appropriately the effects which, in the context of a pharmacological trial, apply as non-specific (placebo effect), though comparably to a psychotherapeutic setting, in the context of an acupuncture treatment, have a specific character. It is the classical "syndrome diagnostics" of Chinese medicine and acupuncture that makes it possible for the patient to interpret his or her symptoms in the context of TCM. Furthermore, the physician-to-patient interaction that results from needling is regarded as specific. The significance of this factor is already referred to in the primary sources of Chinese medicine. Thus, in the most important basic work on Chinese medicine, The Yellow Emperor's Canon of Internal Medicine (*Huang Di Nei Jing Su Wen*), it is said that: "the rotation of the needle must take place in an even and regular way, calmly and atten-

tively observing the patient, see the finest of movements as soon as the *qi* arrives; such changes are so subtle that they are hardly perceptible. When the *qi* arrives it is like a flock of birds (fleeting past) or like the wind, (blowing) over (a) corn (fields)—only too easily can one miss the fleeting moment." Furthermore, the ritualistic character of acupuncture should be mentioned, in which context suggestive elements could play a role. It could be that under certain circumstances acupuncture might resemble some kind of hypnotic induction predisposing patients to be more suggestible during the interaction with the therapist. Future studies will clarify this hypothesis.

2b **Nonspecific, psychological effects** are those that can also be achieved with other therapy methods in a similar way. Here, general factors play a role, such as care and empathy on the part of the physician as well as the expectations of the patient. In addition, non-specific effects of therapy naturally result, also due to the context of repeated treatment, such as the spontaneous process of an illness as well as the statistical regression to the mean.

It must be stressed that the effect categories mentioned here do not naturally run separated from one another. On the contrary, there is a reciprocal effect between all process levels, which finally constitutes the sometimes somatopsychological or psychosomatical character of acupuncture therapy.

Interpretation of the Study Results of ART and GERAC

Is Acupuncture Effective in the Treatment of Migraine, Tension Headache, Osteoarthritis, and Chronic Lower Back Pain?

This question must be permitted, since in view of the extensive discussion around "point specificity," a substantial statement could easily be ignored. The needle therapy (both classical as well as minimal acupuncture) showed a therapeutic effectiveness in the GERAC study, which was clearly superior to the conventional, guideline-oriented standard therapy. This result is supported by previous clinical studies and systematic reviews on the examined indications [17–19]. In the framework of ART and GERAC, the minimal acupuncture was applied to test the relevance of "point-specific" effects. The question of the specificity of acupuncture points is of great interest in understanding the impact of acupuncture. For patients seeking help, however, the general therapy effect (Fig. **1**) is crucial. A representative poll by the Institute for Demoscopy in Allensbach shows that 61 % of the population support a combined treatment of conventional medicine and TCM [20]. More than one-third of those interviewed (35 %) had been treated using TCM (acupuncture 26 %, other TCM treatments 9 %); of those, 89 % voted for the use of Chinese medicine in the context of an integrated therapy concept. This represents a pronounced satisfaction in therapy received by those treated. Therapy satisfaction alone cannot justify the effectiveness of a method, but, in the age of an emerg-

ing consumer-driven healthcare system, attention should be paid to the fact that, apart from a discussion around the "point-specificity" of acupuncture, the data showing therapeutic effectiveness and acceptance of needle therapy are apparent. To neglect this is neither appropriate nor in keeping with the times.

Is the Effect of Acupuncture to be Attributed to a Placebo Effect in the Case of the Examined Indications?

The placebo term originates from pharmacological research where, in the context of double-blind studies, the effectiveness of a test substance is tested against a physiologically inert substance, which is then called a "placebo." In this way the specific pharmacological effects of the test substance are to be differentiated from non-specific effects of the therapeutic situation (placebo effect). While this model is meaningful for pharmacological studies, however, it is problematic for acupuncture studies. This is, on the one hand, because of the fact that no physiologically inert acupuncture placebo exists [21]. On the other hand, the therapeutic processes are clearly more complex than in the context of a pharmacological therapy. In addition to "point-specific" needle effects, different effect categories have here to be considered, which do not arise with pharmacological therapy. The non-specific physiological needle effects described above, as well as the specific psychological effects of acupuncture, are numbered here. For the above-mentioned reasons, it makes sense, in the context of acupuncture studies, to completely forego the term placebo effect. Future research must show by which mechanisms the effect of acupuncture is obtained for individual indications. The placebo effect in this context is not helpful.

Is the Effect of Acupuncture Experienced by the Patient Simply Being Pricked in Any Location, as Opposed to a Specific Location?

It is theoretically conceivable that this statement can be affirmed for different indications in the course of further studies. The results of

ART and GERAC clearly show that the significance of the specific, physiological needle effects for migraines, tension type headache, and chronic lower back pain were overestimated. It would be conceivable that, in the case of these illnesses, rather non-"point-specific" effects, such as the non-specific physiological needle effects described above, as well as the specific psychological effects, are seen [22, 11]. Future studies must examine this. An extrapolation of the GERAC data in the sense of a statement on acupuncture "per se" is, however, scientifically inconclusive. As affirmed by Ots [23], the generalization of "no matter where" would only be possible if repeated studies for the same indication with needling of different areas (in different neural segments), using identical needle techniques, arrive at the same result. In this case, still, this statement would be limited to the examined indication.

Is Acupuncture Training Obsolete?

It is well known that "freshly-baked" acupuncture therapists after their first weekend courses often achieve good therapy results at this early stage. Moreover, as malicious gossip maintains: "the indurance of acupuncture over more than two thousand years, might be due to the fact that also bad or badly trained physicians already show good therapeutic results." The conclusion, however, that the ART and GERAC results indicate that acupuncture training is obsolete is unreasonable. In ART and GERAC, well-trained physicians were treating patients, therefore the achieved data is valid only for a "collective of trained physicians." On the other hand likewise hypothetically is the argument stated from other side, that a low state of training in GERAC would have lead to the fact that the full potency of acupuncture was not employed. In summary yet, the effect of training on the therapeutic outcome has not been examined systematically. It would, however, be interesting to test "physicians without training" versus "physicians with training," with the therapy default "no matter how and no matter where." Should both groups obtain similarly good results, this would be a clear signal to the acupuncture

community to overthink their training guidelines. For research, however, it would remain to be clarified which therapy strategies make the non-trained therapists "successful acupuncturists." A better understanding of the factors influencing the therapeutic effectiveness will help to use these specifically in the treatment, which then should be taught in acupuncture training.

Consequences for Research and Practice

If the therapy effect of acupuncture with certain indications cannot be explained by "point-specific" effects, for example, migraine, the question is posed: by which factors is the therapeutic effect of acupuncture then mediated? Here a challenge exists for basic research into the investigation of the above-described non-specific physiological and specific psychological effects. It is possible that, in this context factors like needling technique, the parameter of stimulation (number of needles, force of the needle manipulation, number and duration of treatments), as well as the physician-to-patient interaction (syndrome diagnosis of TCM, acupuncture as ritual, suggestive elements, etc.), move more into the foreground. In practice and training emphasis would be put on needle technique, as well as on the ability to sense the reactions evoked by the patient. An extension of the practical training in the setting of the in Germany newly introduced auxiliary designation ("Zusatzbezeichnung") "Acupuncture" follows this path and is much welcomed. It appears important to underline that the move to the "how" does not automatically imply "no matter where" acupuncture. The significance of point-exact needling of acupuncture points is secured for different indications as, for example, post-operative nausea [6] or epicondylitis humeroradialis [24]. A task of future will be to uncover still more clearly for what indications the "where" of needling contributes a substantial portion to the therapy effect. Acupuncture research is very much just beginning. This is a long path, aimed at separating the wheat from the chaff of Chinese medicine. Until such time, it is advisable not to be tempted by untenable conclusions.

See also "Comments on the German Acupuncture Studies," p. 37, Research; and "Acupuncture in Western Europe," p. 137; "Acupuncture in Germany in 2006," p. 191, Professional Developments, Legislation, and Regulation.

References

1. Melchart D, Streng A, Hoppe A, et al. Acupuncture in patients with tension-type headache: randomised controlled trial. *BMJ*. 2005;331: 376–382.
2. Witt C, Brinkhaus B, Jena S, et al. Acupuncture in patients with osteoarthritis of the knee: a randomised trial. *Lancet*. 2005;366:136–143.
3. Brinkhaus B, Becker-Witt C, Jena S, et al. Acupuncture in patients with chronic low back pain: A Randomized Controlled Trial. *Arch Intern Med*. 2006;166(4):450–457.
4. Diener HC, Kronfeld K, Boewing G, et al. Efficacy of acupuncture for the prophylaxis of migraine: a multicentre randomised controlled clinical trial. *Lancet Neurol*. 2006;5(4):310–316.
5. Linde K, Streng A, Hoppe A, et al. Treatment in a randomized multicenter trial of acupuncture for migraine (ART migraine). *Forsch Komplementarmed*. 2006;13(2):101–108.
6. Lee A, Done ML. Stimulation of the wrist acupuncture point P6 for preventing postoperative nausea and vomiting. *Cochrane Database Syst Rev*. 2004:CD003281.
7. *Huang Di Nei Jing Su Wen* (The Yellow Emperor's Canon of Internal Medicine). Translation by Paul Unschuld. University of California Press 2003.
8. Ernst M, Lee MH. Sympathetic effects of manual and electrical acupuncture of the Tsusanli knee point: comparison with the Hoku hand point sympathetic effects. *Exp. Neurol*. 1986; 94:1–10.
9. Bäcker M, Hammes MG, Valet M, et al. Different modes of manual acupuncture stimulation differentially modulate cerebral blood flow velocity, arterial blood pressure, and heart rate in human subjects. *Neurosci Lett*. 2002;333:203–206.
10. Andersson S, Lundeberg T. Acupuncture—from empiricism to science: functional background to acupuncture effects in pain and disease. *Med Hypotheses*. 1995;45(3):271–281.
11. Bäcker M, Gareus IK, Knoblauch NT, et al. Acupuncture in the treatment of pain—hypothesis to adaptive effects. *Forsch Komplementarmed Klass Naturheilk*. 2004;11(6):335–345.
12. Bäcker M, Dobos GJ. [Psychophysiology of acupuncture in the treatment of pain.]. *Dt Z Akup*. 2006;49(3):6–17.
13. Bäcker M, Hammes M, Sander D, et al. Changes of cerebrovascular response to visual stimulation in migraineurs after repetitive sessions of somatosensory stimulation (acupuncture): a pilot study. *Headache*. 2004;44:95–101.
14. Bäcker M, Grossmann P, Schneider J, et al. Vegetative effects of acupuncture in migraine—analysis of heart rate variability. ICMART International Medical Symposium of Acupuncture and Related Techniques (Abstract), Prague, 2005.
15. Schandry R. *Lehrbuch Psychophysiologie. Körperliche Indikatoren psychischen Geschehens*. 3rd ed. Weinheim: Beltz Psychologische Verlagsunion; 1998:60–70.
16. Paterson C, Dieppe P. Characteristic in incidental (placebo) effects in complex interventions such as acupuncture. *BMJ*. 2005;330:1202–1205.
17. Vas J, Méndez C, Perea-Milla E, et al. Acupuncture as a complementary therapy to the pharmacological treatment of osteoarthritis of the knee: randomised controlled trial. *BMJ*. 2004; 329:1216.
18. Vickers AJ, Rees RW, Zollman CE, et al. Acupuncture for chronic headache in primary care: large, pragmatic, randomised trial. *BMJ*. 2004; 328:744.
19. Furlan AD, van Tulder M, Cherkin D, et al. Acupuncture and dry-needling for low back pain: an updated systematic review within the framework of the Cochrane collaboration. *Spine*. 2005;30:944–963.
20. Chinesische Medizin—Bei den deutschen beliebt. *Dtsch Arztebl*. 2005;102:B2584.
21. Vincent C, Lewith G. Placebo controls for acupuncture studies. *J R Soc Med*. 1995;88:199–202.
22. Bäcker M, Hammes, M. *Akupunktur in der Schmerztherapie – ein integrativer Ansatz*. Munich–Jena: Elsevier; 2004.
23. Ots T. Egal-Wohin-Akupunktur? Gedanken zur aufgeregten Diskussion der letzten Wochen um die Punktgenauigkeit in der Akupunkur. *Dt Ztschr f Akup*. 2004;47:58–59.
24. Trinh KV, Phillips SD, Ho E, Damsma K. Acupuncture for the alleviation of lateral epicondyle pain: a systematic review. *Rheumatology* (Oxford). 2004;43:1085–1090.

Acknowledgements

This work was supported by the Ministry of Research of North Rhine-Westphalia. We thank Rainer Luedtke for his critical examination of the manuscript.

This article has previously been published in German in the Deutsche Medizinische Wochenschrift: *Dtsch Med Wochenschr*. 2006; 131:506–511.

Contact Details

Corresponding author: Dr Marcus Baecker
Chair of Complementary and Integrative
    Medicine
University of Duisburg-Essen
Department of Internal Medicine V
Kliniken Essen Mitte
Am Deimelsberg 34a
45276 Essen
Germany
+49-201-80531
marcus.baecker@uni-essen.de

Comments on the German Acupuncture Studies

Stephen Birch, PhD, LAc, Amsterdam, the Netherlands

The clinical research on acupuncture may be critical for how acupuncture is accepted by society. A number of large controlled trials of acupuncture have been completed in Germany, some of which have recently been published [1, 2, 3]. Several of these studies are perhaps the largest controlled trials of acupuncture to date [for example, 4]. These studies were conducted as a means for determining whether acupuncture should be retained under the national health insurance system in Germany. Two different groups conducted parallel studies. There was collaboration between researchers in Berlin and Munich (the Acupuncture Randomized Trials [ART] group), and a university-based doctor–practitioner group collaboration known as the German Acupuncture Trials (GERAC). The ART studies have been published, while the GERAC studies have been announced in press releases but have not yet been published in medical journals.

The ART group conducted four randomized controlled trials of acupuncture that were compared to sham acupuncture and no acupuncture (standard care only). There were about 300 patients in each of these trials [1, 2, 3]. The ART group also conducted a large open trial to see how patients fared in normal clinical practice if they received acupuncture, and more than 200 000 patients participated in this trial. The third study looked at adverse effect rates in normal clinical practice, and data from almost 100 000 patients was collected [5]. The general conclusion from these various studies is that acupuncture appears to be safe and effective for the primary conditions for which it was tested: migraine, tension headache, low back pain, and arthritis of the knees.

The GERAC group conducted four very large randomized controlled trials with 900 patients in each trial for the same conditions: migraine, tension headache, low back pain, and arthritis of the knees. At present (July 2006) it is hard to state clearly what the results of these trials have been as the results have not yet been published. It would seem, however, that they draw similar conclusions to that of the ART group, which is that in some studies acupuncture appears to be effective (see "Acupuncture Quo Vadis?—On the Current Discussion Around its Effectiveness and 'Point Specificity'," p. 29, Research).

Although these studies have in the main been discussed within Germany as showing that acupuncture is effective, especially when compared to standard medical interventions, this is not always the case outside Germany [6, 7]. Why are these studies generally viewed as positive for acupuncture inside Germany, but negative for acupuncture outside Germany?

The debate focuses on the results of acupuncture compared to sham acupuncture in the various randomized controlled clinical trials. In many, but not most, studies, the acupuncture was not more effective than the sham. The inclusion of the sham treatment method in each of these studies is of interest to academics [8], but it is not the usual method of answering the particular social medical question that the researchers started with [9]. Since the studies were conducted to address the question of whether acupuncture should continue to be included in the social health care reimbursement system, this is naturally the focus of the researchers and scientists in Germany. The fact that acupuncture often did not perform better than sham acupuncture, however, has been interpreted as meaning that it doesn't make a big difference where the needles are inserted in acupuncture. Therefore, students don't need to study very much, and traditional theories are thought to be irrelevant [6, 7]. This is seen as being bad news for acupuncture outside Germany.

While some of the studies have been explicit in their description of the sham as not being an inert placebo [1, 2, 3], we have yet to see how the other studies describe this. The sham intervention used shallowly inserted needles in non-points. As many readers no doubt know, shallowly inserted needling is a common form of acupuncture in many parts of the acupuncture community. The doctors that conducted these studies, however, chose to ignore this fact in favor of testing the Traditional Chinese Medicine (TCM) style needling with its characteristic *de qi* sensations, and thus selected shallow needling as the control for this. Acting in this way, this poses certain methodological risks.

All is not lost for acupuncture, though. Conducting sham acupuncture studies is very complicated, as it requires many more controls and measures than were used in these studies [10, 11]. Without attempting these controls and measures, the studies risked muddying the waters of the sham treatment, making it very hard to interpret results in these treatment methods [10, 12]. The claim that acupuncture theory is dead, and that it makes no difference where one inserts the needles [6, 7], is both wrong and absurd. In any treatment by acupuncture there are at least two main variables: the location of needling and the method of needling. The sham acupuncture would need to apply the same method of needling at different sites if it wanted to test the hypothesis of whether it makes a difference as to where the needles are inserted. Similarly, it would need to apply a different method of needling to the same sites of insertion if it wanted to test the hypothesis of whether it makes a difference as to what technique of needling is applied [10]. These studies carried out neither of these controls, and thus conclusions cannot be drawn about either sites of insertion or techniques of treatment. In fact, an alternative and equally (non)valid conclusion (in contradistinction to that of Ernst and Henderson [6, 7]) is that shallow needling is a powerful treatment method, regardless of where it is applied. Curiously, this was not the conclusion of acupuncture's detractors. The studies show that it

is difficult to conduct sham acupuncture trials, and when the methodological problems involved are not adequately addressed, the results of the "real versus sham" comparison become confusing and hard to interpret.

The results of these studies, however, also showed that the various acupuncture interventions that were applied were highly effective, and much more so than the standard care usually given to patients with the same symptoms. Additionally, there is evidence that the studies found a high degree of cost-effectiveness [13]. These facts are very good news for acupuncture, especially in light of the dawning recognition that placebo (sham) trials of acupuncture are extremely hard to undertake [10], as shown by the almost complete lack of any trials trying to deal with all the complex issues involved.

It is very likely that these big studies will be discussed for a long time to come. Further strengths and weaknesses will emerge in the ensuing discussions. Eventually we will find that these are important studies with significant implications, but that it will be necessary to be cautious regarding the interpretation of the comparison of the results from the different treatments given. I would not want to be in the shoes of the systematic review methodologists trying to incorporate these trials into their studies. Do they compare the acupuncture with the sham intervention, which is a highly problematic comparison? Or do they compare the acupuncture with the standard care intervention, which is a relatively straightforward comparison? Perhaps Ockham's razor will help*.

---

* Ockham's razor: a principle applied in logic, essentially implying that when there are different solutions for complex problems, the simplest should be chosen.

References

1. Linde K, Streng A, Jürgens S, et al. Acupuncture for patients with migraine: a randomized controlled trial. *JAMA*. 2005;293(17):2118–2125.
2. Melchart D, Streng A, Hoppe A, et al. Acupuncture in patients with tension-type headache: randomised controlled trial. *BMJ*. 2005;331(7513):376–382.
3. Witt C, Brinkhaus B, Jena S, et al. Acupuncture in patients with osteoarthritis of the knee: a randomised trial. *Lancet*. 2005;366(9480):136–143.
4. Haake M, Müller HH, Schade-Brittinger C, et al. The German multicenter, randomized, partially blinded, prospective trial of acupuncture for chronic low-back pain: a preliminary report on the rationale and design of the trial. *J Altern Complement Med*. 2003;9(5):763–770.
5. Melchart D, Weidenhammer W, Streng A, et al. Prospective investigation of adverse effects of acupuncture in 97 733 patients. *Arch Intern Med*. 200;164(1):104–105.
6. Ernst E. Medicine man: an end to "free" acupuncture sessions? No wonder doctors and patients got the needle. *The Guardian*. 16 March 2004.
7. Henderson M. Junk medicine. Complementary therapies. *The Times* (Body and Soul Supplement). 7 May 2005.
8. van Haselen R. The importance of clearly defining the perspective of CAM research. *Complement Ther Med*. 2005;13(3):153–154.
9. Thomas KJ, Fitter M. Possible research strategies for evaluating CAM therapies. In: Lewith G, Jonas WB, Walach H, eds. *Clinical Research in Complementary Therapies*. Edinburgh: Churchill Livingstone; 2002:59–91.
10. Birch S. Clinical research of acupuncture: part two—controlled clinical trials: an overview of their methods. *J Altern Complement Med*. 2004;10(3):481–498.
11. Margolin A, Avants SK, Kleber HD. Rationale and design of the cocaine alternative treatments study (CATS): a randomized, controlled trial of acupuncture. *J Altern Complement Med*. 1998; 4(4):405–418.
12. Birch S, Hammerschlag R, Trinh K, Zaslawski C. The non-specific effects of acupuncture treatment: when and how to control for them. *Clin Acup Orien Med*. 2002;3(1):20–25.
13. Bovey M. Effectiveness and cost-effectiveness. *British Acupuncture Council News*. 16–17 November 2005.

Both the GERAC and the ART/ARC studies were designed to provide an answer to the question: does acupuncture work better compared to placebo? But instead of providing us with answers, both studies have generated even more questions about the nature of research, study design, placebo, doctor–patient interactions, and the healing arts in general. I find the discussions surrounding both these studies and their results exhausting, and for me, as a practitioner, these studies are of NO clinical consequence whatsoever. Whether or not they are published in the *Lancet* or in *Forschung Komplementärmedizin* does not change the way I perceive or practice Traditional Chinese Medicine.

Velia Wortman Chow, MD, Fuerth, Germany

Acupuncture Research Resource Centre

Mark Bovey, MSc, MBAcC, London, UK

The Acupuncture Research Resource Centre (ARRC) was set up in 1994, a joint venture by the British Acupuncture Council (BAcC), the main UK professional body for practitioners who are neither doctors nor physiotherapists, and the Foundation for Traditional Chinese Medicine (a research charity). They had recognized the need for a research profile if acupuncture were to get wider acceptance within the UK. Research priorities and existing obstacles were identified. Initiatives were begun on several fronts: education, strategic planning, funding for small projects, liaison with other organizations—together with the ARRC's information and support role.

Aims

- To provide good quality information on research into acupuncture.
- To promote research amongst acupuncture practitioners and others.
- To increase awareness of the role and effectiveness of acupuncture, and hence help to gain wider acceptance for the use of acupuncture within the UK healthcare system.

Funding

The ARRC is funded entirely by the BAcC, from the pool of members' subscriptions. The main expense is the salary of its coordinator, a half-time post. This person is a practicing acupuncturist and has some research expertise. A management committee oversees the activities of the coordinator and reports to the BAcC.

Location

Originally located in-house, ARRC subsequently moved to a university setting, first Exeter, then Thames Valley. Whilst increasing the overhead costs, this positioned the organization more firmly within research circles, provided access to university facilities, and conferred the stamp of authenticity that comes with university association. The particular university had to be carefully chosen; we looked for emerging complementary and alternative medicine (CAM) activity without the orthodox medical presence that might be off-putting for BAcC members. Most importantly, we wanted to see some degree of enthusiasm for having us on campus.

Database

In order to have a readily accessible source of acupuncture research information, the ARRC began to compile its own electronic database of literature references, subject headings, abstracts. The details have been published elsewhere [1]. For many years the bulk of the records came from Medline (access to which originally required a subscription, but is now free to all) and the British Library's ancillary medicine database, AMED (subscription only). Subsequently, another commercial database, EMBASE, was also incorporated. Each month, relevant records were extracted, re-formatted and imported into the ARRC's own bibliographic database (ARRCBASE). This now contains in excess of 16 000 records, some of which relate to herbs or other aspects of Chinese medicine rather than specifically acupuncture. BAcC members can access the database themselves on the organization's website.

Information Service

Where others have opted for a fee-based service, the ARRC's information provision has remained largely free. Certainly this applies to BAcC members, since their fees ultimately fund it. Acupuncture college students are future members, and their research aspirations are to be encouraged. Members of the public are potential patients, journalists are potential publicists, National Health Service (NHS) workers are potential associates—would they be put off if they had to pay for their inquiry? We look at each request individually, and for some we charge a small amount.

Most questions can be answered with a fairly simple literature search, or by using our own review papers (of which more below). Some clients are happy to receive just a list of database records, others need the output to be filtered, summarized, and presented in language that is easy to understand. Today, many people have the capability to search for acupuncture research literature themselves on the internet, though they may need pointing towards the most appropriate sources and/or help with interpreting the results. Some members of the public are looking for the personal perspective of an independent expert rather than for research results per se.

Requests for information may be taken by email, phone, or letter. Turnaround is usually within one week.

Who Uses the Service and for What?

For the four years 1998–2002, an audit of service user records showed that there were 1333 requests from 960 different clients [2]. More than 60% were either acupuncture practitioners or acupuncture students; other significant groups were other students, the public, journalists, and orthodox health service professionals (see table).

ARRC Service Users

Users	%
Acupuncturists	42.1
Acupuncture students	19.5
Other students: nursing, medical, other health and non-health-related courses	12.2
Members of the public	7.5
Journalists	5.4
NHS: nurses, midwives, doctors, and managers	4.1
Researchers	2.6
Others: other therapists, charities/support groups, and educational institutions	6.5

We try to find out why people want the information that they're asking for; this helps to direct the literature search more precisely, and it may provide us with useful data for the future. Sometimes the purpose is self-evident: students want literature for their course project/dissertation. Acupuncture practitioners' needs are more varied but are usually within four main categories:
1. To help them treat a particular patient, often one with a rather unusual condition.
2. To help a particular patient get treatment paid for by the NHS.
3. To help promote their practice, or set up an acupuncture service within the NHS.
4. To help them carry out some research.

Requests of type 1 would largely indicate articles written by fellow acupuncturists. A high proportion would be from China. For 2 and 3, by contrast, we look for the sort of evidence that doctors and medical researchers like to see, especially evidence from controlled trials.

Help for Research Projects

The ARRC provides a point of contact within the profession for those practitioners involved in, or interested in, research projects. Activities include:

- Encouraging greater participation.
- Helping to generate topic ideas.
- Advising on methodology, ethical issues, and funding.
- Assisting with protocol production.
- Giving technical support for data analysis and presentation.
- Providing literature and contacts.

The ARRC does not usually carry out its own research projects; instead, it is a service organization.

Symposia

Each year, the ARRC organizes an acupuncture research symposium in London. This provides the opportunity for practitioners both to hear from the experts and to report on their own projects.

Papers

The ARRC has produced a series of briefing papers, reviews of the evidence for the effectiveness of acupuncture for particular conditions. So far, there are 13, covering migraine, stroke, arthritis, gynecological complaints, menopause, HIV, asthma, anxiety and depression, obstetrics (two), infertility, and sports injuries. These have been written to an agreed format by different authors, and then edited and published by the ARRC. They provide fairly objective summaries of the available evidence, but are not systematic reviews in the strict sense of the term. In addition, there are a

number of shorter, looser, papers, more directly oriented for publicity purposes, and regular newsletter pieces to inform and inspire the BAcC membership.

For the Future

We are currently moving to place as much as possible of our information service on to a new website, thus freeing up time for the more proactive and creative aspects of the ARRC's activities.

References

1. Gould AJ. Review and description of ARRCBASE: A bibliographic database of acupuncture practice and research. *Complementary Therapies in Medicine.* 1997;5(3):168–171.
2. Bovey M, Ward T. Patterns of demand and supply for an acupuncture research information service. *Focus on Alternative and Complementary Therapies.* 2003;8(4):484.

Contact Details

Acupuncture Research Resource Centre
Coordinator: Mark Bovey
Thames Valley University
Faculty of Health and Human Sciences
4th Floor
Walpole House
18–22 Bond Street
Ealing
London W5 5AA
UK
+44 20 8280 5277
arrc@tvu.ac.uk

Acupuncture and Traditional Chinese Medicine: Researching the Practice

Hugh MacPherson, PhD, MBAcC, York, UK

Introduction

A small group of enthusiasts based in York, England, has been conducting research into acupuncture and, to a lesser extent, Chinese herbal medicine, for over 10 years. It all started in the early 1990s when Richard Blackwell, Mike Fitter, and Hugh MacPherson set up the Foundation for Traditional Chinese Medicine as a vehicle to promote high-quality research. From the outset, the foundation provided an organizational base for promoting research into acupuncture and aimed: "… through research and education, to bring the traditional Chinese system of acupuncture more centrally into the national health care system." By developing the evidence base for Chinese medicine, whether acupuncture or herbs, we hoped to widen access to these modalities in the UK, where the provision by the National Health Service (NHS) is, and always has been, patchy. Given the inherent resource constraints of nationally funded health care, and the need for evidence that is persuasive, we have focused more on pragmatic health service-oriented research, so that our results can feed directly into policy decisions about who and for what conditions patients should be offered a direct referral from primary care. Our research activities and projects have mainly focused on evaluating the benefits, cost effectiveness, and safety of acupuncture.

The Foundation for Traditional Chinese Medicine is a research charity (a not-for-profit organization) with Lord Colwyn as Patron, together with a board of trustees and a board of advisors. As a result of a personal award from the Department of Health, our research director, Hugh MacPherson, recently took up a joint appointment with the Department of Health Sciences at the University of York, where he is working closely with Pro Vice Chancellor Professor Trevor Sheldon.

This has opened up new avenues of research and funding, and so a raft of new projects has recently been started. Several projects of the foundation continue to be undertaken, in close collaboration with other researchers, in particular Professor Kate Thomas who is based at the University of Leeds. Funding has come from a combination of core funding from grant-making trusts and project funding from statutory and other sources. Donations from individuals and grant-making trusts have been a valued source of funding for the work of the foundation.

Acupuncture for Chronic Low Back Pain

Back pain is a major cause of ill health and time lost from work. Conventional medical treatments often have limited success and the NHS has identified back pain as a priority condition for research. In preparation for a randomized controlled trial, we carried out a feasibility study [1] followed by a larger pilot study [2], which together provided a platform for an application for funding a large-scale trial. With Kate Thomas, then of the Medical Care Research Unit at Sheffield University as principal investigator, and funded by the Department of Health R&D Health Technology Assessment Programme, we conducted a pragmatic randomized controlled trial to evaluate the clinical impact and cost-effectiveness of acupuncture for chronic low back pain, publishing the protocol in 1999 [3].

In the trial, we recruited 43 general practitioners who referred 241 patients for up to 10 acupuncture treatments, provided by six local acupuncturists. Both groups continued to receive conventional primary care from their general practitioner. The key outcome measure was bodily pain, as measured by the SF-36, at 12 and 24 months after randomization. The results were in favor of the acupuncture group at 12 months and became significant at 24 months: analysis of covariance, adjusting for baseline score, found a positive effect for acupuncture of 5.6 points on the SF-36 pain dimension (95 % CI 1.3 to 12.5, p = 0.11), increasing at 12 months to eight points (95 % CI 0.7 to 15.3, p = 0.03) at 24 months. Acupuncture patients also reported a significantly greater reduction in worry about their back pain. In addition, the acupuncture service was found to be cost effective. It is hoped that these results will be published soon in a major medical journal. The full report is now published as a monograph by the Health Technology Assessment Programme [4].

In a sub-study we also explored the traditional acupuncture diagnostic concordance between the six acupuncturists. The acupuncture diagnosis was based on up to three predefined low back pain syndromes, for which inter-rater reliability was assessed. The most commonly diagnosed syndrome was *qi* and blood stagnation (88 % of patients), followed by kidney deficiency (53 %) and bi syndrome (28 %). Where patients were rated twice, 47 % to 80 % of classifications were congruent, and Cohen's Kappa was between 0 ("same as chance") and 0.67 ("good"). These results, along with a full description of treatment, have recently been published [5].

The Safety of Acupuncture

The safety of acupuncture has come under scrutiny in the UK over the past five years. As part of establishing the evidence on safety, the foundation researched the medical literature and published a series of review articles. These papers sifted the evidence, examined the quality of reporting, and made proposals for prospective studies to evaluate risks and safety for acupuncture patients. Building on these reviews, in 1999 the British Acupuncture Council (BAcC) commissioned the foundation to undertake a nationwide prospective survey of practitioner reports on adverse events. The survey involved 574 practitioners, who reported for four weeks during May 2000

on all the significant events, as well as any minor transient reactions that took place as a result of the treatment they provided. Between them, the practitioners reported events covering over 34 000 acupuncture treatments. There were no serious adverse events, and forty-three significant minor adverse events. A short report was published in the *British Medical Journal* [6], followed by a full report [7].

As an extension of this work, the BAcC funded a follow-up survey of adverse events as experienced by patients. One-third of all BAcC members helped us recruit 9408 patients, of whom 6348 (67 %) completed three-month questionnaires. At three months, 682 patients reported adverse events, caused directly by the needling process. The most common were severe tiredness and exhaustion. Three events were serious, defined as requiring hospitalization, causing permanent disability, or being life-threatening. There was no evidence that patients not funded by the NHS, or not in contact with their general practitioner or hospital specialist, were at greater risk. Six patients reported a worsening of symptoms after taking advice on medication, and two patients reported delayed conventional treatment. Our recently published results show that acupuncture is a relatively safe intervention when practiced by qualified and regulated practitioners [8]. Two sub-studies, one on the profiles of these patients [9] and one on the short-term reactions to treatment that they experienced, [10] have been recently published.

Acupuncture for Menorrhagia

With over 40 000 hysterectomies being performed every year in the UK, the need for women to have a less invasive and more supportive treatment for heavy menstrual periods continues to be an important issue. Because women can be on an NHS waiting list for a hysterectomy for between one and two years, and many would rather not have one, there is an opportunity to evaluate acupuncture as an alternative treatment. Research in China suggests that around two-thirds of women with heavy menstrual periods can be significantly helped with acupuncture. Based on these findings, and the experiences of patients and practitioners in the West, the Acupuncture for Menorrhagia (ACUMEN) Project was designed by Alison Gamon, a PhD student at the Department of Health Sciences at the University of York, in collaboration with the foundation and Professor Kate Thomas. Funding has come from an independent grant-making trust and the Department of Health Sciences, University of York.

The initial phase of this project involves an exploratory trial, designed to explore a possible role for acupuncture in the treatment of menorrhagia, as a preparation for a full-scale randomized controlled trial. In the exploratory trial, 40 patients were randomized to the offer of acupuncture, in conjunction with normal GP care, while the other half received normal GP care only. The acupuncture group received up to 20 acupuncture sessions on a weekly basis. This trial is now being written up and will be published in 2006. This research has aimed to explore the feasibility of the design and acceptability of acupuncture to patients, as well as testing referral and other procedures, assessing outcome measures, and monitoring costs and safety.

The Safety of Chinese Herbal Medicine

With the aim of providing information about adverse events associated with herbal medicine, we conducted a pilot for a national survey project to assess the level of safety for patients receiving treatment with Chinese herbs. Our wider goal is to help patients make informed choices about treatment and provide policy-makers with robust evidence on safety as a contribution to decision-making on widening access within the NHS.

MSc student Bin Liu has worked with the research director in conducting this pilot. We invited practitioner members of the Register of Chinese Herbal Medicine to participate, and 72 practitioners helped us recruit 170 patients, of whom 126 (74 %) have provided us

with details of adverse events that they associated with taking Chinese herbal medicine over a four-week period [11].

STandards for Reporting Interventions in Controlled Trials of Acupuncture (STRICTA)

The need for better standards of reporting of controlled trials of acupuncture is evident from the difficulties associated with their interpretation and analysis. Hugh MacPherson has worked with an international group of acupuncture researchers and the editors of several leading journals in the field to address this issue. As a result, a set of recommendations for better reporting of trials was developed, called the STRICTA recommendations (STandards for Reporting Interventions in Controlled Trials of Acupuncture.) The guiding principle was a commitment to achieving a broad enough set of recommendations that would cover the most common approaches to both acupuncture and research design.

These recommendations were published in parallel by the key journals in the field [12]. Participating journals are *Acupuncture in Medicine, Clinical Acupuncture and Oriental Medicine, Complementary Therapies in Medicine, Journal of Alternative and Complementary Medicine*, and *Medical Acupuncture*. These journals are committed to adding the STRICTA recommendations to their instructions for authors. Translations and republication in Japan, China, and Korea have been of value in broadening their impact. Further investigations in this area have been initiated elsewhere, and we continue to be involved in extending the influence of these recommendations internationally.

Acupuncture for Depression

This program of research is being conducted jointly between the Foundation for Traditional Chinese Medicine and the Department of Health Sciences at the University of York, where the research director holds a Department of Health post-doctoral fellowship. The aim of the research is to determine acupuncture's potential role as a treatment modality in primary care.

Depression is the second most common cause of disability in the world, and in the UK it is the third most common reason for consulting in primary care. The limited evidence from the medical literature suggests acupuncture may be effective in the treatment of depression, and some patients see it as an attractive non-drug option. A small study we conducted with an uncontrolled case series of ten patients has recently been published [13]. However the controlled trial evidence on the clinical effects of acupuncture is weak, in contrast to its increasing popularity. As a next step, some feasibility and piloting work is now required.

This program is initially tackling a series of methodological challenges associated with design and implementation of a trial of acupuncture for depression (Phase 1), leading to the implementation of an exploratory randomized controlled trial (Phase 2), followed by an optimally designed multi-center trial (Phase 3), to evaluate the clinical and economic impact of offering acupuncture for primary care patients with depression. We are developing specific methodological tools for the evaluation of acupuncture in real-life settings, in order to generate meaningful and credible evidence that can inform decision-making.

The five methodological challenges in Phase 1 are:

- Investigating acupuncture's potential therapeutic niche in primary care.
- Establishing by consensus a protocol for the treatment of depression.
- Identifying and testing a measure of the therapeutic relationship.
- Identifying outcome measures sensitive to acupuncture's broader effects.
- Exploring how trial evidence may influence GP referral for acupuncture.

This program of research is supported by two PhD students, Sylvia Schroer, who is a Department of Health award-holder, and Beverley

Lawton, who has a Department of Health Sciences, University of York scholarship.

Acupuncture for Non-Cardiac Chest Pain

Patients with chest pain commonly present in primary care, followed by referral to cardiac clinics in secondary care. However as many as 50 % of patients referred to such cardiac clinics are found to have no problem with their heart. The causes of non-cardiac chest pain are not always clear, but there is evidence that they could be musculoskeletal, gastrointestinal, respiratory, or psychiatric, the commonest cause being musculoskeletal. Non-cardiac patients are usually referred back to primary care, where they often continue to experience chest pain, with as many as three-quarters experiencing limitations in activities, concern about the cause of their symptoms, and dissatisfaction with medical care. Acupuncture is increasingly being used to treat non-cardiac chest pain, despite an absence of research into effectiveness.

We are undertaking this research in two phases. In the first phase we have surveyed patients who attended the Rapid Access Chest Pain Unit at York Hospital, but whose chest pain was non-cardiac in origin. The survey has captured vital information about this population, including their diagnosis and treatment, their chest pain levels, and, if still in pain, their interest in receiving acupuncture. In this first phase, our collaborators include Dr Jo Dumville, a Research Fellow at the University of York, and Dr Kathryn Griffith, a general practitioner (GP) and Clinical Assistant in Cardiology at the York District Hospital where she works at the Rapid Access Chest Pain Clinic two days a week. At the University of York, Bob Lewin, Professor of Cardiac Rehabilitation and Dr Jeremy Miles have provided important input. This study will inform our design for the second phase, which will be a pilot for a pragmatic randomized controlled trial.

Acupuncture for Chronic Neck Pain

Chronic neck pain is a prevalent problem in general practice, and conventional treatments have limited success. Patients are seeking acupuncture outside the NHS in increasing numbers, yet the current evidence on acupuncture for neck pain is inconclusive. As a result, there is a growing public and scientific imperative to know whether acupuncture is worth offering as a referral option in primary care. In this project, we plan to conduct an open pragmatic randomized controlled trial of acupuncture for patients with neck pain, evaluating the clinical and economic impact when it is provided as an adjunct to normal GP management. As well as informing decisions made by patients and general practitioners, the knowledge gained on cost-effectiveness will contribute to policy decisions on widening access to acupuncture within primary care. In this project we are working with Gemma Salter, an MRC funded MSc student, and Professor David Torgerson, Director of the York Trials Unit. A small pilot has been conducted in which we recruited 24 patients and provided those randomized on acupuncture with ten sessions of acupuncture. We have recently completed the three-month follow-up for this study and are writing up a paper outlining the findings in the context of designing and conducting a large-scale trial.

Neuroimaging of Acupuncture

Even with a growing body of evidence for acupuncture, there are many skeptics who would like to see "objective" evidence of acupuncture's impact on biological correlates. One new area of research, where such "objective" evidence has now become possible, is in the mapping of the effect of acupuncture techniques on regionally specific structures within the brain. Such specific and quantifiable data could extend the evidence base for the mechanisms underlying acupuncture, and potentially contribute to the explanations of its clinical impact. Some recent studies have suggested the remarkable possibility of correlations between classical acupuncture points and cerebral activity not linked by known neural pathways. This research points to exciting opportunities to map the impact of needling specific acupuncture points on brain structures.

We are now working closely with the York Neuroimaging Centre to investigate the impact on brain images of needling *he gu* (LI-4). Our primary aim is to investigate the extent of activation and deactivation of the brain associated with both deep and superficial needling. Secondary objectives are to explore variations on the brain images associated with the participant's sex, prior belief about acupuncture, and the sensation felt at the site of needling. We have conducted experimental trials with using both MRI and MEG scanners. We hope that the first results will be available soon.

References

1. Fitter M, MacPherson H. An audit of case studies of low back pain: a feasibility study for a controlled trial. *European Journal of Oriental Medicine*. 1995;1(5):46–55.
2. MacPherson H, Gould AJ, Fitter M. Acupuncture for low back pain: results of a pilot study for a randomised controlled trial. *Complementary Therapies in Medicine*. 1999; 7(2):83–90.
3. Thomas KJ, Fitter M, Brazier J, et al. Longer term clinical and economic benefits of offering acupuncture to patients with chronic low back pain assessed as suitable for primary care management. *Complementary Therapies in Medicine*.1997;(2):91–100.
4. Thomas KJ, MacPherson H, Thorpe L, et al. Longer term clinical and economic benefits of offering acupuncture to patients with chronic low back pain. NHS Health Technology Assessment Programme monograph, 2005. www.hta .nhsweb.nhs.uk.
5. MacPherson H, Thorpe L, Thomas KJ, Campbell M. Acupuncture for low back pain: traditional diagnosis and treatment of 148 patients in a clinical trial. *Complementary Therapies in Medicine*. 2004;12(1):38–44.
6. MacPherson H, Thomas K, Walters S, Fitter M. The York acupuncture safety study: prospective survey of 34 000 treatments by traditional acupuncturists. *BMJ*. 2001; 323:486–87.

7. MacPherson H, Thomas KJ, Walters S, Fitter M. A prospective survey of adverse events and treatment reactions following 34 000 consultations with professional acupuncturists. *Acupuncture in Medicine.* 2001;19(2):93–102.

8. MacPherson H, Scullion T, Thomas K, Walters S. Patient reports of adverse events associated with acupuncture: a large scale prospective survey. *Quality and Safety in Health Care.* 2004;13:349–355.

9. MacPherson H, Sinclair-Lian N, Thomas KJ. Patients seeking care from acupuncture practitioners in the UK: a national survey. *Complementary Therapies in Medicine.* 2006;14:20–30.

10. MacPherson H, Thomas KJ. Short-term reactions to acupuncture: a cross-sectional survey of patient reports. *Acupuncture in Medicine;* 2005,23(3):112–120.

11. MacPherson H, Bin Liu. The safety of Chinese herbal medicine: a pilot study for a national survey. *Journal of Complementary and Alternative Medicine;* 2005, 11(4):617–26.

12. MacPherson H, White A, Cummings M, Jobst K, Rose K, Niemtzow, R. Standards for reporting interventions in controlled trials of acupuncture—the STRICTA recommendations.

Complementary Therapies in Medicine. 2001; 9(4):246–49. [Co-published in *Journal of Alternative and Complementary Medicine.* 2002; 8(1):85–89; *Acupuncture in Medicine.* 2002; 20(1):22–25; *Clinical Acupuncture and Oriental Medicine.* 2002; 3(1) 6–9, and *Medical Acupuncture.* 2002; 13(3):9–11.]

13. MacPherson H, Thorpe L, Thomas K. Acupuncture for Depression: first steps in a clinical evaluation. *Journal of Alternative and Complementary Medicine.* 2004, 10(6): 1083–1091.

Contact Details

Hugh MacPherson, PhD, MBAcC
Senior Research Fellow
Department of Health Sciences
Seebolm Rowntree Building
University of York
Heslington
York YO10 5DD
UK
+44 1904 321394
hm18@york.ac.uk

Using Herbs in Cancer Treatment and Cancer Research: A Review

Isaac Cohen, OMD, LAc, San Francisco, USA

Introduction

There were close to 560 000 deaths due to cancer in the USA in 2002, amounting to almost 23 % of all deaths. The age-adjusted cancer death rates were 193.9 per 100 000 in 1950 and 193.4 per 100 000 in 2002. The American Cancer Society estimates that in 2005 there were 570 000 deaths as a result of cancer; lung, prostate, and colon cancer with the highest rate in men, and lung, breast, and colon cancer with the highest rate in women. Although the numbers appear to be the same, cancer deaths have witnessed a decline (Fig. 1). Researchers believe that the decline is the result of improvement in early

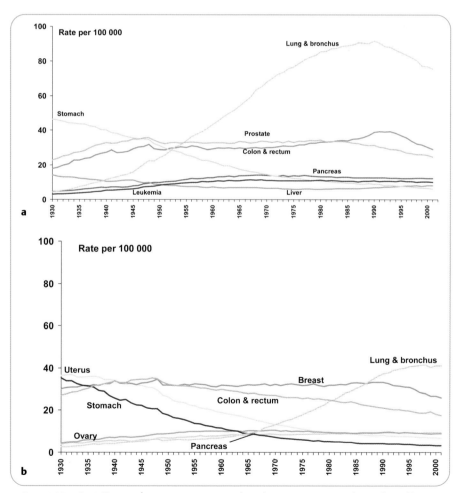

Fig. **1a** Cancer death rates* for men, USA, 1930–2001.

Fig. **1b** Cancer death rates* for women, USA, 1930–2001.

* Age-adjusted to the 2000 US standard population.

Source: US Mortality Public Use Data Tapes 1960–2001, US Mortality Volumes 1930–1959, National Center for Health Statistics, Centers for Disease Control and Prevention

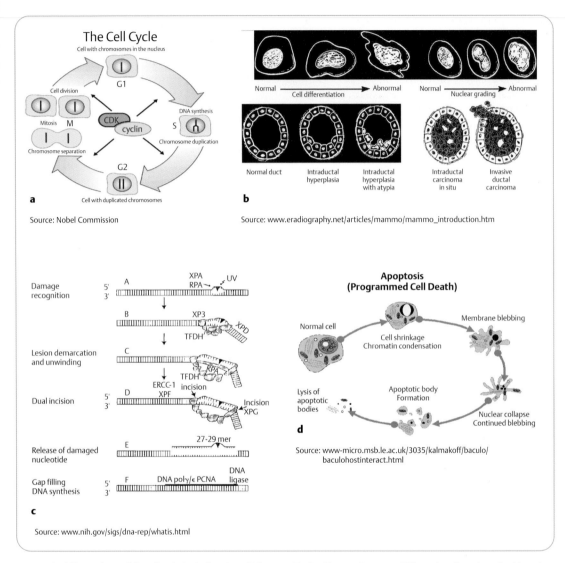

The Cell Cycle

Cell with chromosomes in the nucleus

G1

Cell division

Mitosis M

Chromosome separation

CDK cyclin

S

DNA synthesis

Chromosome duplication

G2

Cell with duplicated chromosomes

a

Source: Nobel Commission

Normal ⟶ Abnormal
Cell differentiation

Normal ⟶ Abnormal
Nuclear grading

Normal duct | Intraductal hyperplasia | Intraductal hyperplasia with atypia | Intraductal carcinoma in situ | Invasive ductal carcinoma

b

Source: www.eradiography.net/articles/mammo/mammo_introduction.htm

Damage recognition — 5' 3' — A — XPA RPA UV

B — XP3 XPD TFDH

Lesion demarcation and unwinding — C — TFDH RPA

Dual incision — 5' 3' — D — ERCC-1 incision XPF — Incision XPG

Release of damaged nucleotide — E — 27-29 mer

Gap filling DNA synthesis — 5' 3' — F — DNA poly/ε PCNA — DNA ligase

c

Source: www.nih.gov/sigs/dna-rep/whatis.html

Apoptosis (Programmed Cell Death)

Normal cell

Cell shrinkage Chromatin condensation

Membrane blebbing

Lysis of apoptotic bodies

Apoptotic body Formation

Nuclear collapse Continued blebbing

d

Source: www.micro.msb.le.ac.uk/3035/kalmakoff/baculo/baculohostinteract.html

Fig. **2a** The different phases of the cell cycle. In the first phase (G1) the cell grows. When it has reached a certain size it enters the phase of DNA-synthesis (S) in which the chromosomes are duplicated. During the next phase (G2) the cell prepares for division. During mitosis (M) the chromosomes are separated and segregated to the daughter cells, which thereby receive exactly the same chromosome set up. The cells are then back in G1 and the cell cycle is completed.

Fig. **2b** Microscopic cell differentiation on a scale from normal to abnormal. Top left illustrates the morphological changes that occur to cells. Top right illustrates the changes that occur to the nucleus where DNA synthesis has lost its regulation. The bottom panel shows the loss of cellular architectural organization in a ductal tissue.

Fig. **2c** The most important DNA repair pathway is **nucleotide excision repair**, which fixes the majority of bulky lesions in DNA. Nucleotide excision repair involves recognition, incision, degradation, polymerization, and, finally, ligation.

Fig. **2d** Apoptosis is a cellular response to a cellular "insult," such as UV light, chemical or physical damage, or a viral infection. This insult triggers a cascade of events that lead to the destruction of the cell. This mechanism is often called "programmed cell death," as it is an innate response of the cell, which protects the rest of the organism from a potentially harmful agent.

detection, more universal access to treatment, and moderate improvements in treatment.

In modern medicine, cancer is viewed as a disease resulting from mutations of normal cells that lose some of their important controls in relation to growth regulation and repair abilities. There are four major aspects in normal cell function that can be mutated and will result in cancer. These are initiation or carcinogenesis, differentiation, repair of DNA damage, and the balance of promotion or growth regulation and death or apoptosis (Fig. **2**). Cell division (proliferation) is a physiological process that occurs in almost all tissues and under many circumstances. Normally homeostasis, the balance between proliferation and programmed cell death, usually in the form of apoptosis, is maintained by tightly regulating both processes to ensure the integrity of organs and tissues. Mutations in DNA that lead to cancer disrupt these orderly processes by disrupting the programming regulating the processes.

Initiation (*carcinogenesis*) is caused by this mutation of the genetic material of normal cells, which upsets the normal balance between proliferation and cell death. This results in uncontrolled cell division and tumor formation. The uncontrolled and often rapid proliferation of cells can lead to benign tumors, some types of which may turn into malignant tumors (cancer). Benign tumors do not spread to other parts of the body or invade other tissues, and they are rarely a threat to life unless they compress vital structures or are physiologically active (for instance, in producing a hormone). Malignant tumors can invade other organs, spread to distant locations (metastasize), and become life-threatening. The features important to cancer cells in order to metastasize are their loss of architectural regulation. They tend to invade their normal surroundings and grow outside of their genetically appropriate place. They can also dislodge from the tissue of origin, travel in the body, bypass immune surveillance, anchor in other tissues, and colonize and create a tumor.

More than one mutation is necessary for carcinogenesis. In fact, a series of several mutations to certain classes of genes is usually

required before a normal cell will transform into a cancer cell. Only mutations in those certain types of genes, which play vital roles in cell division, cell death, and DNA repair, will cause a cell to lose control of its proliferation (Fig. **3**).

It has been the subject of much research and drug development to control these processes in an attempt to treat cancer.

In Eastern medicine, what we call cancer was not clearly defined until the advent of modern pathology. It was clinically well

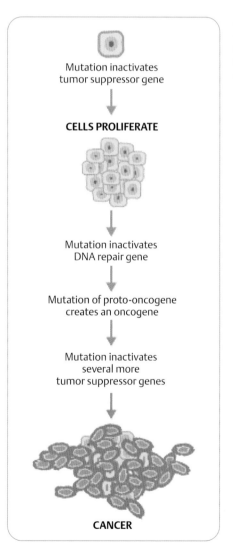

*Fig. **3** Cancers are caused by a series of mutations. Each mutation alters the behavior of the cell.*

Mutation inactivates
tumor suppressor gene

↓

CELLS PROLIFERATE

↓

Mutation inactivates
DNA repair gene

↓

Mutation of proto-oncogene
creates an oncogene

↓

Mutation inactivates
several more
tumor suppressor genes

↓

CANCER

understood that there are a variety of tumor types, some of which can be lethal and cause wasting and death. Yet it was mostly relevant to advanced forms of the disease where a tumor could be palpated or observed with the naked eye.

A variety of diseases are clumped with cancer, but cannot be viewed under this singular category since they do not have one etiology or pathological path ascribed to them. In more recent times, several conceptual and theoretical approaches have been developed to explain cancer etiology and progression with Chinese medical tenets.

In short, there were mainly three schools of thought that developed. The first school viewed cancer as a result of long-standing *qi* deficiency. Long-standing *qi* deficiency evolves over time to create stagnancy of *qi* and an inability to transform and transport nourishment for the tissues. Also, it results in an inability to both produce and separate fluids, resulting in various forms of dampness. The low levels of *qi* lead to slow but significant loss of vital functions. When vital functions are lost, as a result of the *yin* and *yang* interplay, there is loss of regulation and controls that are assumed by *qi*. Also, *yin* functions transform to *yang*, such as damp cold becoming damp heat, or *yang* functions transform to *yin*, such as *qi* accumulations or conglomerations becoming tumors.

The second school viewed cancer as a result of long-term blood stagnation. This view was a hybrid of the modern observation that in advanced cancer there is a significant increase in blood viscosity and coagulation, and the view that "senility," or aging, in Chinese medicine, is associated with the blood not being invigorated, for which the category of "blood-enlivening, stagnancy removing drugs" are used. The mechanism is that the blood loses its innate vitality, or *qi*, over time. When blood is produced in the body it has to have several components that are beyond simply being the plasma for transporting nutrients. It has to have the capacity to diffuse throughout the body, to carry *qi* of all types, to communicate among all organs and tissues, to help regulate and sustain temperature in the body

and facilitate the function of the sense organs. Blood stagnancy is therefore not the physical stoppage of blood flow, but rather the loss of the "lively" function of this essential fluid. Aging and therefore diseases of aging, such as cancer, are a direct result of the blood's loss of innate mobility and capacity to carry everything to everywhere in the body. This results in the lack of nourishing ability and accumulations.

The third view is that cancer is a result of heat toxin accumulation. Heat toxins are originally external and are the outcome of the interaction of the body with pathogenic factors of this kind. Cancer is thought to be the outcome of long-standing, untreated, or wrongly treated, febrile disease. There are many forms of febrile disease, for which we employ the various categories of "heat clearing drugs." Heat toxins are a result of exposure to poisons and infections (viral, bacterial, or otherwise) that result in the build-up of abscesses, purulent fluid, dark green mucus, severe swelling, etc. If they remain untreated they can transform to virulent accumulations and growth. It should be made clear that the emphasis of this school is not only on the toxic but also on the heat side of the equation. Heat causes hyperactivity and a depleting activity. The lethal combination of heat toxin is that the hyperactivity, depletion effect of heat, combined with the accumulation, purulence, and swelling of the toxin, is what results in cancer.

In 2004, over 60 % of cancer therapies employed by allopathic medicine were derived from natural products. Most of the chemotherapeutic agents are derived from microorganisms such as doxorubicin, toxic ores such as the platinum drugs, or plants such as the taxanes and vinca drugs. To date, only 5 % of the world's plants have been studied for their potential pharmacological applications. Since so many oncological drugs are derived from nature, it is relevant to review the progress in both the use of complementary and alternative (CAM) modalities, as well as the basic studies.

Method

The review was done using the National Library of Medicine, PubMed database. The key words in the search were botanicals and cancer, herbs and cancer. The search was limited to publications in 2005. I also added the early results of my own group's clinical and basic research, since it has potential clinical relevance to Traditional East Asian Medicine (TEAM) practitioners.

Clinical Studies

In the past decade there has been an increased interest on the part of the public and among researchers to weigh in the degree of use of CAM in medicine, and in cancer in particular. In 2005 there were some disease-specific reports, as well as general studies, concerning the use and preferences for CAM among cancer patients.

Hyodo et al. conducted a nation-wide survey of CAM use among cancer patients in Japan [1]. Of 3100 cancer patients who responded to the survey, 1382 (44.6%) used CAM. Of these, 96.2% used herbs or TEAM-derived products. The main motivation for use was a personal recommendation. Interestingly, the main motivations for use of CAM were history of chemotherapy, institute (palliative care units), higher education, an altered outlook on life after cancer diagnosis, primary cancer site, and younger age. Among the CAM users, 24.3% experienced positive effects from their treatment and only 5.3% reported adverse reactions.

In a study of the predictors of use of CAM among cancer patients in urban and rural USA, Fouladbakhsh et al. found similar trends as in the Japanese group [2]. They interviewed 968 lung, breast, colon, or prostate patients. In this study, significant predictors of CAM use were gender, marital status, cancer stage, cancer treatment, and the number of severe symptoms experienced.

Trevena and Reeder from New Zealand studied the perceptions regarding CAM treatments for cancer [3]. They conducted an anonymous telephone interview among 438 randomly selected citizens with no particular history of any disease. Most of the patients (63%) felt that complementary therapies might be beneficial to people who were also receiving conventional cancer treatment. When asked if they agreed with the statement that "alternative therapy for cancer has an equal or better chance of curing cancer as medical treatment," 28% agreed, 34% disagreed, and 38% said they did not know. One of the main conclusions of this study is that New Zealanders know very little about CAM therapies for cancer.

At the University of California, San Francisco, Chan et al., the team who conducted the clinical trials for PC-SPES, attempted to assess specific CAM use in the Cancer of the Prostate Strategic Urologic Research Endeavor (CaPSURE), a large, community-based national registry of men with prostate cancer [4]. They asked about more than 50 types of CAM modalities and treatments in a biannual survey within two years of prostate cancer diagnosis. One-third of 2582 respondents reported using CAM. Common practices included vitamin and mineral supplements (26%), herbs (16%), antioxidants (13%), and CAM for prostate health (12%; saw palmetto, selenium, vitamin E, lycopene). In an analysis of other potential variables, users were more likely to have other comorbid conditions, worse cancer grade at diagnosis, a higher income, be more educated, and live on the West Coast of the USA.

Shu et al. conducted a meta-analysis of randomized controlled trials of Chinese herbal medicine and chemotherapy in the treatment of hepatocellular carcinoma (HCC) [5]. They found that 26 studies representing 2079 patients met the inclusion criteria of well-conducted and reported trials. Chinese herbal medicine combined with chemotherapy, compared to chemotherapy alone, improved survival at 12 months (relative risk [RR], 1.55; 95% confidence interval [CI], 1.39–1.72; $P < .0001$), 24 months (RR, 2.15; 95% CI, 1.75–2.64; $P < .0001$), and 36 months (RR, 2.76; 95% CI, 1.95–3.91; $P < .0001$). Tumor response increased (RR, 1.39; 95% CI, 1.24–1.56; $P < .0001$). These results are suggestive of the usefulness of an integrated Chinese herbal treatment with chemotherapy. In my opinion, it is important to state that although these results need to be validated in randomized studies for the oncology community to include herbal treatments for HCC, it is easy to recommend to patients the use of Chinese herbs since chemotherapy alone provides a very poor outcome for this disease.

Our group at Bionovo, Inc, the University of California, San Francisco and the University of Texas, Southwestern, Dallas, reported the results of a phase I trial of an extract of *Scutellaria barbata* (*ban zhi lian*) (BZL-101) for metastatic breast cancer. Twenty-one eligible patients [6] with confirmed metastatic breast cancer and measurable disease, who were not able not receive any other chemotherapy, hormone therapy, or herbal medicine, were treated. Patients received BZL-101 extract daily until there was disease progression, toxicity, or a personal preference to discontinue. The primary endpoints were safety and toxicity and tumor response, defined by Response Evaluation Criteria in Solid Tumors. There were no hematologic or grade III or IV non-hematologic adverse events (AEs). The most frequently reported BZL-101-related grade I and II AEs included nausea (43 %), diarrhea (20 %), headache (20 %), flatulence (14 %), vomiting (10 %), constipation (10 %), and fatigue (10 %). Sixteen patients were evaluable for response. Four of the 16 patients had stable disease (SD) for >90 days (25 %) and three of the 16 had SD for >180 days (19 %). Five patients had objective tumor regressions, of which one patient was 1 mm short of a PR based on RECIST criteria. In conclusion, BZL-101 had a favorable tolerability profile, and demonstrated encouraging clinical activity in this heavily pretreated population of women. Future studies in women with advanced breast cancer are required to confirm the efficacy of *ban zhi lian* as a sole therapy.

Basic Studies

Basic studies are carried out in order to learn about the potential effects as well as the mechanism of action of compounds. These are a prelude to potential specific clinical application. Since herbs were used for centuries in Chinese medicine for the treatment of cancer, it is important to try to identify therapies that can be used for this disease.

Franek et al. selected four compounds from a panel of herbs used in TEAM, representing two functional classes of botanicals [7]. These were the purified plant flavins scutellarin (a circulatory stimulant) and baicalin (antipyretic) from *Scutellaria baicalinensis* (*huang qin*), and two extracts purified from *Salvia miltiorrhiza* (*dan shen*) (SM-470, circulatory stimulant) and *Camellia sinensis* (green tea) (Cam-300, antipyretic). Their anti-proliferation effects on the human breast cancer cell lines were examined. All four compounds inhibited cell proliferation, baicalin being the most potent inhibitor. A synergistic inhibitory effect on cell proliferation was also observed when SM-470 and baicalin were applied together. The anti-proliferative effects of these compounds can be extended to other cancer types: the human head and neck cancer epithelial cell lines.

Peng et al. studied the effect of berberine, a compound isolated from *Coptis chinensis* (*huang lian*) and other plant species such as Goldenseal, on the metastatic potential of lung cancer cells [8]. Berberine exerted a dose- and time-dependent inhibitory effect on the motility and invasion ability of a highly metastatic A549 non-small lung cancer cells under non-cytotoxic concentrations. In cancer cell migration and the invasion process, matrix-degrading proteinases are required for metastasis. The cells treated with berberine at various concentrations showed reduced matrix metalloproteinase-2 (MMP2) and urokinase-plasminogen activator (u-PA). Moreover, berberine also exerted its action via regulating tissue inhibitor of metalloproteinase-2 (TIMP-2) and urokinase-plasminogen activator inhibitor (PAI). These findings suggest that berberine possesses an anti-metastatic effect in non-small lung cancer cells and may, therefore, be helpful in clinical treatment.

The aqueous extract exopolysaccharide fraction (EPSF) of a cultivated *Cordyceps* sinensis (*dong chong xia cao*) fungus (Cs) has been studied by Yang et al. for its effect on the variety of genes that regulate cell growth and proliferation in mice implanted with melanoma [9]. The mice (C57BL/6) were administered three different doses of EPSF peritoneally every two days, starting from the day of implantation of B16 melanoma cells through their tail veins for 27 days (14 times). Sections from mouse paraffin-embedded liver and lung tissues were subjected to immunohistochemical analyses. The genes c-myc, c-fos, and VEGF levels in the lungs and livers of EPSF-treated mice were found to be significantly lower than those of untreated mice ($p < 0.05$). This suggests that EPSF had inhibited tumor growth in the lungs and livers of mice through down-regulation of the growth-promoting genes, and that it might be a potential adjuvant in cancer therapy. (See also "Cordyceps *sinensis*: Mushroom of Stamina and Longevity," p. 101, Clinical Practice.)

Park et al. investigated the effects of the Korean formula Geiji-Bokryung-Hwan (GBH) [10]. This consists of the herbs *Cinnamomi ramulus* (*rou gui*), *Poria cocos hoelen* (*fu ling*), *Moutan cortex radicis* (*mud an pi*), *Paeoniae radix* (*bai shao*), and *Persicae semen* (*tao ren*). They examined its effects on growth-inhibitory activity and cancer chemopreventive activity in assays representing three major stages of carcinogenesis. GBH showed an inhibitory effect on the growth of cancer cell lines such as HepG2 cell and Hep3B cell. GBH was also found to act as a potent inhibitor of cyclooxygenase (COX)-1 involved in growth promotion.

Our group at Bionovo, Inc. and UCSF, Mt. Zion Cancer Research Center, reported on the effect of aqueous extracts of 12 Chinese medicinal herbs [11]. These were: *Anemarrhena asphodeloides* (*zhimu*), *Artemisia argyi* (*xian he cao*), *Commiphora myrrha* (*mo yao*), *Duchesnea indica* (*lou lu*), *Gleditsia sinensis* (*zao jiao ci*), *Ligustrum lucidum* (*nu zhen zi*), *Rheum palmatum* (*da huang*), *Rubia cordifolia* (*qian cao gen*), *Salvia chinensis* (*shi jian chuan*), *Scutellaria barbata* (*ban zhi lian*), *Uncaria rhynchophylla* (Cat's Claw), and *Vaccaria segetalis* (*wang bu liu xing*). They were evaluated for their anti-proliferative activity on eight cancer cell lines, as well as on normal human mammary epithelial cells. Five human and three murine cancer cell lines, representing different tissues (breast, lung, pancreas, and prostate), were used. All the crude aqueous extracts demonstrated growth inhibitory activity on some or all of the cancer cell lines, but only two showed activity against the normal mammary epithelial cells. These results indicate the potential use of traditional Chinese medicinal herbs as anti-neoplastic agents, and suggest that further studies evaluating their mechanism(s) of action and the isolation of active anti-tumor compounds are warranted.

Conclusion

Although many advances have been made in recent years in the understanding of cancer, new safe and effective therapies have lagged behind. People encountering advanced cancers have very little hope of surviving the disease. It is therefore important to find new therapies and delineate the effect of existing therapies.

Since the evolution of cancer is dependent on many regulatory aberrations, the control of the disease may involve many targeted therapies. The regulation of genes and proteins involved in the cells cancerous process and substances found in botanicals may influence its growth control. It is possible that a combination of such compounds with cell-killing therapies will result in more effective, longer-lasting survival for cancer patients.

References

1. Hyodo I, Amano N, Eguchi K, et al. Nationwide survey on complementary and alternative medicine in cancer patients in Japan. *J Clin Oncol*. Apr. 2005;23(12):2645–54. Epub 22 Feb. 2005.
2. Fouladbakhsh JM, Stommel M, Given BA, Given CW. Predictors of use of complementary and alternative therapies among patients with

cancer. *Oncol Nurs Forum*. Nov. 2005;32(6): 1115–22.

3. Trevena J, Reeder A. Perceptions of New Zealand adults about complementary and alternative therapies for cancer treatment. *NZ Med J*. Dec. 2005;118(1227):U1787.

4. Chan JM, Elkin EP, Silva SJ, Broering JM, Latini DM, Carroll PR. Total and specific complementary and alternative medicine use in a large cohort of men with prostate cancer. *Urology*. Dec. 2005;66(6):1223–8.

5. Shu X, McCulloch M, Xiao H, Broffman M, Gao J. Chinese herbal medicine and chemotherapy in the treatment of hepatocellular carcinoma: a meta-analysis of randomized controlled trials. *Integr Cancer Ther*. Sept. 2005;4(3):219–29.

6. Tagliaferri M, Cohen I, Vogel C, et al. A phase I trial of Scutellaria Barbata (BZL101) for metastatic breast cancer. San Antonio Breast Cancer Symposium, Dec. 2005.

7. Franek KJ, Zhou Z, Zhang WD, Chen WY. In vitro studies of baicalin alone or in combination with Salvia miltiorrhiza extract as a potential anti-cancer agent. *Int J Oncol*. Jan. 2005; 26(1):217–24.

8. Peng PL, Hsieh YS, Wang CJ, Hsu JL, Chou FP. Inhibitory effect of berberine on the invasion of human lung cancer cells via decreased productions of urokinase-plasminogen activator and matrix metalloproteinase-2. *Toxicol Appl Pharmacol*. July 2006;214(1):8–15. Epub 4 Jan 2006.

9. Yang J, Zhang W, Shi P, Chen J, Han X, Wang Y. Effects of exopolysaccharide fraction (EPSF) from a cultivated Cordyceps sinensis fungus on c-Myc, c-Fos, and VEGF expression in B16 melanoma-bearing mice. *Pathol Res Pract*. 2005;201(11):745–50. Epub 19 Oct 2005.

10. Park WH, Lee SK, Oh HK, Bae JY, Kim CH. Tumor initiation inhibition through inhibition COX-1 activity of a traditional Korean herbal prescription, Geiji-Bokryung-Hwan, in human hepatocarcinoma cells. *Immunopharmacol Immunotoxicol*. 2005;27(3): 473–83.

11. Shoemaker M, Hamilton B, Dairkee SH, Cohen I, Campbell MJ. In vitro anticancer activity of twelve Chinese medicinal herbs. *Phytother Res*. July 2005;19(7):649–51.

Contact Details

Bionovo, Inc.
5858 Horton Street
Suite 375
Emeryville, CA, USA
www.bionovo.com

Hierarchy of Chinese Medicine Research Methodologies: A Brief Overview

Arnaud Versluys, PhD, MD (China), LAc, Portland, Oregon, USA

Chinese medicine was formed during the four non-industrial millennia BCE as the result of very many eclectic experiences that had been guided by a selection of philosophies derived from natural observation. Around the year 200 CE, these philosophies were consolidated into medically applied theories, and the conclusions drawn from these theories were collated to form the empirical threshold of Chinese medical practice.

Chinese medicine is not an exact science, and therefore quantitative measurements of its efficacy, conducted along current biomedical research models, yield not only poor but questionable results. Chinese medicine research cannot be rigidly structured to fit the hierarchical, linear pyramid of conventional research. Nevertheless, investigation shows that the structure of the pyramid is fully incorporated into the cyclical spectrum of Chinese medicine research.

The hierarchy of Chinese medicine research methodologies can be represented by a flowchart (see Fig. below), which complies with the developmental stages of any science. The stages begin with the lower realms of the experimental stage. This evolves into the empirical stage, which gathers the reproducible

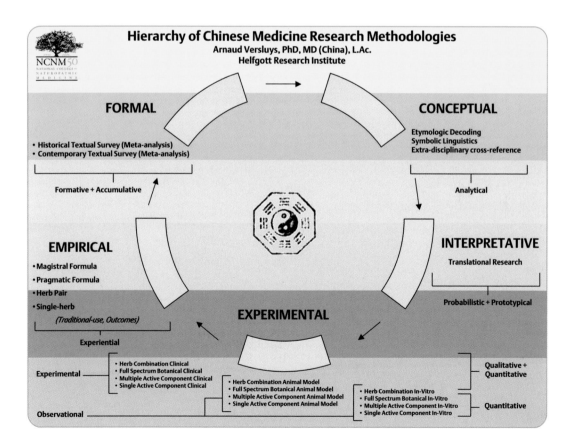

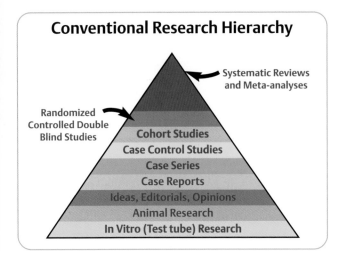

Conventional Research Hierarchy

Systematic Reviews and Meta-analyses

Randomized Controlled Double Blind Studies

Cohort Studies

Case Control Studies

Case Series

Case Reports

Ideas, Editorials, Opinions

Animal Research

In Vitro (Test tube) Research

results of the experimental stage. The latter is succeeded by the formal or formative stage of standardization, categorization, and publication of protocols at the apex, comparable to conventional meta-analysis. This is followed first by a conceptual stage of subjective analysis, often by means of extra-disciplinary cross-reference, and then by the final interpretative stage of probabilistic and prototypical translational research, in order to create future experimental methodologies.

It is therefore clear that the crucial stage before the design of modern Chinese medicine research is the adequate understanding of the existing spectrum of its methodologies.

Contact Details

Arnaud Versluys, PhD, MD (China), CAc
National College of Natural Medicine
Portland, OR, USA
www.ncnm.edu

Clinical Practice

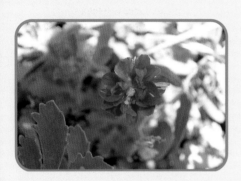

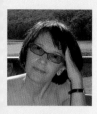

Jane Lyttleton

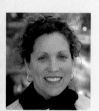

Mary Tagliaferri

Introduction

In this, the first issue of the Almanac, the Clinical Practice section is rather small, but we hope it will expand in future issues as Chinese medicine practitioners feel inspired to contribute articles that come out of their own clinical experience. These will be especially interesting to the international Chinese medicine community if the articles reflect disorders or symptoms that are particularly relevant to a certain country, race, or social or environmental condition. So many of us work in relative isolation in our field, especially in countries that do not have large numbers of complementary medicine practitioners or educational institutions, seminars, or local publication channels. We hope that this Almanac, which has no national boundaries, may become a voice-piece for those of you who have valuable clinical experience, gathered over many years of practice. As the practice of Chinese medicine becomes more popular and prevalent in the West, it is vital that we document its evolution in its new environment. Nowhere can this be done more authentically than at the "coal face" of the clinic—case histories, patient-data collection and analysis, small trials, etc, all contribute to furthering our understanding of how Chinese medicine is taking shape in a non-Asian context. Out of such reflective practice, confidence in ourselves as effective and necessary health-care providers will develop, and the next step is acceptance and integration into the prevailing medical orthodoxy, which, in most Western countries, is scientifically based bio-medicine. At this point, having reached maturity and confidence, the two systems can work side by side, both in the research and clinical arenas.

To begin the Clinical Practice section, we have a short address given by Professor Dr Gustav J. Dobos of the Universitätsklinik Duisburg–Essen to the German–Chinese Society for Medicine in 2005, outlining the importance of integrating Chinese and Western medical systems. He offers this as a model of a health-care system of the future.

This is followed by a report given by an acupuncturist who ran a small research trial in her own clinic in London. Marian Fixler looks at how we might assess the prognosis for a given patient and makes us think a bit more about what exactly we are doing in the clinic. The research she presents examines one part of what it means to be a good practitioner, that is, knowing where you are going with a given patient, and why. Not every patient will get better, and it is important to know why—whether it is the nature of the disease, the combination of the disease with constitutional factors, or the combination of several disparate disease processes that is preventing recovery.

The author examines ancient classics such as the Nei Jing in her exploration of the concepts of prognosis—especially as regards the diagnostic skills of pulse taking and observation. In her clinic she uses Japanese acupuncture (representative of the principles of acupuncture treatment in general) to achieve good improvements in her patients' health and to test her predictions.

An interesting and sad story of a very sick child follows. This clinical case, although it describes a very unusual disease that none of us is likely to see in our professional lifetimes, nevertheless shows us that improving the qi with acupuncture or related techniques can have some positive outcome, even in dire circumstances.

Stephen Birch, in a scholarly discussion of qi, presents a convincing argument (and clinical example) for the importance of enhancing vitality in a patient.

Gabriel Stux does something similar in his article "Acupuncture for Spiritual Opening," as he presents a way of using acupuncture, combined with the chakra system of Indian philosophy and medicine, to treat the essential vitality of a patient rather than specific symptoms.

As a fascinating contribution to our understanding of Traditional Chinese Medicine (TCM) diagnostic skills, Claus Schnorrenberger gives us a description of the tongue from another angle. Rather than merely detailing the meaning of different tongue features in terms of TCM pathology or pattern, this article makes us think more deeply about the meaning of changes in the tongue, as we are asked to examine them from anatomical and physiological points of view. In future, this type of examination might be taken further into other diagnostic areas, such as the pulse and other aspects of human physiology, for which we have excellent scientific understanding, and which could add new dimensions to our Chinese medicine diagnostic skills.

Amir Kalay shares his experience with us in his clinic in Israel, where he treats skin disorders such as atopic dermatitis and psoriasis. His case histories clearly show just how effective Chinese herbal medicine can be in treating what Western specialists would deem to be very intractable conditions. His clinic has developed and marketed cleansers, creams, and shampoos made from Chinese herbs to treat these conditions.

Finally, we have included an article about one of the herbs that is very much in the news at the present time: Cordyceps. This is a fungus that grows on a larva native to the mountainous regions of Tibet, Nepal, and China, which you may well have read about. It first came to the attention of many people in the West in 1993, when Chinese Olympic athletes proved its powers with their outstanding aerobic endurance. Cordyceps became more popular when doctors in Hong Kong and China recommended it as the best defense against the recent SARS outbreak. Very recent research shows that it might have application in reproductive medicine, as it appears to stimulate the activity of ovarian tissue. It may be of use in the treatment of dementia in the elderly, and claims have been made for its positive effect on libido! As you may imagine, all of this creates a great deal of pressure on a little mountain caterpillar and its strange parasitic companion. Prices for Cordyceps have climbed up to US$7050 per kilo (half the price of gold). And a gold find it certainly has been for the Tibetan farmers and nomads who collect and trade the fungus. Suddenly these farmers can afford the latest and most prestigious of their traditional costumes, the chuba, which is decorated with animal skins. A sad result has been the hunting of the snow leopard to furnish this demand, almost to the point of extinction.

As Stephen Birch mentions in his introduction to the Research section (p. 27), there is inevitably some crossover between the Clinical Practice and Research sections of this publication. For a discipline such as Chinese medicine this is entirely appropriate, since so much of the relevant research in this area will be based in the clinic. To conclude, I would like to reiterate Stephen's words: "international collaboration works!" In this spirit I would strongly like to encourage practitioners to support and contribute to local and international networks to facilitate this collaboration. Future editions of the Almanac will, it is hoped, be able to report on and further such collaboration.

Jane Lyttleton, BSc Hons, MPhil, Dip TCM, Cert Acup
Paddington Medical Centre, Sydney, Australia

Combination of Chinese and Western Medicine: A Model for the Future?

Lecture at the Annual Meeting of the German–Chinese Society for Medicine, 8th–10th September, 2005

Professor Gustav J. Dobos, MD, Essen, Germany

Traditional Chinese medicine (TCM) is steadily gaining popularity in the Western world. The author addresses the questions as to whether a combination of Chinese and Western medicine is likely to be a model for a future health care system. The answer to this question is very closely linked to whether there is a need for a combination of Chinese and Western medicine, and whether there is scientific evidence for Chinese medicine.

What are the major health problems facing the Western world in the future? Because of demographic developments, there will be an increase in age-related health events, such as low back pain, osteoarthritis of the knee, falls, and dementia.

Acupuncture is by far the most popular method of TCM used in the Western world. It is now a firmly established and well-recognized alternative therapy. In Germany more than 40 000 physicians practice acupuncture. Although this popularity does not reflect the situation in China, where herbal therapy is applied more frequently than acupuncture, Chinese herbal therapy is also gaining popularity in Germany. At present, approximately 2000 physicians prescribe between 500 and 800 tons of herbs per year in the country. A similar increase in popularity can be observed with *tui na* massage therapy; the specific Chinese exercise therapies *tai ji quan* and *qi gong* are already being practiced by a wide range of people with many kinds of health problems, or for relaxation and meditation purposes.

In a consumer-driven health-care system, it is most important to know about patients' demands. To answer this question, in August 2005 the Institute for Public Opinion in Allensbach, Germany, undertook a survey. The question "If you were sick, would you prefer a therapy consisting only of Western medicine or of a combination of Chinese and Western medicine?" was asked of 772 German citizens.

Interestingly, only 18 % preferred a strictly Western treatment. Thirty five percent of the persons asked had already experienced methods of Chinese medicine (26 % acupuncture and 9 % other therapies).

Most significantly in this poll, 61 % of all people asked, and 89 % of those who had undergone some form of TCM treatment, preferred a combination of Chinese and Western medicine. These data imply that the majority of the German population is in favor of a combined therapy, especially if the people concerned have already experienced TCM.

More than 25 % of the population aged over 65 suffers from osteoarthritis of the knee. Because of the many side effects conventional treatment (non-steroidal anti-inflammatory drugs [NSAID]) causes, there is an interest in acupuncture. According to Wolfe et al., more than 16 000 people in the USA die every year as a result of the side effects of NSAIDs [1]. Recently the ART (Acupuncture Randomized Trials) study, focusing on osteoarthritis of the knee, compared acupuncture with sham acupuncture treatment, using a waiting list group (see also "Comments on the German Acupuncture Studies," p. 37, Research, and "Acupuncture in Germany in 2006," p. 191, Professional Developments, Legislation, and Regulation). The results indicated that 50 % of the acupuncture group had a decrease of 50 % in the WOMAC[1] index at eight weeks [2]. There was a significant difference between the results obtained with acupuncture and sham acupuncture. Good clinical evidence for the effect of *Ginkgo biloba* (*bai guo*) is seen in the treatment of dementia

---

1   Western Ontario and McMaster Universities Arthritis Index Questionnaire. The questionnaire is used to assess the symptoms of pain, stiffness, and physical function in patients with osteoarthritis of the hip or knee.

in Alzheimer disease [3]. A further example is Huperzine A and E (*Huperzia serrata; qian ceng ta*); as cholinesterase blockers in animal experiments, these substances have been shown to improve the memory of rats. The Cochrane database systematic review of Furlan et al. (2002) found clear evidence to show that acupressure massage is more effective than classic massage for low back pain [4]. There is evidence that *tai ji quan* reduces blood pressure and the risk of falls in the elderly [5, 6].

In summary, we may postulate a need to integrate Chinese and Western medicine, primarily because of its partly proven efficacy in the treatment of age-related health problems. Studies suggest that combined therapy has fewer side effects. Consumer demand also reflects a high acceptance of Chinese medicine. There is good clinical evidence for the efficacy of Chinese medicine in pain relief, reduction of falls, therapy of dementia, and other age-related conditions.

References

1. Wolfe MM, Lichtenstein DR, Singh G. Gastrointestinal toxicity of nonsteroidal antiinflammatory drugs. *N Engl J Med*. 1999;340(24):1888–99. Review.

2. Witt C, Brinkhaus B, Jena S, et al. Acupuncture in patients with osteoarthritis of the knee: a randomized trial. *Lancet* 2005;366:136–143.

3. Le Bars PL, Katz MM, Berman N, Itil TM, Freedman AM, Schatzberg AF. A placebo-controlled, double-blind, randomized trial of an extract of Gingko biloba for dementia. North American Egb Study Group. *JAMA*. Oct. 22–29,1997; 278(16):1327–32.

4. Furlan AD, Brosseau L, Welch V. Massage for low back pain (Cochrane Review). *Cochrane Database Syst Rev*. 2000; Issue 4. Art. No. CD001929.

5. Young DR, Appel LJ, Lee S, Miller ER. The effects of aerobic exercise and Tai Chi on blood pressure in older people: results of a randomized trial. *J Am Geriatr Soc*. 1999;47(3):277–84.

6. Gillespie LD, Gillespie WJ, Robertson MC, Lamb SE, Cumming RG, Rowe BH. Interventions for preventing falls in elderly people. *Cochrane Database Syst. Rev*. 2006; Issue 2. Art. No. CD000340.

Contact Details

Faculty for Integrative Medicine
Kliniken Essen Mitte
Essen, Germany
gustav.dobos@uni-essen.de
www.uni-essen.de/naturheilkunde

An Evaluation of Prognosis and its Correlation with Patient-Centered Outcome Measures

Marian Fixler, LLB (Hons), DipAC, MBAcC, London, UK

Preface

Marian Fixler wrote the following paper as a partial requirement for completion of the Advanced Toyohari Program (Amsterdam, March 2004–November 2005). I asked Marian to submit the paper for two reasons. First, it provides a good summary of some of the key traditional features involved in formulating a prognosis. Second, Marian undertook this project as a study for investigating whether, or how well, predictions based on the prognosticated factors she describes in the first part of the paper from within the Toyohari acupuncture system correlated with actual outcome. It was thus a small-scale clinical trial. The beauty of this is that Marian is not a researcher; she is a clinician. She conducted the study within her own clinical practice. Marian utilized a very useful and easy-to-apply validated outcome tool, the "Measure Yourself Medical Outcome Profile" (MYMOP). This measurement allows patients to describe their health in their own terms. Although this was only a pilot study, with the results included in summary form only, Marian has clearly shown how clinicians can, with relative ease, undertake basic research within their clinical practice.

Stephen Birch

Abstract

Prognosis is an important aspect of the treatment process, both for the practitioner and the patient. It is an area that is taken for granted as an integral part of the therapeutic process, yet not much has been written about it in acupuncture textbooks.

This research aims to bring together all the strands for consideration that are relevant to making a prognosis within East Asian medicine (EAM), and to examine whether there is any correlation between an assessment of prognosis and treatment outcomes.

Information relevant to prognosis was gathered at the initial consultation with patients who met the criteria for the study. Semi-qualitative methodology was used in the form of a patient-centered outcome measure to provide an objective comparison by which to assess prognosis.

A large proportion of patients in the study benefited from the acupuncture treatments, showing clinically significant improvements. Of the diagnostic markers examined, some proved to be more useful than others in assessing prognosis as shown by their correlation with treatment outcomes. Owing to the small sample size, however, this cannot be seen as statistically conclusive.

Suggestions are made for the inclusion of further markers that could be analyzed in a larger, future study.

Introduction

"In the practice of any medical discipline, the ability to formulate a prognosis is important, in relation to the modification of the selected treatment for that patient, and in efforts to convey accurate information to the patient. Forming a prognosis involves making a judgement about the nature and severity of a patient's condition, understanding the course of that condition both with and without treatment, and selecting treatment to produce the maximum outcome for that patient" [1].

Many factors need to be considered, even after a diagnosis has been made, prior to starting treatment. This includes an overall assessment of the patient's condition, including a judgement about the balance between the *sei qi* (right *qi*) of the patient, the *jya qi* (pathogenic or evil *qi*) present, and the relativity of each, thus enabling the practitioner to make informed decisions regarding dose and the techniques to use. An evaluation of the prognosis is important for all of the reasons outlined above by Stephen Birch.

Yet, as Birch makes clear, "Few textbooks on acupuncture explicitly discuss the concept of, need for, and methods of forming a prognosis" [1]. This subject, however, is an integral part of each of the diagnostic systems within acupuncture.

In a comparison between Western medicine and Chinese medicine, Ted Kaptchuk claims that Chinese medicine is weak on prognosis [2]. He substantiates this statement by referring to Western medicine's ability, for example, to identify tumors, determine whether they are malignant or benign, and act accordingly by isolating and removing them when necessary. He claims that Chinese medicine cannot attempt to offer a quantifiable prognosis in the way that Western medicine can in such a situation. This statement is part of a bigger discussion on the strengths and weaknesses of each system of medicine, the strength of Chinese medicine being its emphasis on the body as a whole, rather than on its individual parts. Disappointingly, there is no further discussion on how Chinese medicine does form a prognosis. As Birch states above, this is an area that is not covered in most acupuncture textbooks, though practitioners do have an understanding of this concept, mainly through an understanding of *qi* in its broadest sense.

Aims and Objectives

The aim of this study was to bring together many of the factors considered relevant to the forming of a prognosis in EAM, and to evaluate whether the practitioner's prognosis assessment was consistent with the patient's own perception of his or her progress during treatment.

Through an examination of relevant chapters of the classics, and information gathered from acupuncture textbooks, together with articles and individual teachers of Japanese acupuncture, various criteria were identified as important considerations for forming a prognosis. This information was collated as part of the initial consultation with new patients.

A patient-centered outcome measure, MYMOP, served as the primary outcome to compare the prognostic criteria, in order to ascertain whether there was a correlation between criteria observed in clinical practice and outcomes in treatment. An analysis of these outcome measures would provide a mean profile score from which individual patients' progress could be assessed for clinical significance.

Literature Review

Prognosis

In order for a prognosis to be made before treatment commences, the practitioner strives to assess how a patient is likely to respond to treatment. In his article on prognosis, Birch gives the definition of prognosis, from the Greek word meaning foreknowledge, as: "The prospect of recovery as anticipated from the usual course of disease or the peculiarities of the case" [1, 3].

In Western medicine, prognosis is usually based on an evaluation of the progression of disease and the pathological changes that have occurred, rather than an assessment of an individual's particular condition. In EAM we are not only looking at the Western disease condition and what course this may take, but are also making an assessment of all the signs and symptoms within the paradigm of *yin* and *yang* and the *qi* system. Kodo Fukushima talks about the extreme end of the spectrum where it may not be possible to help someone when the disease is too severe or the patient is too weak [4, 5]. Within each of the four diagnostic systems, indications are given of what constitutes good or poor prognosis.

Four Diagnoses

Within the Toyohari system of Meridian Therapy, it is taught that the four diagnoses are more relevant for prognosis than for diagnosis. For example, if the color or odor does not correspond to the primary pattern as identified by the pulse, abdomen, and symptoms, then it may be ignored; that is to say, it does not influence the diagnosis. If the signs and symptoms correspond more closely to the *sho* (also known as *akashi*—"the fundamental nature of the disease and the goal of its treatment" [6]), this is indicative of a better prognosis.

It might be that this is because it indicates that fewer channels have been affected, and that there is less disturbance, and thus more order, within the system. The more internal systems in the body that are disturbed—for example, digestion, sleep, etc—the worse the prognosis.

1 Touching: Pulse Diagnosis

In general terms, the more balanced the pulse in each of the six positions, the better the prognosis. This means that the better the balance between the *yin* and *yang* positions, the better the prognosis. A firm pulse, with clear definition in the middle pulse, with a soft, springy quality that has luster, is a sign of good prognosis [1].

Fukushima (1991) discusses the feasibility of treatment when there is the appearance of one of the seven terminal pulses in which the stomach *qi* is exhausted [4]. There is no further explanation of these qualities.

1.1 Pulse Diagnosis and the Complexion

The *Nan Jing* (Classic of Difficult Issues) in Chapter 13 states:

If one sees a [person's] complexion and cannot feel the corresponding [movement in the] vessels, but rather feels a [movement in the] vessels [indicating dominance of a superior phase according to the order of] mutual destruction, the [respective person] will die. If one feels a [movement in the] vessels [indicating dominance of a superior phase according to the order of] mutual generation, the illness will come to an end by itself. Complexion and [movement in the] vessels must be compared as to their mutual correspondence [7].

The five *yin* organs each have corresponding complexions and pulse qualities. If the pulse

Table 1 Organ correspondences

Depot/Organ	Complexion	Pulse quality
Liver	Blue-green	Stringly, tense, wiry, tight.
Heart	Red	Surface, strong, dispersed, floating, big, scattered.
Spleen	Yellow	Center, relaxed, strong, middle, moderate, or big.
Lung	White	Surface, rough, short, floating.
Kidney	Black	Deep, soft, smooth, sinking, soggy, or slippery.

does not correspond to the complexion but instead relates to the "superior phase" in the *sokoku* cycle (cycle of "mutual destruction"), it is a poor prognosis, which might result in death. If, however, the pulse corresponds to the "superior phase" in the *sosho* generating cycle (cycle of "mutual generation"), the illness will resolve itself on its own.

Matsumoto and Birch (1983) discuss comparing not only the complexion but also the body types, so that a liver-deficient type person should manifest a liver-type quality for a better prognosis [8]. If, instead, the pulse is floating and rough (metal pulse), this would indicate a worse prognosis, as the disharmony is on the *sokoku* cycle.

This further illustrates what the *Nan Jing* says about prognosis. If only a single element or channel is imbalanced, this makes for a better prognosis. If two elements or channels on the generating cycle are imbalanced, this becomes more complicated. The worst prognosis, and the most difficult to treat, is when two or more elements or channels are affected that are in *sokoku* relationship to each other [9].

1.2 Pulse Diagnosis and Symptoms

The *Nan Jing* in Chapter 17 discusses prognosis through the relationship of the pulse to the symptoms. The scripture states:

In case of an illness one may die, or a cure will occur by itself without any treatment, or the [illness] will continue for years and months

Table 2 *Nan Jing* 17 correspondences

Depot/Organ	Symptom presentation	Expected pulse
Liver	Eyes kept closed, doesn't want to look at anyone.	Vigorous, tense, extended; same as stringy, tense.
Heart	Eyes are open, thirst, with a firm area below the heart.	Tight, replete, frequent.
Lung	Spits blood, with repeated sniffles and nose bleeding.	Deep and fine.
Heart	Speaks incoherently, utters nonsense, body should be hot.	Vast and strong.
Spleen	Large abdomen with diarrhea.	Slight, fine, and rough.

without remission. Is it possible, by feeling the [movement in the] vessels, to know whether the respective [person] will die or survive, will continue to exist or will perish? [7]

These descriptions are slightly confusing, as the correspondences are not always consistent. For example, there are two descriptions for the heart but none for the kidney. For the liver symptoms, the pulse should be that of the liver. If the pulse is short, rough, and at the surface (lung pulse), this signals death, as metal is subduing wood. For the heart symptoms, the pulse should be that of the heart. If, instead, it is deep, rough, and slight (kidney pulse), this signals death as it is a *yang* illness with a *yin* pulse quality.

For the lung symptoms, the pulse should be that of the kidney (not, as you might expect, the lung), following the mutual generating cycle. If the pulse is at the surface, strong, and firm, this signals death as it is fire overpowering metal.

For the second heart symptoms, the pulse should be that of the heart. If it is deep, fine, and slight, this signals death, as water is overpowering fire.

For the spleen symptoms, the pulse should be that of the lungs; again, not what you might expect. If it is tight, strong, and smooth (liver), this signals death, with wood overpowering earth.

1.3 Touching: Abdominal and Channel Palpation

The luster of the skin indicates prognosis. If the skin is moist, this indicates vacuity; if a patient becomes moist very easily, this is indicative of a sensitive patient. It is also a guide for treatment dose and points to the importance of checking the abdomen and *naso* area during treatment. If the patient starts to become moist, this can indicate over-treatment.

In a relatively healthy patient, only one area of the abdomen may be deficient. A general springiness in the musculature, especially in the abdomen, is a sign of good prognosis. The temperature should be the same throughout the entire surface of the abdomen, however, the lower abdomen may be slightly warmer. In many patients, the small belly is cooler, indicating a weakness in the kidney area.

Accumulation of fluid in the stomach region, with a "sloshing" sound (felt on tapping) is a sign of extreme spleen *qi* weakness, and indicates a poor prognosis, resulting in a prolonged course of treatment [1].

Fukushima (1991) talks about strong and irregular palpitations involving the heart and kidney *qi* as being indicative of poor prognosis [4].

2 Looking Diagnosis

Birch says there is a better prognosis if there is no dominant color or complexion visible on the face, especially in the area between the eyebrows (*yin tang*), and if there is an absence of pigmentation or other skin changes [1].

The colors corresponding to each of the elements are differentiated into life-like colors and death-like colors in the complexion. These are indicators of prognosis.

The greater the correlation between the *sho* and the complexion, the better the prog-

Table 3 Colors

Phase	Life-like color	Death-like color
Blue-green	Lustrous, like a kingfisher (swimming bird).	Lusterless, like the juice from crushed grass.
Red	Lustrous, like a cockscomb.	Lusterless, like dried blood.
Yellow	Lustrous, like the belly of a crab.	Lusterless, like the fruit of a trifoliate orange.
White	Lustrous, like the fat of pork.	Lusterless, like dried bones.
Black	Lustrous, like the feathers of a wet crow.	Lusterless, like soot.

nosis. A person presenting with a lung *sho* with a white or yellow complexion (following the generating cycle) has a better prognosis than if the complexion is blue/green or red (*sokoku* cycle).

Birch emphasizes the importance of structural integrity—including symmetry of the shoulder and hip girdles, limb lengths, distribution of muscle tonus, and spine alignment.

3 Listening and Smelling

A dull, weak, scratchy voice, with improper vocalization or poor tone quality, indicating a lack of vital energy, implies a poor prognosis.

Proper breathing, that is, abdominal breathing, is a sign of good prognosis.

If the sound of the voice relates to the *sokoku* cycle, this is a poor prognosis, following on from the same principles as described above.

Yukata Shinoda (2003) differentiates between the five sound qualities, which he says are used to judge the constitution, and the five speaking qualities, which he says are useful to see the change of the condition of the disease [10]. In his opinion, the former does not change so easily with disease. In his experience, however, the speaking quality changes more rapidly, even after needling a single point. This is a helpful way to monitor changes in the disease condition. Once again, a correlation between the five sound qualities and the five speaking qualities with the *sho* indicates a better prognosis.

Birch says that the absence of a clear body odor is a sign of good prognosis. Fukushima (1991) talks about foul-smelling mixtures of

the *sokoku* relationship as signifying death; for example, a sweet (earth) smell with a putrid (wood) smell [4].

4 Asking

4.1 General

The greater the disruption within the system, the worse the prognosis. For example, if appetite, sleep, and bowel movements are all disrupted, this indicates a poorer prognosis.

Other factors possibly affecting prognosis include: the patient's age and duration of the condition, how quickly the patient has recovered from past illnesses, if illnesses are still affecting him or her, and/or a complex medical history.

4.2 *Nan Jing* Chapter 49

This chapter of the *Nan Jing* [7] indicates how channels can become spontaneously diseased or be harmed by one of the five "evils." For channels to fall ill by themselves, they come under the influence of the following: grief and

Table 4 Sounds

Phase	Sound qualities	Voice qualities
Wood	Sharp	Shouting
Fire	Solemn	Muttering
Earth	Sacred	Humming
Metal	Entreating	Whining
Water	Bass	Groaning

anxiety; thoughts and considerations (heart); cold body and chilled drinks (lung); hate and anger causing counter-flow *qi* (liver); drinking and eating in excess; weariness and exhaustion (spleen); exposure to humidity; over-exertion; and going into water (kidney).

The five "evils" are wind, heat, excessive drinking and eating, cold, and humidity.

The chapter goes on to describe how each of the organs rules one of the diagnostic categories:

- Liver rules colors, irrespective of what the color is.
- Heart rules odors, irrespective of what the odor is.
- Spleen rules one's preference for a specific taste, irrespective of what the taste is.
- Lung rules sounds, irrespective of what the sound is.
- Kidney rules liquids, irrespective of what the liquid is.

Although this chapter is not explicitly about prognosis, the correspondences above will be examined to see if there is any congruence between the presence of these categories and the *sho*, and whether this can be an indicator of prognosis. For example, if a patient has a particularly strong odor, does he or she also have a heart *sho*?

Constitutional Diagnosis

In his lecture, Shinoda sensei (2003) says, "the goal of treatment should be to get the *sho* stable, and then keep it that way for good health maintenance. … If the presenting *sho* is the constitutional *sho*, then the prognosis is good." He gives the example: "If you diagnose a patient with a Spleen constitution with either a Spleen *sho* or a Lung *sho*, the prognosis is good, but if you diagnose the same patient with a Liver *sho* the prognosis is poorer" [11]. A discussion regarding the constitution is beyond the remit of this project.

As an overall assessment, a *kyo* (*xu* or vacuous) person, presenting *jitsu* (*shi* or replete) symptoms, or, conversely, a *jitsu* person with a presentation of *kyo* symptoms, also shows inconsistency, and thus a poor prognosis.

Conclusion

The greater the consistency between all the patient's signs, symptoms, and the diagnosis, the better the prognosis. The more out of balance or chaotic the system is, the less normal rules of physiology are followed.

In his article on prognostication, Shinoda (2004) talks about the responsibility practitioners have to their patients when deciding whether they can help them [10]. He emphasizes the need not only to make a careful diagnosis according to the principles of EAM, but also to improve skills in Western medicine, so that a decision can be made as to when it is more appropriate to refer on to a doctor.

By integrating all of the above information, practitioners are better able to provide an indication to patients of what they might expect regarding response to treatment and length of treatment.

Methodology of the Study

A semi-qualitative study was chosen that could compare an assessment of the prognosis by the practitioner with the treatment outcomes as assessed by the patient. This would be qualitative in nature, as the information gathered from both the patient and the practitioner would be subjective. It would be based on each of their perceptions, using specific criteria for recording this information. It was hoped that comparing information from both perspectives would introduce an element of objectivity. Using a patient-centered outcome tool with a numerical scale would also introduce a quantitative element, as this information would be collated and the data analyzed in order to gather statistical information.

Measure Yourself Medical Outcome Profile (MYMOP2)

MYMOP has been available for use since a paper was published in the *British Medical Journal* in 1996. This was revised as MYMOP2 after the second validation study in 1999.

An outcome questionnaire that is patient centred should encompass the aims, values and treatment effects that are prioritised by individuals, and should enable each individual to provide an unambiguous assessment of change over time [12].

The MYMOP form asks the patient to identify one or two related symptoms that relate to the same condition for which they are seeking treatment.

MYMOP is a problem-specific measure. The reason that all items should relate to the same problem is that the scores are going to be amalgamated into the profile score (the mean of the scored items) then it doesn't make sense for them to relate to different things. For example if symptom 1 is headache and symptom 2 is a painful toe, then the intervention may cure the headache, but the toe may get worse. In this scenario, the profile score would show no change and this would not be a useful measure of treatment outcome. So MYMOP is a problem-specific measure, but the patient decides what constitutes the parameters of the problem [13].

Patients are also asked to identify an activity of daily living—which can be physical, social, or mental—that is important to them, and which their problem limits or prevents them from doing. Finally, patients are asked to rate their general feeling of well being. All of these issues have to be assessed in the week prior to treatment.

The form also asks for information regarding the length of time the patient has had the condition. Finally, details of medication can be recorded, and whether cutting down this medication is important to the patient. The reason that this section can be valuable is that the priority of some patients may be to cut down or cut out their medication, even though this might result in an increase in their symptoms. If this section were not included, it would be an incomplete reflection of the treatment outcome.

For the purposes of this study, emphasis was not placed on the medication part of the questionnaire, as this was not relevant in all cases. It was intended to look at scores across the board. As the medication questions are

scored separately from the main MYMOP scores, it was possible to leave them off.

Patients were asked to complete the MYMOP form at the initial consultation prior to receiving treatment, and again at the sixth session as part of a review process routinely carried out with new patients. Patients gave verbal consent to this information being used as part of an audit tool. The nature of the research was not discussed, as it was felt that if patients were told that the project was related to an examination of prognosis, this might in some way influence their scores.

Criteria for Inclusion in the Study

Criteria for inclusion in the study were the following:

- New patients or existing patients who were coming for new conditions, and had not been seen for a minimum of six months prior to the study.
- Patients being treated with Toyohari as the main root treatment.
- Patients being treated for a minimum number of six sessions.

For this reason it was deemed inappropriate to include conditions such as induction treatments and breech presentation in pregnant women, where on average fewer than six sessions were routinely carried out. Patients with fertility issues were also not included, as treatment outcome in such cases could not readily be assessed using a scale. Treatment was either successful or not with regard to a positive pregnancy test.

Nineteen patients were included in the study.

Prognosis Form

The second part of the study involved developing a prognosis form that could be completed at the initial consultation. Information would be recorded using the four methods of diagnosis: looking, listening and smelling, touching, and asking. This would include information that is discussed in the classics as indicators of prognosis.

This information falls into three main categories:

1. Asking questions:
   - age of the patient
   - duration of the condition
2. Diagnostic signs that are consistent with the *sho* or main complaint:
   - *Nan Jing* 49 characteristics
   - color, taste, sound, and odor
   - abdominal findings and their correlation with the main complaint
3. Assessment of the patient's *sei qi* (right *qi*), as judged by the following:
   - assessment of luster of the face and abdomen as judged by looking and touching
   - quality of the voice
   - abdominal tone

The initial form was revised to include more information that would be useful for assessment purposes.

Summary of Findings

Information was recorded as percentage scores for comparison purposes, even though it is recognized that this data is not necessarily of statistical significance because of the small sample involved.

Age

With a mean age of 48 years, it was found that patients who were younger than the mean overall scored higher than those who were older.

Duration of the Condition

The largest number of patients fell within the 1–5-year category, indicating that a higher proportion of patients (47 %) came with more chronic conditions. Although there was a slightly higher number of patients within the 0–4 week group who showed a higher than mean score, and a slightly lower number within the 1–5 year group who showed a lower than mean score, overall, the numbers were fairly evenly spread. This is promising, as it shows that duration of the condition alone cannot determine outcome, and that even patients with chronic long-term conditions show significant clinical improvement with acupuncture.

Nan Jing 49 Characteristics

Nan Jing characteristics were recorded for 10 of the 19 patients. Of these 10 patients, six of the characteristics correlated to the *sho* presentation. Of these six, two were higher than the mean, two were the same as the mean, and two were lower than the mean. Of the four where there was no correlation, two were higher than the mean and two were lower.

Overall, where there was correlation with the *sho*, two-thirds of the patients (four out of the six) showed clinically significant changes. This indicates that this information may well be relevant in assessing prognosis, but cannot be seen to be conclusive.

Color, Sound, Taste, and Odor

As the evidence gathered in these categories was quite limited, no conclusive patterns emerged. For both color and sound, a correlation with the *sho* did not necessarily correspond to a better treatment outcome. With regard to taste, very little information was recorded, and nothing was recorded for odor.

Strength of Voice

This finding showed more conclusive evidence that patients with a weak (*kyo*) voice, irrespective of the particular sound emitted, had a poorer prognosis than those patients whose voice was more "normal." This is indicative of the overall state of the *qi* that is likely to affect prognosis.

Abdominal Luster and Tone and Facial Luster

The largest group of patients comprised those who had no luster in the face and abdomen, and poor abdominal tone. These patients showed poorer prognosis overall. The next largest group had a positive response to only one of these three categories, and they all showed higher than mean scores. Only a small number of patients had a positive response for two or all three of these categories, so the information was inconclusive. When each of these categories was analyzed separately, in each case where luster or good tone was present, these patients had higher than mean scores, or the same as the mean scores. Interestingly, of those who did not have luster or who had poor tone, the spread was more even and thus inconclusive.

Abdominal Areas Showing *Kyo*

Information was not only recorded regarding the areas on the abdomen that were *kyo*, but also whether the big or little belly was more *kyo*. This information was then compared to the primary complaint to see if there was any correlation, and to see how this related to the mean score. Once again, it was found that where there was correlation, the prognosis was overall marginally better. Where there was no correlation, however, there was an even spread.

Conclusion

Most patients in the study (approximately 75 %) showed an improvement to their symptoms that could be classified as clinically significant (with a MYMOP mean profile of 1 or greater). In spite of certain limitations that have been discussed, the MYMOP form is a useful tool for obtaining a standardized and quantifiable gauge of response to treatment.

In order to be able to more effectively include patients with conditions of a more cyclical nature, it might be more appropriate to ask questions such as: "Overall, how would you class your symptoms?" and at the end: "Overall, how has this changed?". Paterson, however, suggests that it is difficult for patients to analyze their symptoms beyond the time frame of a week. Because of the validation studies that apply to the use of MYMOP, it is not possible to adapt or change the wording or layout. If this were to be done, it could no longer be called a MYMOP study and would require a new process of testing and validation [13].

Not all prognostic markers mentioned in the literature review were analyzed in this study. This was partly owing to the time and resources available. Areas that were not examined included a correlation between pulse and complexion (*NJ* 13). This was because detailed information about the pulse qualities is not routinely recorded beyond speed, strength, and depth, and recording of color was also not consistently recorded in all instances. For simi-

lar reasons, a comparison of symptoms and pulse (*NJ* 17) was also not used. The symptoms listed for each organ are quite limited, and did not correspond to patients' presenting conditions. Although information was recorded about which channels showed weakness, this was not used. Some patients showed several areas of weakness while others showed fewer; it was beyond the resources available to analyze this data.

Although the prognosis form included a category for *yin* and *yang* as an assessment of constitution, and *kyo/jitsu* for an assessment of symptoms, recording this information was found to be problematic as patients did not consistently fit into one or another category, particularly with regard to *yin* and *yang*. An examination of constitution and its relationship to the *sho* could be the subject of another study.

The prognostic markers that were examined can be classified into three broad categories:

1. Factual information—Asking diagnosis:
   It seems that age and whether the condition is functional or organic in nature does have a bearing on treatment outcome. The duration of the condition, however, does not necessarily conclusively indicate a better prognosis, though a condition of shorter duration does suggest a better prognosis.
2. Diagnostic information—Congruence with the *sho*:
   Congruence was examined between the presenting *sho* and the diagnostic markers, in particular *NJ* 49 characteristics, color, sound, and taste, and abdominal areas of weakness in relation to the region of the symptoms. A positive correlation between the *sho* and the presence of a *NJ* 49 characteristic did indicate a better outcome, though conversely, where there was a lack of correlation, this was inconclusive. Unfortunately, insufficient information was gathered under the category of color, sound, and taste to sufficiently ascertain any patterns. This was in part owing to the practitioner's lack of training in these areas of diagnosis. From the information that was gathered, correlation between color and

sound, in particular, did not seem to indicate a better outcome. Where the abdominal areas of weakness correlated to the region of the symptoms, for example, weak upper abdomen with cough, there was a better treatment outcome. Where there was no correlation, however, this was inconclusive.

One recurring pattern emerging from the findings was that a positive correlation between the diagnostic markers and the *sho* was generally indicative of a better outcome, though a lack of correlation did not necessarily indicate a poorer outcome.

3. Assessment of the *sei qi* (right *qi*):
   The third area was an examination of quality of voice, abdominal and facial luster, and abdominal tone. These markers were used as a measure of the overall quality of the patients' *sei qi*. Patients who had an absence of luster and tone did have a lower mean profile; however, surprisingly, patients who had better tone and luster did not necessarily have a better treatment outcome. Abdominal luster did marginally show a better outcome, yet lack of luster did not indicate a worse outcome. This was also true for facial luster. Abdominal tone, however, seemed to be a more reliable indicator of outcome, with consistency both ways.

It can be concluded that any one area of diagnosis cannot by itself be an indicator of prognosis, and even where patients' signs and symptoms seem to suggest a poorer prognosis, this is not always reflected in the treatment outcomes. Conversely, not all patients whose signs and symptoms seem to suggest a better prognosis necessarily respond as well as might be expected to treatment. In this study, a thorough analysis of other relevant information taken during the initial consultation was not included. In particular, a disruption to appetite, sleep, and bowel movements are also seen to be important considerations. Other relevant medical conditions, both past and present, in particular hypertension and other circulatory disorders, may well have an important impact on treatment outcomes. A future, larger study should consider these fac-

tors. The exclusion of these areas and the limitation in patient numbers might well explain the areas of inconsistency within each prognostic category.

References

1. Birch S. Forming a prognosis—perspectives from the works of Japanese acupuncturists: A preliminary compilation of ideas. *North American Journal of Oriental Medicine*. 1997;4(10):4–8.
2. Kaptchuk TK. *The Web that has no Weaver: Understanding Chinese Medicine*. London: Rider publications; 1983:260.
3. *Webster's Ninth New Collegiate Dictionary*. Springfield: Merriam-Webster Inc; 1983.
4. Fukushima K. *Meridian Therapy*. Tokyo: Toyo Hari Medical Association; 1991.
5. See ref 4, Chapter X1, p. 135.
6. See ref 4, Chapter V111, p. 74.
7. Unschuld PU. *Medicine in China. Nan-Ching* [The Classic of Difficult Issues]. Berkeley, CA: University of California Press; 1986.
8. Matsumoto K, Birch S. *Five Elements and Ten Stems*. Brookline, MA: Paradigm Publications; 1983.
9. See ref 8, p. 122.
10. Birch S, Ida J. The translation project: prognostication. From the first four lectures by Yukata Shinoda on the selection of *sho, published in Keiraku Shinryo. Keiraku Chiryo. European Toyohari News*. July 2004;1(2).
11. Craig J, Young M. Constitutional diagnosis and its effects on treatment and selection of *sho*. A summary from a lecture by Shinoda sensei. April 2003, Japan. *Keiraku Chiryo. European Toyohari News*. July 2003;1.
12. Paterson C. MRC health services research collaboration, University of Bristol. Seminar held at the University of Westminster, 2005.
13. www.hsrc.ac.uk/mymop/main.htm

Further Reading

Guyatt GH, Juniper EF, Walter S, Griffith LE, Goldstein RS. Interpreting treatment effects in randomised trials. *BMJ*. 1998;316:690–693.

Juniper EF, Guyatt GH, Willan A, Griffith LE. Determining a minimal important change in a disease-specific quality of life questionnaire. *J Clin Epidemiol.* 1994;47(1):81–87 .

Shudo D. *Introduction to Meridian Therapy.* Seattle: Eastland Press;1990.

Acknowledgements

My thanks go to Stephen Birch for helping me to formulate the study theme and providing advice along the way; to Charlotte Paterson who provided valuable suggestions for implementing and analyzing the MYMOP data; to Oran Kivity, my colleague and valued friend, for his feedback on my initial ideas; to Katherine Klinger, my partner and constant support, for her proofreading skills and patience; and finally to Raphael, who is a constant reminder of the vibrance of *sei qi.*

Contact Details

Marian Fixler, LLB (Hons), DipAc, MBAcC
Highgate Acupuncture Practice,
London, UK
www.toyohari.org.uk

Acupuncture for Spiritual Opening:
Chakra Acupuncture—An Additional Method of Energy Therapy

Gabriel Stux, MD, Düsseldorf, Germany

Abstract

Chakra acupuncture integrates the Indian chakra system, a system of major energy centers, into the acupuncture practice, expanding and activating the flow of *qi* in the channels and organs. It promotes a significant spiritual opening, through the connection of the soul with the heart chakra and other major energy centers. This method is characterized by focusing the conscious awareness into the major energy centers. The chakras of Indian medicine are energy centers in the center of the body. The most frequently used chakra point is Du-20 (*bai hu*), situated in the center of the crown chakra (Fig. **1**).

Introduction

In addition to acupuncture, moxibustion, laser acupuncture, and herbal treatment, new

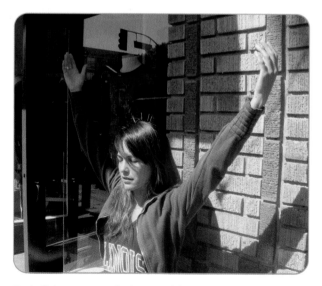

Fig. 1 Chakra acupuncture for the crown chakra with Du-20 and Ex-6.

methods have recently been introduced to intensify the energetic actions of these traditional methods. In this article, a new form of energetic treatment is summarized, which focuses more deeply and directly on the energy bases of body, mind, and spirit.

This method, known as chakra acupuncture, promotes a significant spiritual opening through connecting the soul (which in some literature is considered to be the eighth chakra) with the heart chakra and other major energy centers.

The use of chakra acupuncture helps to open and activate the energy fields of the patient on many levels. The needling of chakra points has a strong effect on the aetheric body level, releasing growth hormones, which activate the life force on this body level. The needling and activation of the second, third, and fourth chakras have a strong releasing effect on emotional levels, freeing the emotional field. The activation of the higher chakras calms mental activity, thus liberating the mind from an overload of thoughts. The connection of the soul with the heart and other energy centers activates the spiritual level in the energy field, promoting more flow of light on all levels.

Chakra acupuncture is characterized by focusing conscious awareness into the major energy centers, by an intensive act of cooperation on the part of the patient in the treatment process, who thus takes more responsibility for the treatment results.

The chakras of Indian medicine are energy centers in the center of the body. Five main spaces are known, located in the pelvis, abdomen, heart, throat, and cranium (Fig. **2**).

These five energy spaces form the system of seven major chakras. Indian chakras are spaces with two openings, one to the front and one to the back. The pelvic space and the cranium both have three openings—one down to the perineum, one up to the crown, and one each to the front and to the back.

In addition, there are a dozen minor energy centers of secondary importance, which in most cases correspond to the location of important acupuncture points. The chakras, similar to the Chinese organs, have certain functions.

The aim of the treatment in Chinese acupuncture is to harmonize the flow of *qi* by dissolving the blockages and stagnations in the channels and organs. Conditions of excess or deficiency are balanced, thus achieving an undisturbed function of the organs by harmonizing *yin* and *yang*. These ideas form the basis of Chinese acupuncture.

In chakra acupuncture, apart from the acupuncture points selected according to Chinese methodology, additional chakra points are needled in the area of the seven energy centers. Thus the chakras are activated, and the energy flow is promoted; this is known as opening of the chakras.

The most frequently used chakra points are Du-20 (*bai hui*), which is situated in the center of the crown chakra, the seventh chakra, and Ex-6 (*si shen cong*), surrounding *bai hui*. Other important chakra points are Ex-1 (*yin tang*), and Du-15 (*ya men*), for the sixth chakra, Ren-17 (*shan zhong*), and Du-1 (*shen dao*) for the heart chakra.

Technique

After all acupuncture points have been needled with the usual technique, including traditionally chosen points and chakra points, the patient is asked to direct his or her awareness toward the relevant chakra (starting, for example, with the crown, where the points Du-20 [*bai hui*], and Ex-6 [*si shen cong*], have been needled). Thus, in addition to needling of the chakra points, the focusing of the conscious awareness, that is, the direction of the patient's attention toward the respective chakra region, is important for the efficacy of this treatment. After a short time the patient should feel a slight tingling or a gentle flow in the given area. The patient should observe

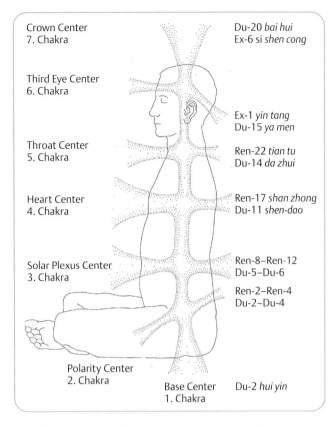

Crown Center 7. Chakra	Du-20 *bai hui* Ex-6 si *shen cong*
Third Eye Center 6. Chakra	
	Ex-1 *yin tang* Du-15 *ya men*
Throat Center 5. Chakra	Ren-22 *tian tu* Du-14 *da zhui*
Heart Center 4. Chakra	Ren-17 *shan zhong* Du-11 *shen-dao*
Solar Plexus Center 3. Chakra	Ren-8–Ren-12 Du-5–Du-6 Ren-2–Ren-4 Du-2–Du-4
Polarity Center 2. Chakra	
Base Center 1. Chakra	Du-2 *hui yin*

Fig. 2 The five energy spaces forming the system of seven major chakras.

this sensation during the course of the treatment session. The therapist, together with the patient, also directs his or her attention toward this region. He or she repeatedly asks the patient to be aware of the area, to "open the area" and to "observe the energy flow from above downward." If the patient does not initially experience the opening of the chakra, the therapist asks the patient to breathe deeply into this area, that is, to focus his or her breath into the chakra. The opening of the chakra, as well as the flow of life force, are thereby intensified.

When the flow through one energy center is clearly experienced by the patient, the patient proceeds to another energy center (e.g., to the heart chakra in the center of the thorax). Here the points Ren-17 (*shan zhong*) and Ren-15 (*jiu wei*) have already been needled. The patient is then asked to breathe into this area, to hold his or her awareness there, and to "observe the opening of the heart chakra," until a sensation of expansion, charge, and flow in this region is felt. Following this step, the patient proceeds to the base chakra, establishing an opening and flow in this chakra, and connecting to the crown, heart, and base with his or her awareness.

The first step is to open and activate the energy centers and to promote the flow of life force in them, thus to establish a strong charge, to raise the awareness of the patient of the energy centers, and to vitalize the energies.

At the beginning of the chakra acupuncture treatment, it is important to focus upon the crown, the heart, and the base energy centers, and to establish a strong and constant flow. The soul, located above the crown, often seen as a ball of light, connects after a few sessions with the heart chakra and later with other major energy centers.

The heart chakra, the fourth, is situated in the center; there are three chakras above and three below. Thus the heart chakra, because of its mid-position, has an important balancing function for the whole energy of the body. Also, the healing quality of the heart energy harmonizes the other energy centers.

After a few treatment sessions, when the flow of energy in these chakras is well established, one proceeds to further chakras, especially to those where the illness of the patient is located. It is not recommended to start with the disturbed region; rather, to begin with, to open and activate the main chakras (crown, heart, and base).

Description of the Major Chakras and Their Relation to Acupuncture Points and Chinese Organs

1. Base chakra: *muladhara*
   Location. The first chakra is situated on the perineum and opens downward. The position corresponds to the point Ren-1 (*hui yin*), the meeting point of the entire *yin*.
   Functions. The *yin* corresponds to earth, and thus the base chakra provides the energetic connection of the human being to the earth.

The opening of the base chakra and the energetic flow through the chakra is responsible for the energetic connection of the body to the earth, which is known as grounding. This chakra corresponds to the kidney *yin*.

2. Polarity chakra: *svadhishthana*
   Location. The second chakra is situated in the pelvis and has two openings, one forward to the acupuncture points Ren-2 to Ren 4 (*guan yuan*), and one backward to the sacrum, Du-2 to Du-4 (*ming men*).
   Functions. The polarity chakra balances the *yin* and *yang*, inside and outside; it forms the base for harmonious sexuality, that is, the *yin* and *yang* balance and exchange outside. The first and second chakras form a unit and correspond to the kidney and the lower *jiao* of the *san jiao* (pelvis). The polarity chakra corresponds to the kidney *yang*, the urinary bladder and the large intestine.

3. Solar plexus chakra: *manipura*
   Location. The third chakra is situated in the abdomen. It opens forward to the navel and backward to the region of Du-5 to Du-6.
   Functions. The Manipura chakra regulates the personal will in the upper part, and emotional expression in the lower part. In case of imbalance, it is responsible for striving for power, anger, rage, and addiction. The Chinese organs spleen and liver correspond to the third chakra.

4. Heart chakra: *anahata*
   Location. The fourth chakra is situated in the center of the thorax, and opens forward to the point Ren-17 (*shan zhong*), and backward to the point Du-11 (*shen dao*).
   Functions. The corresponding functions are friendliness, understanding, compassion, balancing of contrasts, striving for harmony, inner peace, and love. The heart chakra, as the fourth chakra, represents the center of the human being, and it is the most important integrating chakra, located between the three upper and the three lower chakras. The Anahata chakra corresponds to the heart and the upper *jiao*.

5. Throat chakra: *vishuddha*
   Location. The fifth chakra is situated in the throat and opens forward to the larynx and backward to the point Du-14 (*da zhui*).

Functions. The throat chakra produces the strength and expressiveness of speech. Another function is creativity. The throat chakra corresponds to the lung.

6. Third eye chakra: *ajna*

   Location. The sixth chakra is situated at the base of the skull.

   Functions. The functions of the third eye are the ability to focus and expand the mind, deepen understanding, enhance the power of discernment, intuition, and clairvoyance.

7. Crown chakra: *sahasrara*

   Location. The seventh chakra is situated on the top of the cranium.

   Functions. The crown chakra represents the highest *yang* in the body, in contrast to the meeting point of the entire *yin* in the base chakra. The crown chakra is considered to be responsible for the understanding of higher aspects of life; it provides the connection to the soul and the spiritual world. The points Du-20 (*bai hui*) and Ex-6 (*si shen cong*) are particularly important and serve to lighten up and to harmonize the mind, as well as the whole energy field.

Bibliography

Jung CG. *Über psychische Energie und das Wesen der Träume*. Zürich: Rascher; 1948.

Krieger D. *The Therapeutic Touch, How to Use Hands to Help to Heal*. New York: Prentice Hall; 1979.

Stux G. Was ist Energie-Medizin? *Therapeutikon*. 1992;6(4):171–172.

Stux G. Chakra acupuncture. *Pacific Journal of Oriental Medicine* 2. 1994:16–18.

Stux G. Chakra flow meditation. *Frontier Perspectives*. Philadelphia: Temple University; 1996.

Stux G, Hammerschlag R. *Clinical Acupuncture: Scientific Basis*. Berlin, Heidelberg: Springer; 2000.

Stux G, Hammerschlag R. *Acupuntura Clínica*. Tamboré, Brazil: Editora Manole; 2005.

Stux G, Pomeranz B. *Fundamentos de Acupuntura*. Barcelona, Ibérica: Springer; 2000.

Stux G, Pomeranz B. *Basics of Acupuncture*. 5th ed. Berlin, Heidelberg, New York: Springer; 2002.

Contact Details

Gabriel Stux, MD
German Acupuncture Society Düsseldorf
(Deutsche Akupunktur Gesellschaft
    Düsseldorf, DAGD)
Düsseldorf, Germany
www.akupunktur-aktuell.de
akupunktur@arcor.de

Improving Vitality—A Case History

Stephen Birch, PhD, LAc, Amsterdam, the Netherlands

Acupuncture is a complex intervention, involving selection from among a wide range of theories, diagnostic classification systems, and treatment techniques [1, 2]. Over the centuries, many different approaches to using acupuncture have developed [3]. Historically, acupuncture started as a basic method for improving patients by correcting theorized underlying disturbances in physiology, mostly using a *qi*-based model. This approach was later called the "*zhi ben fa*," or "root" treatment. Over time, the focus on correction of underlying physiological disturbances was increasingly complemented by symptomatic treatments, aimed at directly relieving the suffering of the patient. The symptomatic treatment approach came to be called the "*zhi biao fa*," or "branch" treatment approach, in contrast to the "*zhi ben fa*." Today, acupuncture is practiced either as a combination of these approaches (*ben* and *biao*), or uses only one of these approaches (*ben* or *biao*), or combines them with other therapeutic methods such as herbal medicine, Western medicine, etc. (*ben* and/or *biao*, etc. [2, 3, 4]).

While it is difficult to discuss this development and the range of possible treatment approaches [3], it is possible to make very general statements about what the more traditionally based "root" treatment is trying to do. As the earliest acupuncture literature developed, evidence from an analysis of the *Huang Di Nei Jing Su Wen* (The Yellow Emperor's Classic of Medicine), circa 200 CE, shows that the original introduction of a *qi*-based model started with a non-differentiated universal or generic *qi* [5]. Then, owing to the needs of practitioners trying to figure out specific treatment tactics, this undifferentiated *qi* was later differentiated into the multiple forms that have been discussed by various authors since then [5, 6]. It appears to have developed out of a wind-based model, replac-

ing a blood circulation-based model [6, 7]. Despite the needs of clinicians to describe more specialized forms of *qi* in the body in order to posit theories of physiology and patho-physiology, several less well-, or non-, differentiated forms of *qi* continued to be discussed by early medical authors. Among the labels used, we find the four following terms: *yuan qi* ("original" *qi*); *yuan qi* ("source" *qi*); *sheng qi* ("vital" *qi*); and *zheng qi* ("right" *qi*). Although each term has a separate history and usage over the centuries among different authors, when we look back over these usages they are pretty much interchangeable [8, 9]. They refer to a basic idea that I shall simply call the "vitality" of the patient.

The term "vital" *qi* in Chinese is *sheng qi*, literally, "living" *qi*. Wiseman describes the *sheng qi* as associated with the growth of all things, the "original" *qi*, and that it "loosely refers to the life force" [10]; it is the *qi* that sustains life. But the other terms are used to mean or refer to similar concepts. The "original" *qi* (*yuan qi*) is often understood to be the first or primordial form of *qi*, from which all other forms of *qi* are derived [14]; it is sometimes equated with both the "right" *qi* and "source" *qi* [11]. In the body, it is the basic *qi* from which the various subsets of *qi* are derived. The "source" *qi* (*yuan qi*) is said to be a product of the combination of various *qi* from the prenatal–kidney axis—the *qi* derived from digestion and the *qi* derived from breathing— it is "the basis of all physiological activity. All other forms of *qi* inherent in the body are considered to be manifestations or derivatives of source *qi*" [12]. The *zheng qi* ("right" *qi*) is commonly used to refer to the *qi* that combats disease. The "right" *qi* fights the *xie qi*, or "pathogenic" *qi*, (literally, "evil" *qi*). The "right" *qi* is all over the body and in everything, and "stands in opposition to evil *qi*" [13]. Further discussions of these concepts can be found in the context of "that which indicates you are alive," the "*shen jian dong qi*," the "moving *qi* between the kidneys," which is described as the source of "vital" *qi* and "source" *qi*, where the "original" *qi* is rooted [15].

It seems that the four terms "original" *qi*, "source" *qi*, "right" *qi*, and "vital" *qi* are used interchangeably. Certainly, different authors and schools seem to use one or more of these terms to refer to pretty much the same thing. For example, one acupuncture approach in Japan uses the term "*seiki*" (*zheng qi*) or "right" *qi* as the generic form of *qi* in the body [16]. I suspect this is largely due to the emphasis on using appropriate treatment techniques to strengthen the "*seiki*," to help push the pathogenic *qi* out of the body, followed by the use of additional draining techniques to remove the pathogenic *qi* [16].

One aspect of traditionally based systems of acupuncture that is not well developed in much of the modern literature is the idea that an underlying reason for applying the root treatment is to strengthen patient vitality (whether called "original," "source," "vital," or "right" *qi*). A possible reason for this is that most publications relating to traditionally based root treatment models have tended to stress correction of underlying pathologies, imbalances, or syndromes as the purpose of the root treatment [17, 18, 19, 20, 21]. While obviously an important reason for applying the root treatment, the practical emphasis on describing how to do this has tended to obscure the fact that it also triggers, or is accompanied by, a strengthening of patient vitality. This aspect has not tended to be well articulated. Another potential reason for the lack of discussion or de-emphasis of this aspect of root treatment effect is probably the fact that the doctrine of Vitalism was misrepresented and discredited in the West in the twentieth century, and continues to be seen negatively in the more modern period [22]. Modern authors of acupuncture have therefore probably been afraid to associate their therapy with this doctrine.

The case that follows highlights the value of targeting an improvement in the vitality of the patient, and essentially doing nothing

else. It will be seen that the patient presented virtually no opportunity to treat symptoms, and my role was explicitly to administer preventive treatment. The preventive aspect of treatment is also not so well developed in modern acupuncture literature. Focusing on improving the vitality of the patient is a natural means for undertaking preventive therapy.

Interestingly, the medical conditions for which the best evidence from clinical trials exists, is the prevention of future problems such as post-operative dental pain, nausea and vomiting, and chemotherapy-induced nausea and vomiting [23, 24, 25, 26, 27, 28, 29, 30, 31]. While the trials that demonstrate this preventive effect of acupuncture used simplistic non-pattern-based, and thus non-root-based, symptomatic treatments, this does not preclude a more general preventive effect from a properly applied root treatment, regardless of symptoms. Such an approach has not been tested in clinical trials before.

The case below describes treatment of a very sick hospitalized child. The root treatment model that was used was the *keiraku chiryo* or the Japanese Meridian Therapy treatment model [20], in particular the *toyohari* style, where needles are not inserted to obtain treatment effects [16, 32] (see also "Perspectives on Traditional Acupuncture by Senior Blind Practitioners in Japan—Two Interviews," p. 169, Professional Developments, Legislation, and Regulation). A simplified *shonishin*, or Japanese pediatric acupuncture model, was used as well—this involves techniques of lightly rubbing and tapping, usually without inserting any needles [34]. Also note that the only time needles were inserted in the patient (second treatment), it resulted in an immediate, but temporary, worsening of his condition.

Patient: DM, A Five-Year-Old Boy

Main Complaints

DM had been hospitalized for the previous three months with severe gastrointestinal (GI) disturbance. He had chaotic peristalsis in the GI tract, causing fecal matter to pass back up through the intestine to the stomach and out through the nose and mouth. This was life threatening and was due to a birth defect with an irreversible abnormality of the autonomic nerves that regulated the GI tract. To deal with this problem he had a tube placed through his abdominal wall around left ST-26, to drain his small intestine. He had a tube placed down his nose to drain his stomach. He had enemas twice daily to clear out his colon. The name of the diagnosis of this problem is "chronic intestinal pseudo-obstructive syndrome." It is very rare, with only about 20 children throughout the world living with the condition. (I couldn't find any reference to the problem on the Internet, or in any of my textbooks.) Life expectancy is very poor. He could not eat solid food and was fed liquid nutrients through a tube, known as a "porta-cat," in the right thoracic region.

History

It was not until the age of one year that the full extent of the patient's problems was appreciated. Since that time he had spent about half of his life in hospital. He'd had multiple abdominal surgeries to investigate and try to remedy the problem, including multiple surgeries for obstructed bowel. He'd had continuous medical interventions with multiple tests for over four years. He couldn't eat normally. His teeth were abnormal and in poor condition. At this stage, eating solid matter only increased the amount of material drained out into the stomach and small intestine drainage bags. One measure of how well he was doing was the amount of fecal matter drained out of the stomach. He spent most of his time sitting in bed. As a result, he had developed problems of hip dysplasia and had difficulty walking normally. He also had very stiff and, at times, painful back muscles.

A week before my visit to DM, the doctors had decided that probably the best thing to try next was a colostomy, since the colon was the more problematic region of the GI tract. DM was on the waiting list for this surgery. His parents had decided to try acupuncture before the operation, to see if it would help prepare him for, and recover from, the surgery. Following each operation, DM usually spent

around two weeks in a lot of pain and discomfort, and this caused a lot of stress for both DM and his family. His mother would stay with him at the hospital, and this was proving to be very disruptive to family life. DM had had so many medical interventions that he showed fear reactions in the presence of a new therapist, a normal reaction in a small child with his medical history. To support DM through the first visit, a caseworker from the hospital explained the procedures and helped him through the various stages and methods of the diagnosis and treatment.

Diagnosis

DM's face was puffy, probably from the prednisone he was taking. He was generally in a good mood. Sitting on the bed, he had no problem playing and moving around, except to make sure that he didn't pull out any of the tubes to which he was attached. He sat with splayed legs as a result of his hip problems. Once the caseworker had explained what was going to happen, it was possible to get him to strip down to his underwear. Abdominal diagnosis was not possible, because of the numerous tubes and scars and the tape on the abdomen and chest. His arm muscles were very stiff, his back muscles were stiff and jumpy on palpation, and the shoulders and neck were also very stiff. The pulses were difficult to take, as he would not stay still for very long; the quality was overall slightly sinking and weak. Pulse rate was difficult to assess because of his repeated movements. The heart (first left–deep) pulse, the spleen (second right–deep) pulse and the *ming men*/pericardium (third right–deep) pulse were weak.

The symptoms and signs indicated a spleen vacuity pattern in the Japanese Meridian Therapy model [16, 20]. He was not, as I had expected, in an advanced state of vacuity, probably because of the forced nutrition delivered through the portacat. I reckoned that the *yang* channels were all slightly weak. I decided to apply supplementation techniques for the spleen vacuity pattern and the *yang* channels, and to apply techniques to try to release some of the tightness of the muscles. As it was the first visit, and it was possible to schedule the second visit the following day at the hospital, I decided to apply a simple low-dose treatment using the *tei shin* instead of a regular needle.

Treatment

Using a silver *tei shin*, supplementation was applied to left SP-3 and then left PC-7. See Figure **1** for examples of the *tei shin*, which is a round-tipped "needle," used for pressing, or lightly touching, the points. It is one of the original nine needles of the *Huang Di Nei Jing Ling Shu* (The Yellow Emperor's Classic of Medicine); (see [35] for a discussion of the *tei shin*).

The pulses were rechecked, and it was noted that the kidney (third left–deep) pulse was relatively weak. Supplementation was then applied to right KI-3, using the *tei shin*. The pulses were then rechecked. It was not clear whether or how to select any draining techniques on the *yang* channels, which remained slightly weak. Therefore supplementation was applied to bilateral TB-4 and then ST-36, using the *tei shin*. Next, using a *hera bari*, light rhythmic tapping was applied over the back of the neck and shoulder regions (Fig. **2**). To finish, stainless-steel press-spheres were taped onto GV-12 and bilateral ST-36. (For a discussion of the press-spheres, see [36].)

Second Visit: The Following Day

There had been no significant change. There had been no word, as yet, about when the surgery might take place, and since it would be almost a week before the third treatment, it was decided to try to increase the dose of treatment already undertaken. The same basic treatment was applied with the following two changes: a silver *en shin* was lightly rubbed down the back. (See Fig. **3** and [37] for a discussion of the *en shin*, which is another of the original nine needles from the *Ling Shu*.) Intradermal needles were inserted bilaterally to ST-36, with instructions to replace them the following day with press spheres. The intradermal needles were 3 mm long, and inserted horizontally about 1 mm to a depth of less than 1 mm. They were taped to ensure their

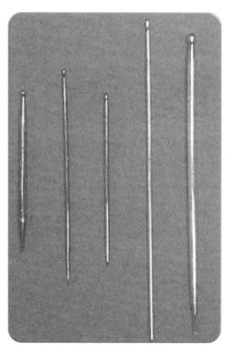

Fig. **1** Tei shin *needles*

safety. (See [38] for a discussion of intradermal needles.) DM's mother was also given appropriate tools to use, and was taught how to apply the light rhythmic tapping over the back, arms, legs, and neck, with recommendations to do this daily for a few minutes.

Third Visit: Five Days Later

DM had suffered a lot of intestinal gas and pain on the day of the treatment, with increased reflux of food and draining of matter into the stomach bag. This had improved the following day. The situation was discussed, and it was decided that while this could happen at any time, it was highly likely that the intradermal needles were probably causing the problem. It was decided to not use them again. DM was scheduled for surgery the following day, so this third treatment was principally to help him prepare for, and recover from, the surgery. To help prepare for the surgery, I decided to apply a little extra treatment to the extraordinary vessels. First, I placed a small copper disc on left KI-6, and a small zinc disc on left LU-7 [16]. These were retained for approximately two minutes. The pulse filled

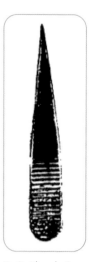

Fig. **2** A hera bari

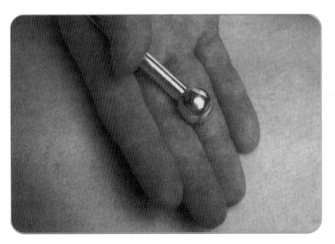

Fig. 3 An en shin

out, and DM became visibly relaxed. Then the same basic treatment was applied, but with stainless-steel press spheres left at bilateral ST-36 instead of intradermal needles.

Fourth Visit: Nine Days Later

DM had recovered remarkably well and quickly from the surgery. Instead of lying in bed and complaining for two weeks, he had been up playing after only two days! He was quite active at this visit. Since the surgery, the stomach drainage had decreased slightly, but not significantly.

The parents had been trying to postpone this surgery for years. Now that they had decided to go ahead with the surgery, they found themselves torn about what to do as far as the acupuncture was concerned. On the one hand, they could see that it had done something for DM. On the other hand, it was very important to see what the surgery could do for their child. Additionally, they had decided to use acupuncture only to help with the surgery, which had now taken place. As a result, they decided to discontinue the acupuncture, so that this would be the last visit. They agreed to call if help was needed in the future.

The same basic treatment was applied, without the additional zinc–copper application.

Seventeen Months Later: First Visit

DM's parents called out of the blue asking for more acupuncture treatments. DM, who was now seven, had recovered well from the colostomy and had been able to go home for a while. Four months previously, however, he had been readmitted with acute abdominal pain as a result of an obstruction in the small intestine. He had required emergency surgery, from which he had spent over two weeks recovering. Ten weeks later he had required further emergency surgery for a similar problem, from which he had also spent weeks recovering. During the last surgery the professor in charge of his case had found that DM's colon was completely abnormal, and after consultation with international experts had decided that the best course of action was to remove the colon completely. It was decided to replace the tube down his nose to the stomach and the tube through the abdominal wall into the jejeunem at the same time. This surgery was planned for ten days following the previous operation, and DM's parents had remembered that he had recovered well after the acupuncture the previous year. Therefore, they called to find out if acupuncture could be used to prepare DM for his operation and help with post-surgical recovery. Two more appointments were scheduled before the surgery.

Diagnosis and Treatment

Despite having been in hospital for the last four months, and having had major surgeries during that time, DM looked quite robust, again probably as a result of the tubal feeding. His flesh was full and strong, but the muscles were still very tight. When I inquired about his walking, his parents told me that DM was scheduled for a brain computed tomography (CT) scan to determine if there was any abnormality of the brain that might be causing the muscle spasticity. The same diagnostic pattern was identified. Treatment was applied as before, with a *tei shin* to the same basic points, with the addition of draining techniques to left SI-7, right LI-6 (decided from the pulse, which was easier to read as he remained still longer than he'd done previously). Using the

tei shin, super light stroking was applied
down the large intestine and stomach channels on the arms. Using a silver *en shin*, very
light rubbing was also applied down the backs
of the arms and legs, and down the back.
Light rhythmic tapping was applied on the
head and over the areas ST-36 to ST-37, using
the *hera bari*. I had forgotten to bring the
press-spheres and was thus unable to leave
them on ST-36 as usual.

One Week Later: Second Visit

Two days earlier, DM's portacat feeding tube
mechanism had failed mechanically. This
meant that he had to have emergency minor
surgery to replace the tube. Following such
minor surgeries with general anesthetic, it
was thought DM would have to spend at least
two days recovering. He was out of bed playing two hours after the surgery! The same
basic root treatment was applied as in the
treatment the week before, with the same
light stroking, rubbing, and tapping over regions of the body surface. Press spheres were
applied to both ST-36.

Two Days Later, One Day Before Surgery: Third Visit

DM was doing well and was ready for the surgery. An identical treatment was applied, except that no draining methods were applied.
Additionally, a press sphere was applied to
GV-12 as well as to the ST-36 points.

Fifteen Days Later: Fourth Visit

Fifteen days later, and just before the summer
vacation, DM had recovered amazingly well
from the long and complicated surgery. The
surgery had gone well and his entire colon
had been successfully removed. It had been
expected that he would be in intensive care
after the operation for three to four days. He
was out of intensive care within 20 hours. It
was expected that he would be laid flat on his
back in bed, complaining for two to three
weeks. In fact, he was sitting and playing
within three days. For the first time, even the
surgeon was wondering about the acupuncture! DM was still on pain medication, and
still had post-surgical pain, but was neverthe-

less doing very well. He was quite active, and
had no difficulties moving around. The CT
scans of his brain had come back negative. It
had been decided to start pediatric physical
therapy as soon as he was able to cope with
this. The parents stated their intention to try
and get DM home as soon as possible, as it
was a very big burden to have him stay in hospital, since one of them had to stay with him
all the time. The same treatment as before
was applied, with the addition of a draining
technique to left SI-7, right TB-5.

Subsequent Treatments

Three more treatments were applied: four,
five, and six weeks later, once DM had come
back home. He had recovered well from the
surgery and was able to go to school and be
off the tubes during the day, but was hooked
up to the gastric and small intestine drainage
tubes each evening at 6 o'clock for the night.
I also had a chance to see him seven months
after the final treatment. DM was still at home
and doing very well. He was going to school
by bus every day. He had not needed to be
hospitalized since then.

Final Thoughts

I chose this case because I could only apply
preventive treatment on this child. It was not
possible to treat the symptoms. The treatment
involved an exclusive focus on improving the
patient's vitality. From this extremely light
treatment approach, this very sick little boy
was able to recover remarkably well from one
minor, and two major, surgeries. I think that
the case illustrates an enhanced recuperative
ability as a result of attempting to increase the
vitality of the patient. The skeptic may feel
that I falsely attribute treatment effects to my
intended treatment, and that the patient simply exhibited a strong placebo effect. To this
end, I raise the following objections. First, this
child was hospitalized for extended periods of
time and was treated by numerous people, especially well-trained nursing staff, yet he had
always had difficulty recovering from the numerous surgeries that he needed. To attribute

superior placebo effects only to me as a thera-pist and not to the much more charming and friendly nursing staff is unrealistic. Second, evidence to date shows that in clinical trials acupuncture therapy that works for adults pre-surgical does not work for children. This suggests the absence of both a specific effect and placebo effect [27, 29]. To suggest that the treatment worked because of a placebo effect is, in my opinion, both unreasonable and non-sensical.

I also included this case as it presents a series of challenges to current thinking about how to test acupuncture in clinical trials. If the target of treatment is the improvement of vitality, how do we know that when we are forced to administer a sham control treat-ment, in order to try to control for a placebo effect, we have not accidentally controlled for precisely that which is the specific target of treatment? This might happen if the placebo effect employs some of the same self-healing pathways that we are trying to target using the root treatment. Thus, if we are forced to control for the specific target of treatment because of the "placebo controlled" model requirements, this is a logical contradiction and impossibility [39]. To date, this issue has been virtually ignored in clinical trials of acu-puncture.

In addition, most trials of acupuncture have incorrectly assumed that one must obtain *de qi*, as defined in China since 1950 [17, 40], for acupuncture to be effective [41], and, therefore, shallowly inserted needles, or non-inserted needles, serve as an appropriate control [42]. In studies using this assumption, the idea that non-*de qi* type needling methods are inert or have minimal effects is highly questionable [39, 43, 44]. In the case outlined above, I gave no treatment to elicit the sensa-tions typical of the modern Chinese interpre-tation of *de qi*; additionally, with the excep-tion of one intradermal needle that seemed to trigger a worsening of stomach symptoms, I did not rely on inserted acupuncture as a healing modality. Even so, the treatment ef-fects were very noticeable.

Finally, to my fellow acupuncturists, I say: "Try it." Try applying your treatment in a sim-ple manner, exclusively targeting the im-provement of patient vitality, and see what happens. This treatment approach works well on adults as well as on children (though the effects are not usually as rapid as we've seen in this child), especially if the adults have chronic symptoms, are run down, tire a lot, and seem to be very sensitive. I hope we re-visit this simple concept in future publica-tions.

References

1. Birch S. Diversity and acupuncture: Acupunc-ture is not a coherent or historically stable tra-dition. In: Vickers AJ, ed. *Examining Comple-mentary Medicine: The Sceptical Holist*. Chelten-ham: Stanley Thomas; 1998:45–63.
2. MacPherson H, Kaptchuk TJ. *Acupuncture in Practice*. New York: Churchill Livingstone; 1997.
3. Birch S, Felt R. *Understanding Acupuncture*. Ed-inburgh: Churchill Livingstone; 1999.
4. Birch S, Kaptchuk T. The history, nature and current practice of acupuncture. In: Ernst E, White A, eds. *Acupuncture a Scientific Appraisal*. Oxford: Butterworth-Heinmann; 1999:11–30.
5. Chiu ML. Mind, body, and illness in a Chinese medical tradition. PhD thesis. Cambridge, MA: Harvard University; 1986.
6. Unschuld PU. *Huang Di Nei Jing Su Wen. Nature, Knowledge, Imagery in An Ancient Chinese Med-ical Text*. Berkeley: University of California Press; 2003.
7. Epler DC. Bloodletting in early Chinese medi-cine and its relationship to the origin of acu-puncture. *Bull Hist Med*. 1980;54:337–367.
8. Birch S. Filling the whole in acupuncture. Part 1: What are we doing in the supplementation needle technique? (In preparation.)
9. Wiseman N, Feng Y. *A Practical Dictionary of Chinese Medicine*. Brookline, MA: Paradigm Publications; 1997.
10. See Ref 9, p. 657.
11. See Ref 9, p. 421.
12. See Ref 9, p. 548.
13. See Ref 9, p. 507.
14. Matsumoto K, Birch S. *Hara Diagnosis: Reflections on the Sea*. Brookline, MA: Paradigm Publications; 1988:83, 84.
15. See Ref 14, pp. 108–129.
16. Fukushima K. *Meridian Therapy*. Tokyo: Toyo-hari Medical Association; 1991.

17. Ellis A, Wiseman N, Boss K. *Fundamentals of Chinese Acupuncture.* Rev ed. Brookline, MA: Paradigm Publications; 1991.

18. Maciocia G. *Foundations of Chinese Medicine.* Edinburgh: Churchill Livingstone; 1989.

19. Manaka Y, Itaya K, Birch S. *Chasing the Dragon's Tail.* Brookline, MA: Paradigm Publications; 1995.

20. Shudo D. *Introduction to Meridian Therapy.* Seattle: Eastland Press; 1990.

21. Wiseman N, Ellis A. *Fundamentals of Chinese Medicine.* Brookline, MA: Paradigm Publications; 1985.

22. Kaptchuk TJ. Historical context of the concept of vitalism in complementary and alternative medicine. In: Micozzi MS, ed. *Fundamentals of Complementary and Alternative Medicine.* New York: Churchill Livingstone; 1996.

23. Acupuncture: NIH consensus development panel on acupuncture. *JAMA.* 1998;280(17): 1518–1524.

24. Birch S, Keppel Hesselink J, Jonkman FAM, Hekker TAM, Bos A. Clinical research on acupuncture 1: what have reviews of the efficacy and safety of acupuncture told us so far? *J Alt Comp Med.* 2004;10(3):468–480.

25. British Medical Association (BMA). *Acupuncture: efficacy, safety and practice.* London: Harwood Academic Publishers; 2000.

26. Ernst E, Pittler MH. The effectiveness of acupuncture in treating acute dental pain: A systematic review. *Br Dent J.* 1998;184:443–447.

27. Lee A, Done ML. The use of non-pharmacologic techniques to prevent postoperative nausea and vomiting: a meta-analysis. *Anesth Analg.* 1999;88(6):1362–1369.

28. Rosted P. The use of acupuncture in dentistry: a review of the scientific validity of published papers. *Oral Dis.* 1998;4(2):100–104.

29. Tait PL, Brooks L, Harstall C. *Acupuncture: Evidence from Systematic Reviews and Meta-analyses.* Alberta, Canada: Alberta Heritage Foundation for Medical Research; 2002.

30. Vickers AJ. Can acupuncture have specific effects on health? A systematic review of acu-

puncture antiemesis trials. *J Roy Soc Med.* 1996;89:303–311.

31. Vickers A, Wilson P, Kleijnen J. Effectiveness bulletin: acupuncture. *Qual Saf Health Care.* 2002;11:92–97.

32. Birch S. Grasping the sleeping tiger's tail: perspectives on acupuncture from the edge of the abyss. *N Amer J Orient Med.* 2004;11,(32):20–23.

33. Yoneyama H, Mori H. *Shonishin Ho:Acupuncture Treatment for Children.* Yokosuka: Ido-no Nippon Sha; 1964.

34. Birch S, Ida J. *Japanese Acupuncture: A Clinical Guide.* Brookline, MA: Paradigm Publications; 1998.

35. See Ref 34, pp. 39–41, 50–54.

36. See Ref 34, pp. 175–180.

37. See Ref 34, pp. 39–41, 48–49.

38. See Ref 34, pp. 139–164.

39. Birch S, Hammerschlag R, Trinh K, Zaslawski C. The non-specific effects of acupuncture treatment: When and how to control for them. *Clin Acup Orien Med.* 2002;3(1):20–25.

40. Vincent CA, Richardson PH, Black JJ, Pither CE. The significance of needle placement site in acupuncture. *J Psychosom Res.* 1989;33(4):489–496.

41. Pomeranz B. Scientific basis of acupuncture. In: Stux G, Pomeranz B. *Basics of Acupuncture.* 4th ed. Berlin: Springer Verlag; 1998:6–72.

42. White AR, Filshie J, Cummings TM. Clinical trials of acupuncture: consensus recommendations for optimal treatment, sham controls and blinding. *Complem Ther Med.* 2001;9:237–245.

43. Birch S. A review and analysis of placebo treatments, placebo effects and placebo controls in trials of medical procedures when sham is not inert. (In submission.)

44. MacDonald AJR, Macrae KD, Master BR, Rubin AP. Superficial acupuncture in the relief of chronic low back pain. *Ann Royal Coll Surg Engl.* 1983;65:44–46.

Tongue Diagnosis in Chinese Medicine

Professor Claus C. Schnorrenberger, MD, Basel, Switzerland

Excerpts from *Pocket Atlas
of Tongue Diagnosis,*
Thieme Stuttgart–New York, 2005

Modern Research on Tongue Diagnosis

Over the last few decades, traditional Chinese tongue diagnosis has been analyzed by the application of modern Western medical theories. Since the mid-1970s, for example, such research has been carried out at the German Research Institute of Chinese Medicine (GRICMED), Freiburg im Breisgau in Germany.

The Appearance of a Normal Tongue

Under normal conditions, the tongue varies in color from pink to red, since the tongue muscles and its mucous membranes are morphologically well supplied with blood vessels. Moreover, the tongue is normally covered with a thin, white coating. This white layer consists of the tips of threadlike filiform papillae (papillae filiformes), often split at their ends, and mushroom-shaped fungiform papillae (papillae fungiformes), in addition to food particles, saliva, and bacteria.

Changes in the Appearance of the Tongue

Changes of the Body

Any change in the color of the tongue body is closely related to the blood circulation within the organ. A whitish tongue indicates a reduction in the amount of blood, an anemia, or edematous swelling of the tongue body. In such cases the blood vessels shrink, the circulation slows down, and there is an insufficient blood supply in general. Chinese medicine denotes this condition as emptiness of *yang*, *qi*, or blood.

In contrast to this, a dark red tongue signals that the blood vessels have enlarged in their capacity and that blood has accumulated in the tongue body. A bluish or purple discoloration of the tongue is related to a venous blood stagnation in the tongue, or a general lack of oxygen in the organism. In such cases, the sublingual veins appear thickened and darker than normal, and the inferior side of the tongue should therefore be inspected during the examination. The purple color can be related to a lack of oxygen within the red blood cells contained in the blood vessels of the tongue. Orthodox medicine refers to this condition as cyanosis.

If a tongue is thick, soft, and swollen, this may be the result of a decrease in plasma proteins. The decrease causes a drop in the colloid osmotic pressure (water–attracting force of the blood). Thus, plasma fluid escapes from the blood vessels into the tongue tissues and forms an edema. This causes an enlargement of the tongue, which swells to the point of touching the teeth, resulting in teeth marks at the edge of the tongue. An increase in the size of the tongue can also be caused by a failure of the tongue muscles to relax. In addition, the lymphatic and venous drainage may be impaired, thus causing a swelling of the tongue body.

Fissures in the tongue occur when the filiform and fungiform papillae separate, or when they form close groups produced by the mucous membranes shrinking. This always corresponds with serious health disturbance in the organism, for example, in cases of internal heat or "*qi* emptiness" in Chinese medicine terminology.

A granular tongue, with rough and swollen papillae, which can sometimes look inflamed and protruding, as much as thorns do on a plant, is the result of a conversion of filiform into fungiform papillae. At the same time, the supply of blood to the mucous membrane vessels increases to the extent that the converted fungiform papillae are congested with blood, and therefore look red and swollen.

A dry tongue is either the result of decreased production of saliva, or the consequence of a diminished aqueous part of the saliva. This can occur when the entire organism is dehydrated or when the blood density increases, that is, with an increased hematocrit. In such cases, the secretion of saliva decreases, resulting in a dry tongue surface and thirst. Chinese medicine maintains that a dry tongue is the most reliable clinical sign of loss of water in the human system, since all kinds of dehydration of various origin can easily be detected by inspecting the tongue.

The term "*yin* emptiness" has its origins in the theory of Traditional Chinese Medicine (TCM). In such cases, the production of saliva is also decreased and, as a result, the surface of the tongue becomes dry. This is a condition that is also well known to Western medicine, indicating physical overexertion, a heat influence, or severe psychological strain.

According to modern Western medicine, the sympathetic tone is elevated in patients with a *yin* deficiency, whereas the parasympathetic tone is lowered. In such a state, the caliber of the blood vessels narrows as the result of an effect caused by the surrounding autonomous nerve fibers. Consequently, additional blood is forced into the tongue and causes its red discoloration. A person with such a reddened tongue may also show symptoms of high blood pressure (hypertension).

A slanting tongue deflected toward the paralyzed side signifies unilateral impairment of the hypoglossal nerve (twelfth cranial nerve), either in its central or peripheral course. This occurs in cerebral hemorrhage (stroke), brain injury, or brain tumors. The visible lesion of the motor innervation of the tongue is caused by a paralysis of the genioglossus muscle on the diseased side, with a preponderance of muscle activity of the genioglossus muscle on the healthy side.

Changes of the Tongue Coating

Changes in the tongue's coating vary according to its color or shape. From the point of view of orthodox medicine, an increase in filiform papillae, especially of the callous ends at their split tips, plays a role in the appearance of the coating. In addition, changes in the moistness of the mucous membranes of the tongue and the amount of fluid available in the mouth are also considered especially important.

A yellowish coating occurs as a result of a further increase in the callous ends of the filiform papillae, and in such cases even a slight inflammation of the surface of the tongue can occur. A yellow discoloration can also be due to bacterial influence.

A black coating is related to a very strong increase in the callous ends of filiform papillae, giving the surface of the tongue a brownish-black appearance, resulting from the massive proliferation of callous protuberances. Black discoloration can also be caused by the growth of certain types of fungi. According to modern medicine, a black coating of the tongue can be related to many different factors. These are, for example, high fever accompanied by dehydration, infectious or chronic diseases, functional disorders in the stomach and intestines, fungus infection, as well as long-term, and thoughtless, application of antibiotics.

If the coating thickens, the reason may be that the patient is eating very little or consuming only liquid or semi-liquid food. The thickened coating decreases the mechanical friction at the surface of the tongue caused by the normal intake of food. A thickened coating can also be due to high fever and following dehydration, when the production of saliva decreases. This, in turn, also impairs the natural cleansing of the tongue. If the filiform papillae become longer, the coating can also become thicker.

Application of Tongue Diagnosis

Albert Einstein, the Nobel laureate, exposes his tongue to the world. Why does he do this? Because the human tongue is an archetypal organ that casts a disarming spell on the observer. Such a spontaneous gesture, as seen here (Fig. **1**), suggests that showing one's tongue has an important function in human interaction, something that adds important and elucidating information to our primarily medical context. Einstein's tongue impercepti-

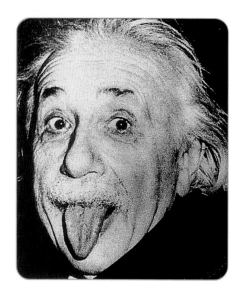

Fig. 1 Albert Einstein

bly closes the gap between body and mind, nature and spirit, the Cartesian split between *res extensa* and *res cogitans* that is still fundamental to the natural sciences and modern medicine. Such an emotional reaction cannot fully be explained by scientific thinking.

Conventional medicine is split up and separated into innumerable heterogeneous subspecialties. No physician or healer in the world of today is able to summarize, let alone control, all the manifold healing methods involved. Thus, the demonstration and evaluation of the tongue might surprisingly lead the practicing doctor of our day back to his or her original task, namely to an understanding and a responsible therapy of his or her individual patient as an integrated whole.

However, there is another aspect to be considered in this context. Poor Einstein is ailing. According to Chinese diagnosis, his tongue reveals *yin* emptiness with empty fire rising. Numerous fissures and creases make the area of the middle burner look chapped. Einstein's tongue is narrow, tense, and slightly shrunken; its edges look puffy and creased. As a result of his weakened *yin*, Einstein has probably suffered from insomnia.
A stomach disorder and constipation may have affected him. The swollen edges signify a liver problem with rising liver *yang*, a con-

dition that presumably urged him to stick his tongue out at obtrusive press and paparazzi.

The appropriate and effective treatment for the Nobel Prize-winner would have consisted of needle therapy by puncturing the foramina Spleen-6, Liver-3 and -14, Kidney-3, Bladder-15, -18, and -23, Conception Vessel-12 (*ren mai*) and Stomach-36.

He would, in addition, have benefited from herbal decoctions such as warm soups made from *Magnolia officinalis*, *Citrus reticulata*, *Glycyrrhiza uralensis*, *Bupleurum chinense*, *Scutellaria baicalensis*, *Pinellia ternata*, *Panax ginseng*, *Zingiber officinale*, and *Ziziphus jujuba*. This might have balanced his disorder and alleviated his scorn.

Einstein's psychosociosomatic problem cannot be properly described according to standard diagnoses of conventional modern medicine. Western physicians would not even interpret his situation as a "disease," because there are no tangible pathological findings involved in the foreground. Only the amazing instrument of tongue diagnosis can show the medical reality and guide us to the right approach to an effective therapy.

The photo of the young chimpanzee shows no sign of a pathological development in his system (see Fig. **2**).

By comparing the two tongues it is easy to realize that our little chimpanzee feels much better, and is probably happier, than the famous physicist.

As pointed out above, the appropriate treatment for Einstein in his time would have consisted of acupuncture and herbal prescriptions according to a differentiating Chinese syndrome diagnosis (*bian zheng*). This treatment is not primarily geared toward a Western diagnosis applying laboratory data and radiographs, or using the reductionist terms of psychology and psychiatry such as neurosis, mental depression, psychopathy, or hysteria. Such suppositions are too inaccurate as far as the patient Einstein as an individual being is concerned. It follows that integrated medical reality is beyond objective measurements, data, and reductionist terms.

The German philosopher Martin Heidegger

explained the term "science" (*Wissenschaft*) in an authentic statement as follows:

*Science in general can be defined as the totality of fundamentally coherent true propositions … within which the objectives of science are presented regarding their **ground**, and this means that they are understood. (From Heidegger's* Being and Time *and* Identity and Difference.*)*

Now, conventional Western physicians have the chance to broaden their outlook by inspecting the human tongue, and by incorporating the result into their medical analysis. The outcome will be a highly personalized diagnosis that corresponds with the individual patient as a whole. This could be the outlook toward a new global medicine: amalgamating the old with the new, as the popular Chinese proverb "*ku wei chin yung*" ("using the past for the present") suggests. Tongue diagnosis was handed down to us by ancient texts such as the *Nei Jing*, and other famous books from early times. But it is not at all antiquated. On the contrary: it can be linked to modern anatomy, embryology, and physiology, as well as to comprehensive clinical experience. Thus, it can be said that tongue diagnosis adds new

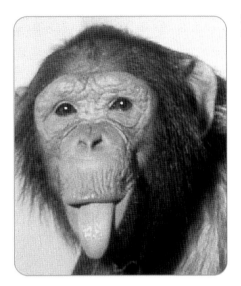

Fig. 2 Young chimpanzee

contrast and deeper insight into Western and Eastern ways of healing.

Contact Details

Professor Claus C. Schnorrenberger, MD
Lifu International College of Chinese Medicine
Basel, Switzerland
www.lifu-college.ch

Atopic Dermatitis and Psoriasis

Amir Kalay, MSc, LAc, Tel Aviv, Israel

The following cases are typical of many patients who come to our clinic seeking treatment for skin disorders. Atopic dermatitis and psoriasis are both chronic ailments that require long-term treatment, and the treatments proposed by conventional medicine are limited, often ineffective, and may be even detrimental. Chinese medicine treatments for these diseases have proved very effective in many cases, applied either exclusively, or in conjunction with conventional medicine treatments.

Atopic Dermatitis (Skin Asthma)

Atopic: allergic (Greek: "in a changed state")
Dermatitis: inflammation of the skin

What is Atopic Dermatitis?

This ailment is also known as skin asthma, because of its frequent incidence in children with a history of respiratory and asthma problems.

In Chinese medicine, the condition is called "Disease of the Four Folds," owing to the frequent appearance of the condition in arm and leg folds. Atopic dermatitis is an allergic inflammation of the skin, characterized by a chronic skin rash and itching. Environmental changes, such as polluted air that contains an increased amount of allergens, and changes brought about by a Western lifestyle (bad nutrition and stress), have in recent years increased the incidence of the disease, which now affects up to 15 % of the population of the United States and Europe.

When Does the Disease Appear and When Will it Disappear?

In 50 % of the cases among young children suffering from the disease, the disease appears within the first year of the infant's life. In 30 %, it appears between the ages of 1 to 5 years.

It is difficult to forecast the development of the condition, but it usually improves as the child gets older and the periods of remission between outbreaks become longer. Around 80 % of the children are cured by the time they reach adolescence.

Chinese medicine therapies accelerate the condition's disappearance and extend remission periods between outbreaks.

What Are the Characteristics of the Disease?

There are four predominant characteristics:

- **Itching**. The disease produces intense itching that affects the quality of life of the patient and his/her family.
- **Skin rashes**. There is redness, accompanied by substantial dryness of the skin. Bacteria, yeast, or fungi play a significant role in staphylocci.
- **Inflamed skin**. This causes chronic skin infections.
- **Additional allergic conditions**. Other conditions, such as allergic rhinitis (hay fever), asthma, conjunctivitis, sensitivity to insect bites and food allergies, are often found in atopic dermatitis patients.

What Causes the Disease?

Chinese medicine attributes the condition to two main factors: heredity and a defective immune system. It also recognizes that conditions of internal imbalance of the body contribute to the disease.

Atopic dermatitis patients are also often diagnosed as having a deficiency in the digestive system, resulting in the accumulation of heat in the body. The heat rises to the skin and causes severe dryness and itching; patients often complain of feeling hot. Adjusting the body's internal balance, therefore, accelerates the process of healing and alleviates this condition.

Hereditary Factors

Around 70 % of atopic dermatitis cases have a family history of the condition. The hereditary disease may not present in the same way with every patient; in fact it may appear in the form of a number of allergy-based conditions (e.g., allergic rhinitis, asthma, and hay fever). Hereditary diseases are not necessarily passed on from parent to child, and may skip one or more generations. Studies have showed that patients with no family history of the condition have a better chance of being cured.

Immune System Deficiencies

The disease is in this instance caused by the body's defective control over its immune system cells, specifically with respect to the activities of its white blood cells (lymphocytes). Environmental factors, however, may also elicit an overactive immune response resulting in, or further exacerbating, the skin inflammation. These factors include:

- **Allergies**. Contact with an environmental factor that elicits an allergic reaction (allergen), such as food or house dust.
- **Skin infections**. Bacteria, viruses, and yeast/fungi.
- **Physical irritants**. Dryness, skin sores, skin chafing, or friction.
- **Emotional stress**. Irritability, restlessness, and scratching may injure the skin and aggravate the disease.

Case Study: Two-Year-Old Girl with Atopic Dermatitis (Asthma of the Skin) (Fig. 2a–d)

Background

The patient was a two-year-old girl, diagnosed with atopic dermatitis. Her mother had suffered from severe dermatitis for 20 years. The girl arrived at the clinic with mild skin rashes on her face and hands that indicated allergic activity (Fig. **2a**). These skin rashes had appeared two weeks previously. The mother had treated the rashes with Elocom cream (a relatively mild steroid ointment). In addition, she had given the child Fenistil (0.1 % Mometasone Furoate) at night to alleviate the itching (the drops contain antihistamine), and had applied an antibiotic cream behind the ears. (In children with dermatitis, the rash usually appears in the ear folds.) Following her own unpleasant experience, the mother had brought her child to the clinic to prevent the disease from spreading further.

Symptoms

The patient had regular, soft bowel movements, with increased frequency over the past month. She had sensitive skin and an allergic reaction to insect bites. She was generally healthy, and not particularly susceptible to the common cold. She was very energetic, with signs of restlessness. The tongue was slightly red, with red edges and white coating. The pulse was slightly rapid.

Diagnosis

There was accumulation of heat and dampness in the spleen and heart that passes to, and eventually accumulates in, the muscles and skin.

Explanation

Most young children with atopic dermatitis have symptoms as listed above. At this age (up to age three or four years), the deficiency generally manifests itself around the spleen. It is only at a later age that other symptoms, such as *yin* or blood deficiency, appear.

Treatment Goals

To eliminate wind–heat, eliminate damp, and inhibit itchiness.

Therapies

Internal Treatment

Plant formula in powder form, daily dosage of 1 g, comprising the following components:

jin yin hua (Flos Lonicerae Japonicae)	8 g
bai xian pi (Cortex Dictamni Dasycarpi Radicis)	6 g
di fu zi (Fructus Kochiae Scopariae)	6 g
shan yao (Radix Dioscoreae Oppositae)	5 g
ku shen (Radix Sophorae Flavescentis)	5 g
ju hua (Flos Chrysanthemi Morifolii)	4 g
chan tui (Periostracum Cicadae)	4 g

The formula works according to the principles of *fu ping yin* (although different plants are used), and is a blend of plants that eliminate hot wind and damp and inhibit itching. This treatment is suitable for relatively acute conditions.

- *Jin yin hua* eliminates wind heat and is very effective in the treatment of various skin inflammations. It has antibacterial activity. This makes it particularly suitable for treating atopic dermatitis, which is often accompanied by bacteria that are secondary to allergic skin inflammations (Staphylococci infections). Especially *bai xian pi* and *di fu zi* eliminate damp and are particularly effective in alleviating allergy-induced itching.
- *Shan yao* contains properties that strengthen and support the spleen.
- *Ku shen* eliminates heat and damp and has anti-fungal action. It is effective in the treatment of yeasts that cause inflammations and are secondary to allergic inflammations. Anti-fungal plants are therefore effective in the treatment of skin asthma.
- *Ju hua* eliminates wind heat and soothes

the liver. Children affected with asthma of the skin tend toward restlessness and irritability, and *ju hua* acts as an effective soothing agent.

- *Chan tui* eliminates wind heat and inhibits itching.

External Treatment

Topic Medis wash cleanser, mainly for soaking in the bath, and Topic Medis light gel to be applied to skin rashes when necessary.

First Follow-up Treatment

The first follow-up treatment was two weeks after the initial treatment. The skin rash had disappeared completely. There was a change in bowel movements; they were no longer soft. (In both children and adults, bowel movements are significant indicators of treatment effectiveness.)

Second Follow-up Treatment

The second follow-up treatment was one month after the initial treatment (Fig. **2b**). There was a short two-day episode of skinrash that had been successfully treated with Topic Medis light gel. Bowel movements tended to be hard, which indicated that the plants had an over-drying effect. This, however, did not warrant amending the original formula.

Third Follow-up Treatment

The third follow-up treatment was two months after the initial treatment (Fig. **2c**). There had been no incidence of skin rashes. The only sign was slightly dry and rough skin. The Topic Medis light gel was replaced by Topic Medis cream, which reduces skin roughness, raises the skin dampness level, and rehabilitates damaged skin. There was no need to prescribe additional herbs, as the child had reached a level of balance and the current activity of the atopic dermatitis was very mild. In this state, external treatments such as the cream and the soaking lotion are sufficiently effective in preventing additional flare-ups. Nevertheless it is necessary to maintain controlled nutrition and to pay attention to any signs of additional occurrences.

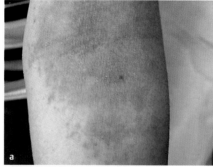
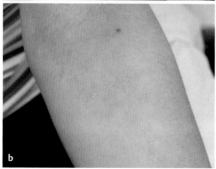

Fig. 1a, b
a Elbow fold of a 20-year-old atopic dermatitis patient.
b Same elbow fold 2 weeks later after treatment with TCM formulas and external application of Kamedis products. The skin is not red and the dryness has disappeared. The patient stops treatment since the dermatitis is cured and completely alleviated.

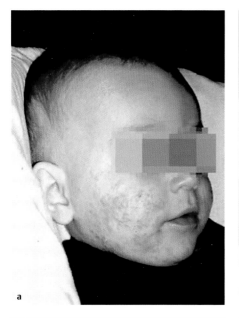

a

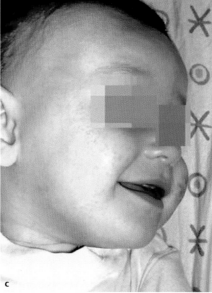

c

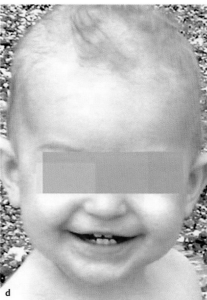

b

d

Fig. 2a–d

a *Severe case of atopic dermatitis.*

b *After 1 month of treatment: fewer red areas and less dryness.*

c *After 2 months of treatment there is more improvement.*

d *After 4 months of treatment the condition is stable and the skin eruptions have cleared up completely. The skin is no longer dry.*

Prognosis

The mother was aware of the problem and brought her child for treatment at the onset of the condition, which was ideal for a positive response to treatment. Had the child received conventional treatment, she would have been subjected to a series of cortisone creams without internal therapies, and it is possible that in the long term the condition might have become more severe. The use of plants for treatment and balance increases the likelihood of the problem disappearing entirely, or of reoccurring in a less severe form that is relatively easy to control.

Psoriasis

What is Psoriasis?

Psoriasis is a chronic skin disease that affects 2 % to 3 % of the total population worldwide. Its name derives from the Greek word *psora*, which means "itching." In Chinese medicine the condition is called *bai bi*—skin rashes with scale-covered patches. The clinical description of psoriasis is symmetric raised layers on the skin, mostly red and covered with a thick layer of white scales, often accompanied by itching. The condition is not contagious.

When Does the Disease Appear and Disappear?

On average, psoriasis affects both men and women equally in the 20–40-year age groups, but also occurs among children and older members of the population. One of the characteristics of the disease is that its appearance is not predictable, as it does not adhere to any set rules. As the disease may also be hereditary, it is difficult to predict when it will pass and whether it may reoccur at any stage in later life.

Chinese medicine therapies will first and foremost alleviate the disease's manifestations on the skin, that is, the redness and scaliness. It will also significantly reduce outbreaks of the disease and in addition will accelerate the recovery process of the body and the skin, thereby enhancing the patient's quality of life.

What Are the Characteristics of the Disease?

There are five predominant characteristics:

- **Skin rash**. This is usually in symmetrical red layers, covered with thick white scales. The rash habitually appears on the scalp, elbows, and knees, but may also appear on the groin, armpits, sex organs, palms, soles, and nails. Skin rashes appear in a variety of shapes, each with a specific name. For example, guttate psoriasis resembles drops spread over the chest, stomach, and back, and is usually triggered by severe bacterial infection (throat infection—streptococcus), and mainly affects children and adolescents.

- **Arthritis**. 10 % to 20 % of patients develop psoriatic arthritis.
- **Itching**. Itching does not affect all patients. Removing scales while scratching often produces blood spots.
- **Seasonality**. In most cases the condition is more serious in the winter, with greater relief in the summer.
- **Stress**. Because of its unaesthetic appearance, the condition is inevitably accompanied by a significant degree of emotional stress.

What Causes the Disease?

The cause of the disease is as yet unknown, but there are several possible explanations.

Chinese medicine recognizes hereditary factors, but also attributes the condition to a physiological and emotional imbalance of the body, which contributes to more serious and recurring outbreaks of the disease. The manifestations of this imbalance are various symptoms, such as heat, damp, the digestive system, enormous stress that harms the energy flow, the blood flow, and the nourishment of the skin. Diagnosis and treatment of the imbalance in body and soul accelerates the healing process and significantly alleviates the symptoms of the disease.

Hereditary Factors

Around two-thirds of all cases are governed by hereditary factors. Hereditary factors are also not ruled out in the remaining third, as information is not always available as regards psoriasis sufferers in previous generations. Also, patients themselves do not always identify dry skin on elbows and knees as a disease.

Physiological and Emotional Imbalance of the Body

Factors include the following:

- **Inflammation and multiplication of blood vessels**. There may be inflammation and multiplication of blood vessels in the dermis, which contains collagen fibers, skin cells, and blood vessels. The inflammation and multiplication of blood vessels cause the skin's redness.

- **Accelerated growth of scale cells**. There may be accelerated growth of scale cells in the external layer of the skin—the epidermis. Normal scale cells are replaced once a month. Psoriasis occurs when the process is reduced to a few days, resulting in a layer of thick, white scales. The number of cells in psoriatic skin is 27 times higher than the number of cells in healthy skin.
- **Emotional stress**. Emotional stress is known to have a negative impact on the disease in approximately 50 % of psoriasis patients, and some claim that in fact emotional stress often precipitates the initial outbreak of the disease.

Chinese medicine regards body and soul as a single, inseparable entity and treatment is therefore designed to calm and restore the patient's emotional balance.

Case Study:
Six-and-a-Half-Year-Old Girl
with Psoriasis (Fig. **3a–e**)

Background
The disease started at the age of one, with flares between the fingers. Initially, it was diagnosed as a fungus and anti-fungal creams were prescribed. These, however, proved ineffective. In the summer the symptoms would disappear. At age two-and-a-half years, the disease started to spread to the legs and around the stomach. At age three-and-a-half years, psoriatic activity in the form of an inflammation and scales appeared on the scalp. The patient arrived at the clinic in a serious condition, with psoriasis that had spread over her entire body and scalp, together with severe hair loss. She had tried a range of conventional therapies, which had proved ineffective, as well as a homeopathic treatment for four months, but this was just as ineffective.

Symptoms
There was widespread psoriasis with red patches, severe and constant itching, a badly affected scalp with redness, and thick, hard scales, together with large, bald patches where the patient's hair had fallen out. The psoriasis had spread all over the girl's body, including her face. The patient was a very active and energetic child, tending towards hyperactivity, who had suffered frequent bouts of streptococcal throat infections. She had also suffered from heat, and drank a lot. She had regular bowel movements. She had sweats at night, in both winter and summer. Her pulse was small and rapid, while her tongue was very red, with a thick, greasy, yellowish-white coating.

Diagnosis
Heat and dampness; heat in blood that consumes *yin*.

Treatment Goals
To eliminate heat and dampness; to cool heat in the blood.

Therapies
Internal Treatment
A formula of raw plants was prescribed—one dose every three days. (Using plants in raw form is essential in this case, as their effect is stronger than that of plants in powder form.) The formula is based on the principles of *yin hua hu zhang tang jia*, comprising the following components:

tu fu ling (Rhizoma Smilacis Glabrae)	10 g
jin yin hua (Flos Lonicerae Japonicae)	12 g
huang qin (Radix Scutellariae Baicalensis)	8 g
huang bai (Cortex Phellodendri)	8 g
ku shen (Radix Sophorae Flavescentis)	12 g
ye jiao teng (Caulis Polygoni Multiflori)	10 g
bai hua she she cao (Herba Oldenlandiae Diffusae)	12 g
ju hua (Flos Chrysanthemi Morifolii)	6 g
chi shao (Radix Paeoniae Rubra)	6 g

- *Tu fu ling* eliminates heat and toxicity and is effective for severe flare-ups of the disease.
- *Bai hua she she cao*, together with *tu fu ling* and *jin yin hua* "extinguish the fire."
- *Huang qin*, *huang bai*, and *ku shen* treat heat and damp, and the upper and lower heaters.
- *Ye jiao teng* nourishes the blood and, together with *chi shao*, also cools the blood.

- *Ye jiao teng* and *ju hua* are plants with soothing properties, aimed at soothing the *shen*, which in such cases is extremely turbulent and restless.

Nutritional Supplements: Omega 3 at a daily dosage of 2000 mg.
Nutrition: based on heat and damp-avoidance principles.

External Treatment
Constant use of Topic Medis wash cleanser and soaking in the bath. Application of Pso Medis night gel at night. Constant use of Pso Medis shampoo and Pso Medis scalp lotion for the scalp.

First Follow-up Treatment
One month after the initial treatment there was decreased itching, and affected areas appeared less red and more soothed. The condition, including on the head and scalp, seemed to be lessening. Severe inflamma- tory activity was still visible, but was relatively moderate in comparison to what it was before treatment. The previous thick coating on the tongue was now a thin coating. The pulse was less rapid.

Second Follow-up Treatment
Two months after initial treatment, there was continued improvement. There was renewed hair growth within the bald patches. (If hair loss is caused by scalp psoriasis, hair is restored to its normal state as soon as psoriasis activity decreases.)

Third Follow-up Treatment
Three months after initial treatment, there was significant improvement in the patient's general condition and continued hair growth. The dosage formula was strengthened as follows:

tu fu ling (Rhizoma Smilacis Glabrae)	15 g
huang qin (Radix Scutellariae Baicalensis)	9 g
jin yin hua (Flos Lonicerae Japonicae)	15 g
huang bai (Cortex Phellodendri)	9 g
ku shen (Radix Sophorae Flavescentis)	12 g
ye jiao teng (Caulis Polygoni Multiflori)	12 g

bai hua she she cao (Herba Oldenlandiae Diffusae)	15 g
lian qiao (Fructus Forsythiae)	9 g
ju hua (Flos Chrysanthemi Morifolii)	4 g
chi shao (Radix Paeoniae Rubra)	12 g

Explanation
As it was apparent that the patient was able to handle strong plants for long periods—in some children the spleen is strong enough and not easily damaged—the dosage of some plants was increased to effect more robust treatment of heat, damp, and toxicity.

Continued Treatment
Treatment has been ongoing for one year, and the patient's condition has greatly improved over the past six months. At the moment the psoriasis has been almost totally alleviated. The girl's hair has grown back fully and the only problem was that she had been taking herbs to eliminate heat and toxicity for too long. Herbs were therefore added to protect the spleen and reinforce the *qi*. These included *gan cao*, *shan yao*, and *huang qi*. The addition of these plants immediately and significantly increased the effectiveness of the treatment, resulting in further improvement in her health. Frequency of treatment was gradually reduced to once in four days, then once in five days, and finally once in ten days. The dose of Omega 3 was reduced from 2000 to 1000 mg daily.

The patient is currently receiving minimal external treatment, which includes the use of Pso Medis shampoo and Pso Medis scalp lotion once a week, and the application of Pso Medis night gel two to three times a week. During treatment, the patient was recommended exposure to the sun and sea (Dead Sea), and this definitely contributed to her general progress.

Prognosis
The case described above represented a severe case of psoriasis, which does not usually respond successfully to conventional treatments and may be subject to very aggressive conventional therapy treatments, such as cortisone creams and other immune system inhibitors.

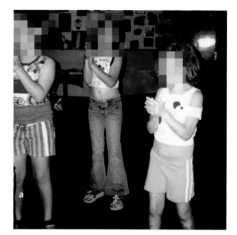

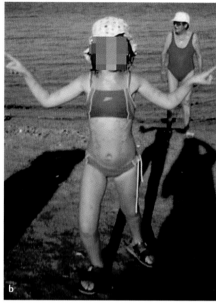

Fig. **3a–e**

a–c *Girl, six and a half years old, with severe psoriasis. Beginning of treatment.*

d, e *After 8 months of treatment the psoriasis is almost completely alleviated (95 % improvement).*

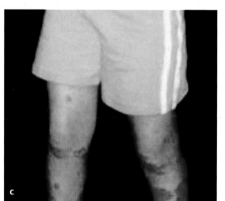

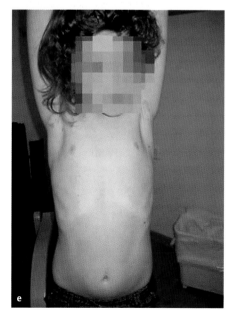

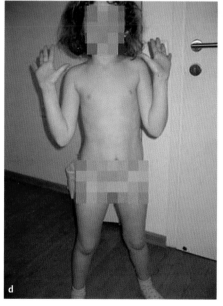

*Fig. **4a–e***

a, b *Severe case of a 35-year-old psoriasis patient. The psoriasis mostly appears on the scalp and there is much scaling and pus. In addition, there are large areas of temporary baldness resulting from long-term inflammation of the scalp.*

c, d *After 2 months of treatment there is much improvement and the inflammation of the scalp has decreased. New hair is already beginning to appear and the bald areas are reduced.*

e *After 4 months of treatment the psoriasis is completely healed.*

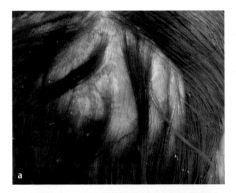

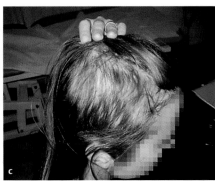

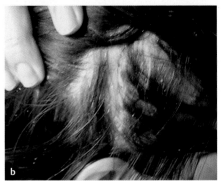

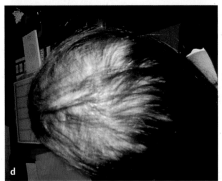

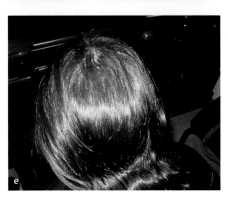

There is a very good chance that the Chinese medicine treatment will prevent further suffering in the future, although psoriasis is a disease that is liable to recur at any stage. Chinese medicine is capable of "controlling" the disease, and contributes to maintaining the disease at a low level of activity, and in some cases to its disappearance for extended periods.

Bibliography

Li Lin. *Practical Traditional Chinese Dermatology.* Hong Kong: Hai Feng Publishing Company; 1995.

Xu Xiangcai (ed.). *The English–Chinese Encyclopedia of Practical TCM. Vol. 16: Dermatology.* Beijing: Higher Education Press; 1991.

Xu Yihou. *Dermatology in Traditional Chinese Medicine.* New York: Donica Publishing; 2004.

Contact Details

Amir Kalay, MSc, LAc
Co-Founder and R & D Manager
Kamedis Laboratories LTD
Tel Aviv, Israel
www.kamedis.com

Cordyceps sinensis: Mushroom of Stamina and Longevity

Beverly Bakken, Dipl Ac (NCCAOM), DOM (NM), Santa Cruz, California, USA
Katie Briggs, LAc, Dipl OM (NCCAOM), Ithaka, New York, USA

Introduction

Cordyceps sinensis (dong chong xia cao) has been in use in China for over a thousand years. It is recognized as one of China's medicinal treasures, a tonic used to reinforce the body's source of vital energy, to increase levels of stamina and enhance the immune system's ability to boost both physical performance and endurance in athletes. In China it is also commonly used for hyperglycemia, hyper-lipidemia, hyposexuality, liver diseases, and heart disorders.

Reference to the mushroom dates back to 620 CE, during the Tang dynasty, and its first written record appears in 200 CE in Sheng Nung's *Classic Herbal of the Divine Plowman*. It was described as transforming from animal to plant and back to animal again, and was named *dong chong xia cao*, or "winter worm, summer grass." Its unique growth process explains this ancient description. The *Cordyceps* mycelium germinates inside a moth larva, the fruiting body spouting up from the head of the caterpillar husk, twig- or blade-shaped, with a dark-brown base and black tip. Though there is debate as to whether the fungus grows outside the caterpillar or in its interior, mycologist Malcolm Clark believes *Cordyceps* spores are actually ingested, then germinate and fully occupy the remains of the caterpillar's body in the formation of this unusual medicine. *Cordyceps* is native to regions of very high altitudes in southern China, Tibet, and Nepal.

Tibetan and Nepalese herdsmen led their yaks to high elevations during the spring snow melt, where the yaks were drawn to the *Cordyceps* mushroom amid snowy grass marshlands. Folklore tells of the herdsmans' awe at the renewed vigor and stamina of their animals after imbibing the mushroom, and of how they began trying it themselves. Legend of their markedly increased stamina and sexual potency and reduced susceptibility to respiratory and other illnesses eventually spread beyond the Tibetan plateau. By the Ming dynasty, the Emperor's court held *Cordyceps* in such high esteem that for a time law dictated that it be the sole beneficiary of its remarkable powers. Due to its rarity and expense, it was long a medicinal for the upper classes. In *MycoMedicinals*, Paul Stamets underscores the metamorphic symbolism of the fungi sprouting from the cadavers of insects, leading the ancient Chinese to believe it granted immortality. He writes that stone effigies of *Cordyceps* "were traditionally used in funeral ceremonies, placed with the deceased to prevent rebirth, or life after death." [22]

Owing to the scarcity of *Cordyceps* in the wild and increasing medical demand, methods of cultivating the mycelia on grains, primarily rice and soybeans, were developed in the 1980s. Tests have shown the potency of the mycelia grown under laboratory conditions to be equal to, or greater than, the wild, caterpillar-body form. Further, purity is assured. Extraction with both water and alcohol access optimal levels of medicinally important compounds, such as polysaccharides.

Pharmacology

The biological actions of *Cordyceps sinensis* are due to a number of constituents in its make-up. Corycepin (cordycepin-3-deoxyadenosine) is its major bioactive substance, found in very high concentrations; 32 % of the fungus by weight. Other important substances include glutamic acid; amino acids (phenylalanine, proline, histidine, valine, oxyvaline, arginine); unsaturated fatty acids (oleic and linoleic acids); carbohydrates (d-mannitol); vitamin B12; glactomannan polysaccharides; Beta

Cordyceps sinensis

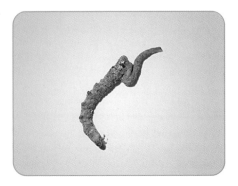

Glucans; and some pyranosides. Polysaccharides such as Beta Glucan have a very powerful biological response modifier that is able to alter the degree to which the immune system responds to a stimulus.

Traditional Chinese Medical Uses

In Traditional Chinese Medicine (TCM), *Cordyceps* is used to tonify the kidney and lung channels, the kidney being the "root of life," and the lung the "*qi* of the entire body." As *Cordyceps* tonifies both *yin* and *yang*, without adverse effects such as increased dampness or heat, it is a very safe, balanced herb, ideal for convalescing, elderly, or extremely weak, patients. Indications include fatigue, spontaneous or night sweating, and neurasthenia. It assists lung and kidney (*xu*) respiratory disorders, such as asthma, shortness of breath, and consumptive cough with blood-streaked sputum. Tonifying kidney *yang* and *jing* (essence), it aids generalized soreness, lower back and knee pain, frequent urination, tinnitus, poor memory, and sexual difficulties such as impotence and premature ejaculation.

The herb can be ingested daily for a long period of time, to remedy chronic weakness, or as a tonic for promoting health. A study showed 92 % of elderly patients in a controlled study reported reduction of fatigue after taking it for 30 days [1]. As in all herbal therapy, dosage is key. In one study, a daily dose of 3 g was shown to create a marked effect in elderly patients [2]. Traditionally, *Cordyceps* was cooked in a duck meat stew as a potent tonic

for the elderly, and depleted patients with weak "protective," or *wei qi*. Cooked this way, 85 g of *Cordyceps* was equated with a 50-g dose of ginseng. Today, the fungus is also cooked with chicken, pork, or fish.

Regulating Immune Function

The ability of *Cordyceps* to immunomodulate is well noted. Cell-mediated immune response and cancer therapy studies have substantiated earlier claims to *Cordyceps* being a powerful immune regulator. *Cordyceps* enhances immunity by increasing the activity of T-cells; this allows a partially suppressed immune system the ability to ward off illness. A study at the Kaohsiung Medical College, Taiwan, found that *Cordyceps* is helpful in treating the autoimmune disease systemic lupus erythermatosus (SLE) in mice [3]. *Cordyceps* anti-viral and antibacterial activity is initiated by two derivatives, cordycepin and cordycepic acid, which work to resist *Staphylococcus*, *Streptococcus*, and other bacterial strains. *Cordyceps* also resists epidermal and ascites warts.

Immune function is often compromised as important biological levels of free radical scavenging enzymes are reduced. The oxidative stress caused by free radicals is viewed as essential to the "aging process," leaving the defense mechanism more prone to illness and degenerative diseases. *Cordyceps* maintains health and delays conditions caused by aging by eliminating free radicals, thereby reducing damage to vital biochemical processes in the human body. It also shows potential in tempering ravages caused by cortisone intake. A Chinese study involving *Cordyceps* and cortisone found that although damage induced by cortisone, such as leukocyte decrease, was countered by *Cordyceps*, the anti-inflammatory function of cortisone was not [4].

Sexual Tonic

Renowned in China for nearly two thousand years as an aphrodisiac, to replenish sperm and relieve impotence, modern clinical studies on *Cordyceps* also show hope for sexual dysfunction and infertility. In Chinese studies on reduced libido involving both men and women, 66 % showed improvement of symptoms and desire [5]. A male fertility study showed that *Cordyceps* increased sperm count, decreased sperm malformations, and increased survival rate after eight weeks of supplementation [6].

Anti-Tumor and Anti-Cancer Activity

Cordyceps' anti-tumor activity and immune stimulant properties have been substantiated by numerous studies in China and Japan [7, 8, 10]. Hot water extract of its mycelium stimulated macrophage activity in mice by 1.7 fold, and after only seven days their bone marrow cells had significantly proliferated, 1.9 fold [9]. A study at Kanazawa Medical University, Japan, found that administration of *Cordyceps sinensis* to tumor-bearing mice, with decreased phagocytic activity, restored macrophage activity to above the normal level, allowing the mice to live significantly longer than the control group [10]. Researchers are intrigued by *Cordyceps*' ability to enhance human natural killer (NK) cell activity, while modulating the overproduction of leukocytes. Studies also suggest hope for leukemia patients, including a study that showed cordycepin to be specifically cytotoxic against leukemia cells [11].

Enhancing Stamina and Endurance

In 1993, *Cordyceps* made international sports headlines when Chinese women runners shattered numerous world records after training with the use of this herb. Suspicions of steroid use were dispelled by tests. One stunning victory, the 10 000-meter race, surpassed the world record by 42 seconds. A 1996 study on long-distance runners using *Cordyceps* mycelium products showed significant improvement in 71 % of the subjects, with evidence of increased respiratory activity and metabolism of lactic acid [12]. Now that it has reached the

mainstream, many marathon runners have incorporated it into their training regimen.

Cordyceps is thought to increase energy by raising plasma cortisol levels, thereby increasing the function of the plasma cortex, and secretion levels of the adrenal gland. This enhanced adrenal functioning strengthens vital energy. The herb also helps to break down waste materials in muscles, such as lactic acid, which creates less fatigue, shorter recovery time, and increased motion potential during times of stress and exertion. A Japanese research group found aqueous extracts of this mushroom significantly dilated the aorta under stress [13], which would benefit muscles in endurance-based athletics.

For athletes who undergo prolonged intensive exertion, overtraining syndrome (OS) is a hazard. In both OS and chronic fatigue (CF) the suppression of the immune system is a contributing factor. This immune deficiency mainly results from a counter regulatory shift in the neuroendocrine system during prolonged or repeated stress. *Cordyceps* works to balance the body's endocrine system, providing hope for OS and CF.

Cardiovascular Tonic

The effect of *Cordyceps* on the heart and cerebral vessels is well noted: it decreases plasma triglycerides, lowers cholesterol and B-lipoprotein levels, prevents thrombosis, resists arrhythmia, and lowers hypertension [14, 15]. *Cordyceps* apparently helps to prevent atherosclerosis by reducing the blood's viscosity, thus lessening the potential for platelets to catch in arterial lesions and abrasions, known as fibrous plaques [16]. *Cordyceps* is known for increasing beneficial cholesterol (HDL), and reducing detrimental cholesterol (LDL) (14). A Japanese study showed that *Cordyceps* inhibited LDL oxidation and, thereby, cholesterol deposition in the aorta [16]. A 1990 study at Beijing Medical University found that a two-month protocol of mycelial extract significantly increased average HDL levels [17]. Research also indicates that *Cordyceps* enhances oxygen uptake by the brain and heart, thereby improving resistance to hypoxia, a condition in which the supply of oxygen to these vital tissues is diminished, even in the presence of adequate blood flow [17].

Improving Respiratory Function

Cordyceps has traditionally been known as a treatment for asthma, and for facilitating the discharge of phlegm from the lungs and trachea; effects have been confirmed by modern science. Compounds in *Cordyceps* relax bronchial passages and loosen bronchoalveolar fluids, allowing for a productive cough and aiding respiration [18]. The preventative effect of *Cordyceps* in asthma is in part due to its action as a smooth muscle relaxant. *Cordyceps* can assist in reducing airway reactivity and inflammatory responses, therefore reducing the incidence of asthmatic attacks. In the elderly, a study found that *Cordyceps* significantly improved the maximum amount of oxygen they were able to assimilate [19].

When to Select *Cordyceps* Over Other Medicinal Mushrooms and How They Can be Combined

Almost all medicinal mushrooms enhance immunity, bolster the body's natural defense system, and, in addition, have outright antibacterial and anti-viral properties. Studies have also shown varying levels of tumor inhibition, especially when a variety of mushrooms are used together.

Cordyceps shares these intrinsic qualities, but is recognized for its ability to increase physical stamina, energy levels, and endurance. *Cordyceps* is also valuable for the elderly and for those who are recuperating from long-term illness, and can be safely taken for extended periods. Its ability to strengthen and restore the body likens it to classic herbal tonics, such as ginseng. It strongly assists the respiratory system by its toning, as well as by its bronchial dilating effect, making it ideal for asthma and conditions with respiratory compromise, such as chronic obstructive pulmo-

nary disease (COPD). Medicinal mushrooms with an anti-inflammatory effect, such as Reishi or Chaga, would compliment the respiratory enhancement of *Cordyceps*, to benefit this type of condition.

Both Reishi and *Cordyceps* modulate blood pressure, reduce cholesterol, balance blood sugar, and assist with cardiovascular health. In TCM differentiation, Reishi is sweet, neutral, and enters the heart, liver, and kidney channels, whereas *Cordyceps* is sweet, warm, and enters the lung and kidney channels. While both herbs address issues of the lung, Reishi stops cough—specifically cough due to cold—and arrests wheezing. *Cordyceps* addresses disorders of the lung and kidney with chronic cough, caused by *yin* or *qi* deficiency. Reishi is noted for its ability to nourish the heart and calm the *shen*, and is excellent for emotional well being; *Cordyceps* tonifies kidney *yang* and augments essence, and is historically noted as a sexual tonic.

It is of note that modern research has borne out the effectiveness of *Cordyceps* for a range of conditions attributed, in Chinese medicine, to the concept of kidney deficiency, including not only some directly related to the kidney, such as chronic kidney failure [20], but also some unassociated in Western medicine, such as impotence and tinnitus [21].

Mycologist, Christopher Hobbs, discussing dosage in *Medicinal Mushrooms*, suggests that *Cordyceps* should be taken as one would any herb—for three to nine months—to fully benefit from its strengthening effects. He makes reference to research that recommends that 3–9 g powdered herb, or 1 g extract, be taken twice daily for weakness and debility. For anemia and impotence he underscores the tradition of stewing it with chicken pork [23].

Cordyceps sinensis has been the subject of considerable research, but merits the focus of continued clinical studies in order to highlight which of its traditional uses holds the most promise for challenging modern conditions and to measure the benefit of its use as a tonic herb for enhancement of health and prevention of disease.

References

1. Cao A, Wen, Y. *Applied Traditional Chinese Medicine.* 1993;1:32–33.
2. Zhu JS, Halpern, GM, Jones, K. The scientific rediscovery of an ancient Chinese herbal medicine: Cordyceps sinensis. Part I. *Journal of Alternative and Complementary Medicine.* 1998; 289–303.
3. Chen JR, Yen JH, Lin CC, et al. The effects of Chinese herbs on improving survival and inhibiting anti-ds DNA antibody production in lupus mice. *Am J Chin Med.* 1993;21(3–4):257–262.
4. Zang, QZ, He, GX, Zheng, ZY, et al. Pharmacological action of the polysaccharide from Cordyceps. *Chinese Traditional Herbal Drugs.* 1985; 16:306–311.
5. Wan, F, Guo, Y, Deng, X. *Chinese Traditional Patented Medicine.* 1988;9:29–31.
6. Guo, YZ. Medicinal chemistry, pharmacology and clinical applications of fermented mycelia of Cordyceps sinensis and JinShuBao capsule. *Journal of Modern Diagnostics and Therapeutics.* 1986;1:60–65.
7. Kuo YC, Lin CY, Tsai WJ, et al. Growth inhibitors against tumor cells in Cordyceps sinensis other than cordycepin and polysaccharides. *Cancer Invest.* 1994;12(6):611–615.
8. Xu RH, Peng XE, Chen GZ, Chen GL. Effects of Cordyceps sinensis on natural killer activity and colony formation of B16 melanoma. *Chinese Medical Journal.* 1992;105(2):97–101.
9. Koh JH, Yu KW, Suh HJ, Choi YM, Ahn TS. Activation of macrophages and the intestinal immune system by an orally administered decoction from cultured mycelia of Cordyceps sinensis. *Biosci Biotechnol Biochem.* 2002; 66(2):407–411.
10. Yamaguchi N, Yoshida J, Ren LJ, et al. Augmentation of various immune reactivities of tumor-bearing hosts with an extract of Cordyceps sinensis. Kanazawa Medical University. *Biotherapy.* 1990;2(3):199–205.
11. Liu C, Lu S, Ji MR, Xie Y. Effects of Cordyceps sinensis (CS) on in vitro natural killer cells. *Zhong-guo Zhong Xi Yi Jie He Za Zhi.* 1992;12(5): 267–269.
12. Hiyoshi T, et al. Cordyceps effects on cardiopulmonary function of long distance runners. *Japanese Journal of Physical Fitness and Sports Medicine.* 1996;45:474.
13. Naoki T, et al. Pharmacological studies on Cordyceps sinensis from China. From the *Fifth Mycological Congress Abstracts.* Vancouver, BC, August 14–21, 1994.
14. Koh JH, Kim JH, Chang UJ, et al.. Hypocholesterolemic effect of hot-water extract from mycelia of Cordyceps sinensis. *Biol Pharm Bull.* 2003; 26(1):84–87.
15. Yamaguchi Y, Kagota S, Nakamura K, Shinozuka K, Kunitomo M. Inhibitory effects of water extracts from fruiting bodies cultured *Cordyceps Sinensis* on raised serum lipid peroxide levels and aortic cholesterol deposition in atherosclerotic mice. *Phytotherapy Research.* 2000; 14(8): 650–652.
16. Zhao Y. Inhibitory effects of alcoholic extract of *Cordyceps sinensis* on abdominal aortic thrombus formation in rabbits. *Chung-Hua Hseuh Tsa Chih* (Chinese Medical Journal). 1991;71:612–615.
17. Lei J, Chen J, Guo C. Pharmacological study on Cordyceps sinensis (Berk.) Sacc. and ze-e Cordyceps, *Zhongguo Zhong Yao Za Zhi.* 1992; 17(6):364–366.
18. Kuo YC, Tsai WJ, Wang JY, Chang SC, Lin CY, Shiao MS. Regulation of bronchoalveolar lavage fluids cell function by the immunomodulatory agents from Cordyceps sinensis. *Life Sci.* 2001; 68(9):1067–1082.
19. Xiao Y, Huang XZ, Chen G, et al. Increased aerobic capacity in healthy elderly humans given fermented Cordyceps Cs-4: a placebo controlled trial. Annual meeting American College of Sports Medicine, June 1999.
20. Chen YP, Liu WZ, Shen LM, Xu SN. Clinical effects of natural Cordyceps and cultured mycelia of Cordyceps sinensis in kidney failure. *Chin Trad Herbal Drugs.* 1986;17:256–258.
21. Zhuang JM, Chen HL. Treatment of tinnitus with Cordyceps infusion: A report of 23 cases. *Fujian Med J.* 1985;7:42.
22. Stamets P. *MycoMedicinals: An Informational Treatise on Mushrooms.* Olympia, WA: Myco-Media Productions; 2002.
23. Hobbs C. *Medicinal Mushrooms: An Exploration of Tradition, Healing, & Culture.* Santa Cruz, CA: Botanica Press; 1986.

Further Reading

Bensky D, Gamble A. *Chinese Herbal Medicine: Materia Medica.* Seattle, WA: Eastland Press, Inc.; 1993.

Chen JK, Chen TT. *Chinese Medical Herbology and*

Pharmacology. City of Industry, CA: Art of Medicine Press, Inc.; 2004.

Gilbert UK. *Immune and Stamina Booster Cordyceps Sinensis*. Pleasant Grove, UT: Woodland Publishing; 2000.

Halpern GM, Miller AH. *Medicinal Mushrooms: Ancient Remedies for Modern Ailments*. New York, NY: M. Evans and Company, Inc.; 2002.

(Original publication of this article: Kan Herb Company's Newsletter *Herbal Crossroads*, September 2005.)

Contact Details

Beverly Bakken, Dipl Ac (NCCAOM), DOM (NM)
Kan Herb Company
beverly.bakken@yahoo.com

Katie Briggs, Dipl OM (NCCAOM), LAc (CA)
Kan Herb Company, Resonation Acupuncture
katie@resonationacupuncture.com

Professional Developments, Legislation, and Regulation

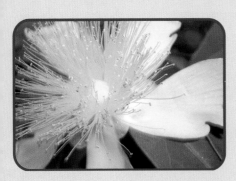

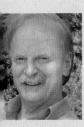

Michael McCarthy

Introduction

One of the purposes of this Almanac is, among other things, to help create a global community of practitioners of the ancient healing arts found in traditional East Asian medicine. This disparate community comprises practitioners within the Asian communities of the medicine's origin and its different branches, as well as practitioners of the Western adaptations that have emerged, especially over the last 40 years in the non-Asian community in the West.

Within its original cultural context, the practice of traditional East Asian medicine has various forms but is generally carried out in combination with allopathic medicine. In the West this is generally not the case, as its acceptance as a serious, efficacious treatment model is taking time. As a result, its emergence has been more as an alternative to allopathic medicine and thus its development has emerged as a totally separate and largely unofficial model of treatment. Separately, allopathic medicine has chosen to develop a hybrid form of East Asian medicine that answers to conventional allopathic investigation and diagnosis whilst retaining the theoretical mapping framework of the traditional Eastern energetic model of the body (Chinese, Japanese, and others).

The traditional medicines of the East Asian countries have a multi-varied genesis and development, no one model of which does total justice to the immense variety of its traditions. In the West the tradition that dominates the field in this particular grouping is the branch that has become known as Chinese medicine, itself a multi-varied traditional development. Standing alongside this are Japanese, Vietnamese, Korean, and other practices, which claim the same root and, notwithstanding their unique cultural and historical contexts, are today mainly separated by artificial geographical boundaries and contemporary legislative practices within the jurisdictions of those boundaries.

The development of the practice of traditional East Asian medicine in the West in the modern era goes back to the 16th century, and other information, though apocryphal, suggests that it even crossed the continents long before. In the 17th century, Portuguese Jesuits returning from China reputedly brought back to Europe some of the then extant teaching manuals on Chinese physical manipulation therapy (tui na). It is suggested that from this, Per Ling developed his Swedish Remedial Gymnastics and Swedish Movement Cure in the 18th century (Swedish Massage). The French Jesuit, Jean-Joseph Marie Amiot (1718–93), published an illustrated work on Taoist physiotherapy (chung fu). This appears to have had some influence on the contemporary development of physical therapy in Europe at that time. Similarities between these exercises and those of Per Ling are also reported (Chinese Medicine, Huard and Wong). In the 1800s, Berlioz's father, a physician, published an account of the positive effects of acupuncture treatment.

In terms of its contemporary development in the Western countries we can look to the French translations of some of the classics. In the 1950s, Soulié de Mourant translated some of the Chinese texts into French. Its worldwide Western expansion is attributed to the visit of the USA's President Nixon to China in 1972 when demonstrations of acupuncture analgesia for surgery during that visit received international attention. Academically, scholars such as Joseph Needham, Lu Gwei-Djen, and Paul Unschuld have contributed hugely to its acceptance and establishment in the West. We also owe much to scholars such as Dan Bensky, Charles Chace and Zhang Ting Liang, Nigel Wiseman and Feng Ye, for their constant interpretation of the classics and the historical, cultural, etymological and semantic context out of which the medicine has emerged. During a time when China was beginning to emerge from its isolation from the rest of the world, their respective in-depth analyses of this and other ancient cultures provided ground for the serious acceptance of traditional Eastern medicine and in particular, Traditional Chinese Medicine.

One way or another the West has seen a dramatic expansion of traditional East Asian medicine over this period to the point where it has become a major player in the global health care delivery system. Put quite simply, its success stands testament to its fundamental capacity as a model of medicine that enables people to recover from illness. This is dramatically exemplified in the outreach volunteer services provided in Asia post-tsunami, in Pakistan post-earthquake with Operation Heartbeat, and in New Orleans post-Hurricane Katrina, where several hundred practitioners of acupuncture under the auspices of organizations such as Acupuncture Sans Frontières and Acupuncturists Without Borders provided and developed services to help alleviate these emergency situations.

The principal purpose of this section of the Almanac is to attempt to map the current worldwide practice of this traditional medicine. Of necessity it must be a work in progress as not all of the information can be gathered in this round and the information is constantly changing. Also, as we will be depending on various sources both official and non-official, it is essential as a professional community that we endeavor to correct any inaccuracies as we go. To facilitate this we have included a form on our website to enable the uniform and accurate collection of this information through the readership. All responses from you the reader will be followed through annually to enable the further refinement of the information as we go. To the extent that resources allow, all information will be cross-referenced and checked against other sources.

This section of the Almanac will give a concise summary of the practice in each country, referring to professional regulation, numbers in practice, and legislative issues. It will include, where possible, tables analyzing how practice is distributed throughout the world and in the various jurisdictions. It will also attempt to give a picture of how some of the various traditions emerged and of the principal developments that have given rise to the contemporary state of East Asian medicine worldwide. This will be done by looking briefly at particular legislative and professional developments in some of the jurisdictions. The fact that some countries have been omitted will mainly be due to the fact that information is either not available or accessible at this time. As a work in progress the hope is that this information will accumulate over a few years, continually yielding a clearer picture of the practice and distribution of traditional East Asian medicine around the globe.

This section will also put useful and informative data in the hands of the practitioner of East Asian medicine so that each can see the nature and extent of the worldwide community to which they belong. We are a global community at the cutting edge of the development of a medical practice that is pushing us beyond the purely scientific into the practice of an art that has attended humanity for aeons.

Michael McCarthy, MA (ThB), LAc, DipCHM
Director of the Institute of East West Medical Sciences, Dublin, Ireland

Bibliography

1. Bensky D and Gamble A. *Chinese Herbal Medicine: Materia Medica.* Revised Edition. Seattle: Eastland Press; 1993.
2. Chace C and Zhang Ting Liang, eds. *A Qin Bowei Anthology, Clinical Essays by Qin Bowei.* Brookline MA: Paradigm Publications; 1997.

3. Chengnan S. *Chinese Bodywork: A Complete Manual of Chinese Therapeutic Massage*. Berkeley: Pacific View Press; 1993.

4. Gwei-Djen L and Needham J. *Celestial Lancets, A History and Rationale of Acupuncture and Moxa*. London: Routledge; 2002.

5. Huard P and Wong M. *Chinese Medicine*. London: World University Library; 1968.

6. Kaptchuk TJ. *Chinese Medicine, the Web that has no Weaver*. London: Rider; 1988.

7. Langevin HM and Yandow JA. Relationship of acupuncture points and meridians to connective tissue planes. *Anat Rec*. 2002;269(6):257–265.

8. Palos S. *The Chinese Art of Healing*. New York: Bantam; 1972.

9. Unschuld P. *Medicine in China, A History of Ideas*. Berkeley: University of California Press; 1985.

10. Wiseman N and Ellis A. *Fundamentals of Chinese Medicine*. Brookline MA: Paradigm Publications; 1995.

11. Wiseman N and Feng Y. *Introduction to English Terminology of Chinese Medicine*. Brookline MA: Paradigm Publications; 2002.

Acurevue

Michael McCarthy, MA(ThB) LAc, DipCHM, Dublin, Ireland

A recent study of the efficacy of acupuncture in the treatment of arthritic pain showed that not only was it more effective than placebo but it was more effective than proprietary pain medications to a statistically significant degree.

In Europe the EATCM had to change its name to ETCMA so that it would not be conflicting with that of a German physicians' acupuncture association.

A study in Vermont University being carried out by a team under Dr. Helen Langevin has designed a protocol for evaluating Traditional Chinese Medicine (TCM). Assistant Professor of Neurology and a licensed acupuncturist, Langevin insists that the key to acupuncture's biomechanical effect is not the insertion of each ultra-fine acupuncture needle, but its manipulation.

In California there seems to be a move to prosecute as fraudulent any health practice not within the conventional system.

In Ireland the three largest acupuncture associations have formed a single association now called the Traditional Chinese Medicine Council of Ireland (TCMCI). Also in Ireland the National Herbal Council (NHC) has been set up comprising the five principal herbal medicine practitioner associations, two of which are Chinese herbal medicine associations. The Council also controls the National Register of Herbalists, which is accessible on the Web at nationalregisterofherbalists.com.

In Holland it is now illegal for anyone other than conventionally trained physicians to diagnose or prescribe medications of any description, whether synthetic or natural.

In post-Hurricane Katrina, New Orleans, after intense lobbying by the Acupuncture Without Borders (AWB) group and others, the Governor of Louisiana instituted an Executive Order that suspended state licensing requirements that allowed licensed out-of-state

medical and health practitioners to practice in Louisiana within the scope of their out-of-state license until 28th February, 2006. There is ongoing trouble with the bureaucracy with no clear answers to questions about the legal status of these volunteers from the Louisiana Recovery Authority, the Louisiana Board of Medical Examiners, and the Department of Health and Hospitals.

In Louisiana, unlike in most states in the USA where acupuncture is its own profession, acupuncturists are considered assistants, unless they are medical doctors. AWB volunteers are all fully licensed in their home states.

University of Pittsburgh School of Nursing researchers are investigating the effectiveness of acupuncture in reducing the severity of menopausal symptoms in women who have breast cancer.

The National Center for Complementary and Alternative Medicine (NCCAM) has launched a clinical trial of electro-acupuncture to determine if it reduces the delayed nausea experienced by cancer patients following chemotherapy. This study marks the first clinical trial for NCCAM's Division of Intramural Research, which was established in April 2001, at the National Institutes of Health (NIH) in Bethesda, Maryland.

We know that in the 1970s, Chinese scientists isolated a compound called Artemisinin from *qing hao*, or *Artemisia annua*, a relative of the sweet wormwood found in North America. *Qing hao* is traditionally used to treat fever but the researchers found that Artemisinin killed even chloroquine-resistant strains of *Plasmodium falciparum*, the malaria parasite transmitted by mosquitoes. Recent research in USA and Europe suggests that Artemisinin may also have anti-cancer properties. Zhou Weishan, chemist at the Shanghai Institute of Organic Chemistry, who led the efforts to synthesize Artemisinin, says they never patented any part of the work.

Under the new Traditional Herbal Medicinal Products Directive (THMPD) regulations in the EU a German company seems to be first out of the blocks with the registration of a complex remedy of 13 herbs called Klosterfrau Melissengeist/Melisana. It has a wide range of applications and is a very old formulation, having been in existence for over 300 years.

Is the randomized, double-blind, placebo-controlled trial a contradiction to the philosophy of Traditional Chinese Medicine, which concentrates on treatments tailored to the individual rather than to the fictional average of a population? Yet more objections could be levelled at the statistical methods of analyzing the data, which are based on an outmoded mechanistic biology totally inadequate to capture the predominantly non-linear behavior of the human. The randomized, double-blind, placebo-controlled trial also excludes the interpersonal relationships between practitioner and patient that are crucial in all holistic health systems.

Irrespective of the many conceptual contradictions with the dominant Western model, TCM has more than 300 000 practitioners in over 140 countries. The first hospital for Chinese medicine in Europe was opened in Germany in 1990. British doctors are increasingly contracting out for acupuncture. Public health-insurance companies in Germany, the UK, and Ireland routinely refund part of the costs of acupuncture treatment provided by trained doctors and acupuncturists, and in France acupuncture is a widely accepted part of the health care provision.

This year the AGTCM, Germany's largest Traditional Chinese Medicine professional practitioner group, held its annual conference which exceeded all records for attendance. We have reports that 930 attended this year. This event, which takes place each year in Rothenburg in Germany, has been going for 37 years and has managed to provide a very high standard of organization, program quality, and consistency over the years. (See "The History of the Rothenburg Conference for Traditional Chinese Medicine,

Germany," p. 10, History, Language, and Culture).

Hong Kong's Chief Executive Tung Chee Hwa has laid out a ten-year plan for making the city an "international center for Chinese medicine." His government is currently funding 18 TCM research projects including clinical trials, developing quality standards, and basic pharmacological studies. The Hong Kong Jockey Club Charities Trust is equipping research labs and donating US$64 million to get research started at a new Institute of Chinese Medicine.

Last year, Taiwan's President Chen Shuibian proposed spending US$1.5 billion over five years to develop the country's Chinese medicinal herb industry, pending a detailed plan.

Speaking about the effect of the globalization of TCM, Dr. Volker Scheid, Academic Director of the European Institute of Oriental Medicine (EIOM) and a practitioner of Chinese medicine, suggests three possible outcomes, both in terms of its widespread adoption in countries across the world and in its entry into the global drugs market (see "Contemporary Education in Chinese Medicine within a Strategy of Standardization: A Response," p. 203, Education). Chinese medicine may be destroyed as an independent medical tradition by the Western biomedical establishment, by assimilating some of the tools, such as acupuncture, massage, and pharmaceuticals, but discarding the core concepts and practices, such as the notions of *yin* and *yang*, and *qi*. Alternatively, it may be institutionalized along the Chinese model, or it may "develop into a heterogeneous vibrant tradition that eschews political and economic power for the sake of clinical efficacy, grounded in personal experience and in modern research."

Dr Joseph Pizzorno, who helped found Bastyr University, Seattle, in 1978 and served as its president for more than two decades, was honored with the "Physician of the Year" award from the American Association of Naturopathic Physicians (AANP). Under Dr Pizzorno's leadership, Bastyr was selected as the first Center for Alternative Medicine Research by the National Institute of Health's Office of Alternative Medicine.

The Macao Special Administrative Region of China has announced the opening of its first Traditional Chinese Medicine hospital. The hospital will be based at the Macao University of Science and Technology in Taipa, and will be run in conjunction with the Nanjing University of Traditional Chinese Medicine.

The American College of Traditional Chinese Medicine has announced that its doctoral program has received approval from the Accreditation Commission for Acupuncture and Oriental Medicine and the California Bureau for Private Postsecondary and Vocational Education, making it the first acupuncture school in Northern California to have its doctoral program receive approval from both agencies. The program will be offered at the college's San Francisco campus and is set to begin in October 2006. In Kentucky, Governor Ernie Fletcher signed the state's first law regulating acupuncture on 26th April, 2006. Kentucky becomes the 44th state to implement laws regulating the practice of acupuncture. The new regulation came into effect on 15th July, 2006 and requires acupuncturists to meet national standards for education and certification.

And finally, as we all know, the first written rules of golf were set down in 1754 CE at St. Andrews Golf Club in Scotland, having been around in one form or another since the 15th century. However, an exhibition of paintings in Beijing from the Ming dynasty (1368–1644 CE) shows Chinese noblemen on the green hundreds of years before. Chinese historians argue that they have been teeing off since 945 CE and that Mongolian travelers brought the game of *Chui Wan* (Hit Ball) to Europe. The rules of the sport were laid down in a book in 1282 CE called *Wan Jing* (Manual of Ball Games). In fact an ancient scroll called *The Autumn Banquet* (1368 CE) shows officials playing *Chui Wan*.

Now we know that the Chinese have given the world the gift of acupuncture. They have also given us gunpowder, pasta, the fork, the compass, the umbrella, the printing press … but golf? Is this possible?

Acupuncturists Without Borders:
Trip to New Orleans, 20th–29th November, 2005

Sachiko Nakano, LAc, MAc, Seattle, Washington, USA

On the 29th August, 2005, Hurricane Katrina changed many people's lives along the Gulf Coast in the USA.

I went to New Orleans with Acupuncturists Without Borders (AWB) in November. This organization was established shortly after the Hurricane Katrina devastation. It has done many things in a short time through direct action and training of locals to provide acupuncture services to help with post-hurricane traumatic stress. I highly recommend their web page (www.acuwithoutborders.org) to find out more about them.

First of all, seeing the large scale of devastation was simply mind-boggling. I hadn't expected it to have such a strong impact on me until I saw the destruction and felt the damage with my own hands. Have you ever lost your favorite or valuable items, or lost a loved one? These people had lost all of their material possessions. They lost their loved ones; they lost their jobs; they lost their beloved pets; they lost their community. They had nothing to eat or drink for several days, and they were abandoned by their government. Many rescue volunteers from all over the country had been turned away by the government officials, and because of what?

The streets of New Orleans were astonishing. They were full of trash, including household electrical items and furniture. There was broken glass everywhere, on every street. Mud and dust-covered cars; I was told that 300 000 cars were abandoned. Many traffic lights were not working. Huge trees were ripped from the ground and boats sat in the middle of the street. Spray paint on the houses said: "u loot, u dead," "1 dog trapped under," "will be back soon," "R.I.P.," and much more.

The 9th ward had a very distinctive smell— it was muddy, moldy, and what else …? Driving in the evening in this ward was very challenging without any streetlights, and often the street signs were gone or facing in a different direction as a result of the hurricane. Military vehicles, police, sheriff's men, and national guards were everywhere in town. It was the creepiest feeling I ever felt. In the middle of the disaster areas someone had remodeled a few houses very nicely. There was a for-sale sign of $169 000. A few beautiful houses sitting in the middle of a town like a graveyard.

Described below are a few of the people I met among many. At the Hyatt Hotel (treating a Federal Emergency Management Agency [FEMA] and 9/11 employee), a female National Guard with a gun greeted us at the front lobby. This was unexpected, but by this time the unusual had become normal. I approached a military policeman to offer him acupuncture and asked if I was scaring him with my needles. Then I realized that he had a gun. I thought, who is more scared now? A couple stood by our treatment area at the FEMA site in the 9th ward. They asked us what we were doing. We explained that acupuncture is good for stress reduction and post-trauma. She immediately started to cry, and he had watery eyes. I said to them, "Would you like to try?" They nodded yes. As soon as the wife sat down on the chair she put her sunglasses on and I saw a few teardrops running down her cheek. I couldn't speak and was about to cry, too. I glanced at her husband. He had tears in his eyes and said, "She's going through a lot." They had lost everything. A female staff member at Covenant House was smiling, although she lost everything. She'd got separated from her daughter and for four days didn't know where she was. After they were reunited it didn't matter what she had lost, as long as she had her daughter. A 9/11 worker at the Hyatt had to stay and work. All of her family except for her father was evacuated safely. She still doesn't know where he is. Another 9/11 worker stayed with a caller until she drowned

… the caller asked to stay with her. A homeless man was obviously drunk and incoherent at Washington Park. He kept mumbling with an alcohol bottle in his hand, "You don't understand, I was swimming … water was coming …"A man living in his home shot and killed two men. When he called the police for help they told him to protect himself. He was a relief worker at Tent City, he said. "There is a reason for every action." It's another challenge that he has to go through in his life. He just has to keep moving forward.

The areas we were going to at that time were the following: Common Ground clinics sites (in Algiers, in the 9th ward and in Kenner), Covenant House (for the homeless), Odyssey House (halfway house), Hyatt Hotel, Tent City, Vietnamese Churches in Baton Rouge and in New Orleans East, Animal Rescue of New Orleans, and Cruise boat. And the clinic sites were still growing because of the local demand.

AWB set up the treatment style based on a National Acupuncture Detoxification Association (NADA) (www.acudetox.com) protocol. It's primarily an auricular acupuncture for stress-related symptoms, post-trauma, and drugs addiction. It's a community-style acupuncture, so that we are able to treat many people at once in a small area while people sit on their chairs or, as in this case, on the ground or floor. This type of treatment was

used for many fire fighters, police, rescue workers, and residents of New York after 9/11. I was able to do a little Japanese Meridian Therapy and Japanese moxa *okyu*, as well as the NADA treatments.

It was hard to explain moxa to people; it was hard enough to explain about acupuncture. But it doesn't make much difference to them. They are desperate for help, and they are very appreciative that people are there to help after they have lost everything and their bodies and minds have been badly injured. In some cases they didn't even receive treatment, but we talked. Mostly, we listened. I believe it was helpful for them to talk.

Case Studies

- I had a lady who just cried continually, didn't stop crying while she was sitting on her chair. She didn't talk much; it was clear what was going on. I checked her pulse: totally weak and deep. I tonified right LU-9 and left SI-4. I checked her pulse again: it was still weak and deep. She had no idea what I was doing. She had four points in each ear. Shortly after, she asked me if she could go smoke a cigarette. I wasn't sure if it was a good sign, but she stopped crying. Her response was that she didn't know what was going on, but that she'd try the acupuncture again.

- The FEMA worker was totally overwhelmed and overworked. Her visions were very disturbed. I did the usual five needles in her ears. Her main issue was insomnia. I checked her pulse. She had a liver pattern. She was a pleasant lady, but I could tell that her smile was coming from hopelessness (if you know what I mean). I tonified on her right PC-7; checked the pulse again; it seemed okay, so I left it there. After the treatment she told me that she'd had many acupuncture treatments just on her ears, but that this time it had been different, her vision had improved. She asked me what the special thing was that I did and that nobody had done it before. I explained what it was. Amazingly she said that she

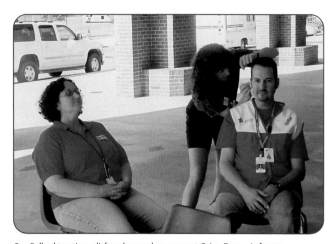

Sue Pollard treating relief workers and evacuees at Cajun Dome, Lafayette.

might talk to her boss in the White House about this!

Although people's initial reaction was often "What? Acupuncture?" they nevertheless tried and liked the treatment. People were open to sharing their thoughts, and we were there to listen and to give them a human touch. There is nothing you can compare to what human hands can do to each other. The people were so appreciative of us. Some gave us a huge hug and even gave us donations that we didn't expect from displaced residents. It was always nice to see their smiles after treatment.

The last day I saw a butterfly flying in Tent City. How peaceful is that? I also saw a lonely flower, and a few sunflowers bloomed by the I-10 ramp in downtown. They were surrounded by the shuttered houses, mud, and dust. How did they survive in this toxic environment? Our *qi* is all connected. As Meridian Therapists, we constantly talk about regulating the *qi*. As long as nature is so imbalanced, how can we keep our *qi* balanced? What can we learn from this?

I have been very humbled by this experience. This trip has taught me about life at various levels. What is it that really matters to you in this life? I was very inspired by these people's courage and strength. That's something you can't describe in words. You have to experience it. Giving is receiving.

I was fortunate that I was able to go to New Orleans and help the afflicted in some way. I'm glad that I could be a part of the healing process.

Epilogue

The end of February 2006: the Louisiana Board of Medical Examiners has forced AWB to immediately terminate all of its humanitarian relief efforts in Louisiana. The Board gave as its reasoning the "absence of a demonstrated need" for relief work by out-of-state volunteer acupuncturists. We have given over 4000 free treatments on people in New Orleans. Six months after the devastation,

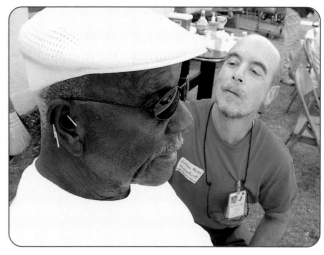

Graham Marks doing acupuncture treatment at Common Ground clinic, New Orleans.

people still live in houses without roofs, without running water, without electricity, and in a toxic environment. Bodies are still found in the neighborhood, and there are many basic living and legal issues still unresolved. The hospitals are not fully functional, and there is a great need for a lot of medical care to be delivered to the residents.

The acupuncture community still has a long way to go to convince the Western medical society of its efficacy.

On 17th May, 2006, Acupuncturists Without Borders issued the following press release:

Diana Fried, Executive Director of Acupuncturists Without Borders (AWB) announced today that the Louisiana State Board of Medical Examiners (LSBME) enacted an emergency regulation on 16th May, 2006 to allow out-of-state licensed acupuncturists to again offer free trauma relief treatment to victims of Hurricanes Katrina and Rita. This was done pursuant to an agreement worked on by AWB, LSBME representatives, and the Louisiana Department of Health and Hospitals (DHH). The rule becomes effective on 1st June, 2006.

Contact Details

Acupuncturists Without Borders (AWB)
National Office
37 Kelly Lynn Drive
Sandia Park, NM 87047
USA

Hurricane Katrina Office
Robyn Mizerrose
ATTN: AWB
341 Verret
New Orleans, LA 70114
USA

For more information contact:
Info@AcuWithoutBorders.org
Or call us at +1 504 232 7091

Other web pages you might want to visit:
Common Ground Clinic
(www.commongroundrelief.org)
NADA (www.acudetox.com)

Acupuncture Sans Frontières—
The Tsunami Relief Project in Sri Lanka

Oran Kivity, BAc, MBAcC, Kuala Lumpur, Malaysia

In the summer of 2005, 21 acupuncturists, three massage practitioners, and a homeopath went to Sri Lanka to offer treatment to tsunami survivors.

"I think we've hit the ground running," said Danny as I climbed out of the bus. It certainly seemed that way. People surrounded us, smiling or just staring. I felt more like a rock star arriving at a gig than an acupuncturist arriving for his first day at work at a temple. "You've missed the speeches, and there are 700 people waiting," he added.

We got straight to work. Our treatment area looked like an unfinished multi-storey car park: a ground-floor space topped with bare concrete, steel reinforcing rods sticking into the air and out to the sides. Orange cloth had been stretched across the window spaces for privacy. The waiting room was partitioned from us by more orange cloth; there was a mud floor, seething with men and women who held their children up to us as we passed by. I put my bag down by a trestle table with a folded blanket on it for padding. An interpreter came up to me. "Can you see this woman now?" We kept going till it got dark.

The team was a diverse bunch, in age, experience, and styles of acupuncture. Most practiced Traditional Chinese Medicine (TCM), some practiced Leamington Five Element style. I practice a Japanese Five Element style called *Toyohari*. We all got on with what we knew, at our own pace. For the first couple of days the situation felt quite pressured. Eight of us working flat out could not see 750 people in a day. Many people were coming early in the morning and leaving untreated at night. The chaos gradually subsided as we introduced more structure to the waiting area. People were given tickets and let into the waiting area, which was cordoned off from the outside. We set up an ear acupuncture clinic there so that, eventually, everyone received

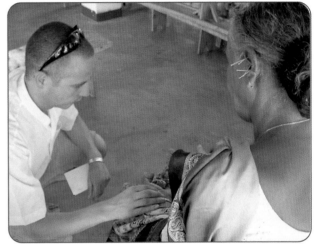

James Unsworth, clinic leader at the Galle Clinic, checks the pulse of an elderly patient.

ear acupuncture, hand acupuncture, or some kind of symptomatic treatment for knee, back, or shoulder pain while waiting to be seen for full body treatment.

The ear acupuncture was performed mainly by local Sri Lankans who had been trained by members of the team to do a simple five-point formula for shock and depression. A remarkable group *qi* developed, and each day the nervous chatter and crying of children subsided to a calm and meditative silence.

In the meantime others ploughed on with individual treatments in the main treatment area. TCM acupuncture is a system designed to treat large numbers of people quickly. This is the kind of situation in which it excels. By contrast I was a bit of a plodder as I worked with *Toyohari*. I watched with some admiration, and sometimes a little envy, as some of the TCM practitioners diagnosed and treated three or four people at a time, but there was no sense of competition, and I was confident that my treatments were doing good.

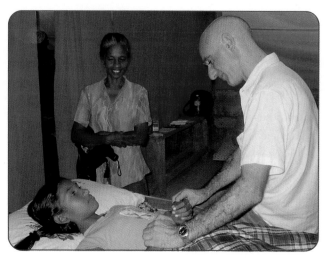

The author Oran Kivity checks the pulse of one of the many young patients.

With such a large group of people waiting, we had to have some difficult discussions with the chief monk about repeat treatments. Clearly, as we were only in the country for three weeks, our therapeutic relationship with our clients was going to be somewhat akin to a holiday romance. Our natural inclination was to see people we had already seen daily, but this would have meant that a large proportion of those as yet untreated would only ever get ear acupuncture in the waiting area. The monks wanted us to give one treatment per person, which to me brought the holiday romance to the level of a therapeutic one-night stand. They saw it as a special honor that these people would be treated by us, even just once: a very special kind of attention from Western "doctors." In the end, we forged a compromise: everyone got at least one treatment; no one got much more than three.

Most of our patients were 40 to 60 years old, and over half the cases we treated were for pain or musculoskeletal problems. These were generally chronic, long predating the tsunami; not surprisingly, as the south of Sri Lanka where the tsunami hit is tea farming land. I will never look at a cup of Ceylon tea in quite the same way again, now that I know how much human toil and suffering has gone into it. We treated endless rows of people

with bad backs, numbness in the feet and hands, swollen knees, sciatic pain. It was really an eye-opener into what a life of hard labor in the sun can do to you.

As the debate about repeat treatments was taking place, we were starting to observe something quite unusual. People were getting better much faster than we had anticipated. Ordinarily we would not expect results after only a few treatments, but people with chronic arthritic pain were showing huge improvements, and this took us by surprise.

This reinforced what the monks were saying. There was an inherent placebo effect in having a group of Westerners working with such zeal and commitment, so that the event itself had its own healing momentum. I think there was also a special group energy that developed, not only in the treatment area but also in the waiting area once people had their ears needled, and this group energy accelerated the healing. So although seeing people once or twice was not ideal it certainly made a big difference to many people.

Some teenagers responded very quickly to treatment. One 20-year-old boy had been blind since an eye infection at the age of four. He'd had terrible headaches and dizziness daily, ever since. The headache stopped during his first treatment and didn't come back during the two weeks I was in Sri Lanka.

Not everyone got better, of course, and many cases were heartrending. On my last day we saw a baby with liver cancer. We weren't able to do much, but we did babysit the wee thing while his mother got some much-needed treatment for stress and depression. The legacy of polio was common in the children I treated, as well as complications after surgery. I got the impression that the standard of Western medicine practiced locally could be improved.

Sri Lankans are really charming. They have the same gentle way of smiling that the Thai have and are extremely stoic. Despite the all-pervasive national trauma of the tsunami, the years of hard labor and physical pain, and the powerful undercurrent of depression and sadness, there was a genuine and palpable inner serenity to many of the people we treated.

Perhaps this is a legacy of the Buddhism they practice, or something inherent in the national psyche.

It was hard work. When my day off came I plunged into the sea, noticing how tense I'd become. But despite its intensity, I had an amazing time. I've done volunteer work back home in the UK, but this was the most fulfilling I have ever done.

The exotic location helped, of course; it's somewhat nicer being in Sri Lanka than in King's Cross, but there was also a powerful human connection. The kind of giving experienced in the country feels to me like what healing should be about. The practitioners were not distracted by any sense of transaction: no bills to pay, no charges to levy. It was just giving, out of a sense of human kindness, of community, and in that giving we received something very special, a sense of worth and purpose that I, for one, had never experienced before.

Fieldwork like this is not for the faint-hearted, or for those who like their creature comforts, or, most critically, for those who need daily certainties. The whole project was a moving target: we had to think on our feet the whole time, improvise systems, design research forms, and scavenge stationary on the hop. The teams chopped and changed and were kept on the move: it wasn't always clear which clinic or what part of the island we would be in, from one day to the next. A night's fatigued group discussion and decision would be overturned in the morning by new information.

We set up a simple clinical audit, which showed that 77% of those asked about their treatment reported positive benefits [1]. The provision of acupuncture in the various temples was clearly of great benefit to the people who came. The administration of ear, hand and symptomatic acupuncture as a "holding" treatment, or as a treatment in itself, was also clearly a resounding success, and took the burden off the others doing full body acupuncture. It's clear to me that acupuncture of all

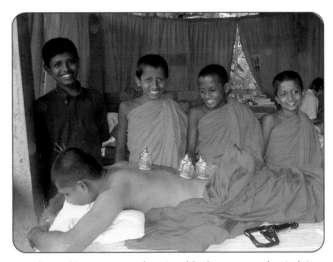

A monk enjoys his acupuncture and cupping whilst the younger monks enjoy being photographed.

kinds has a huge role to play in future relief operations: in Sri Lanka, in New Orleans, and perhaps in the future in Pakistan.

Reference

1. Maxwell D, Kivity O, Cassidy M. Acupuncture sans Frontières. *Journal of Chinese Medicine.* February 2006;80.

Contact Details

Acupuncture sans Frontières

Collective of Acupuncturists and Herbalists (with selected other therapists) committed to providing treatment to people affected by disaster, trauma, and poverty.

First project in Sri Lanka 2005 (Galle, Matara, Negombo).
Second trip to Sri Lanka (Ampara) 2006.
Future work planned for Pakistan.

For more information about volunteering in Sri Lanka or other destinations, please contact: info@danielmaxwell.com.

Humanitrad

Patrick Shan, Valence Cedex, France

Humanitrad on mission in Piatra Neamt, Romania.

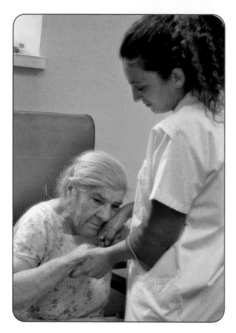

Based in France and Switzerland, Humanitrad are providers of Chinese medicine outreach services and training to ethnic minorities and underprivileged peoples.

Humanitrad is a legally constituted humanitarian Chinese medicine healthcare mission, whose purpose is to:

- develop the practice of Chinese medicine through humanitarian health missions to ethnic minorities or underprivileged populations;
- work toward collaboration between ethnomedicine and modern medicine in humanitarian and healthcare programs;
- promote exchange between medicines from different cultures;
- contribute to the preservation of traditional, autochthonous, and ancestral medical knowledge.

Patrick Shan in Benin.

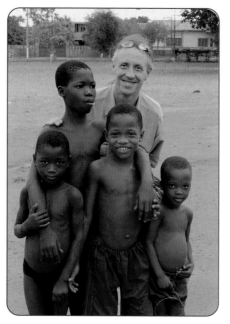

Humanitrad is based in Valence, France and organizes its missions together with the Center for the Development and Research in Ethnomedicine (CEDRE), which trains practitioners of Chinese medicine in France and Switzerland. Humanitrad manages the missions from the organization of the trip and accommodation for the participants to on-site logistical aid.

For each mission the CEDRE provides a team of students and practitioners doing their internship in Chinese medicine. The team operates under the supervision of experienced practitioners. In order to ensure the autonomy and continuity of the treatment, CEDRE also trains local healthcare personnel interested in the simplified treatment methods in Chinese medicine.

Example of a Mission: Romania

Humanitrad's missions in Romania take place twice a year. A team of around 10 practitioners carry out an average of approximately 1000 consultations in two weeks. The healthcare personnel from the Foundation for Intercommunity Healthcare, who receive the Humanitrad teams, are gradually being initiated into simplified treatments based on acupuncture and pharmacopoeia. The Humanitrad team also teaches a form of *qi gong*, which has been adapted for the treatment of rheumatic illnesses.

Contact Details

humanitrad@free.fr
www.humanitrad.org

Operation Heartbeat—
Caring for the Victims of the Pakistan Earthquake

Marc O'Regan, PA-C, LAc, CMT, Santa Barbara, California, USA

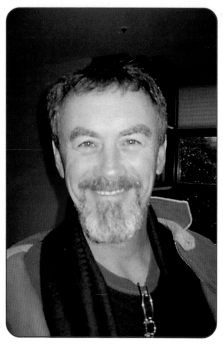

Marc O'Regan

Obituary

Sadly Marc O'Regan passed away suddenly on Friday 17th February, 2006 at 53 years of age. Marc had recently returned from an extended trip to Pakistan, where he went specifically to help earthquake victims, as a result of which he wrote the following article for *Acupuncture Today.*
Just prior to that, we learned that he'd been on the front lines in New Orleans, after Hurricane Katrina hit. He was involved in house to house search and rescue, and the provision of massages to other aid workers. As a former Navy Seal, Marc was an activist, always trying to be where he could do the most good. He was also a qualified physician's assistant, acupuncturist, and trained diver. His passion for life and his concern for his fellow human beings is a lesson for us all. He was an acupuncturist who took his art and skill to help provide for those less well off than himself at a time of crises in their lives. As practitioners we owe him our deep gratitude. May he be at peace.

Michael McCarthy, August 2006

I don't think you can find land more idyllically beautiful than the high mountains and passes of Kashmir in Pakistan. It was during the holy week of Ramadan, on 8th October, 2005, at approximately 9 a.m. while most women and young children were at home, school-age children were in class, and the men off to work in the fields or offices, that Kashmir was struck by a magnitude 7.9 earthquake.

The epicenter was near a town called Gori, 60 miles (approx. 95 km) north of the major city of Islamabad, and not all that far from the line of control. In a matter of 80 seconds, and in the days that followed, an estimated 87 350 people died; 2.5 million were left homeless, and the number of injured grew (as did the bacteria in their wounds). This earthquake was a "shallow" one, beginning only six miles under the earth's surface, thereby making it more deadly while being felt in three different countries. What was considered one of the most beautiful places in the world now lay in ruins, as whole villages were covered with tons of dirt, and shattered houses, schools, and shops lay beside and on top of crushed corpses.

As an acupuncturist/physician assistant/ bodyworker, I wanted to do something for the refugees, to help them rebuild their lives and assist in their medical needs. My Western medical training and experiences working in other natural disasters came in handy, but what excited me most was using acupuncture in the midst of this crisis.

Prior to these events I had the fortune of meeting Wendy Henry, LAc, of Community

Relief and Rebuilding through Education and Wellness (CRREW) while spending some time training to be a National Acupuncture Detoxification Association (NADA) instructor in New York City. Dr. Mike Smith, one of the co-founders of NADA, knew of my interest in bringing the NADA protocol into the military for its use, not just in addiction rehabilitation, but for the treatment of acute anxiety disorder, post-traumatic stress disorder (PTSD), and helping the civilians affected by combat and natural disasters. Dr. Smith hooked me up with Wendy, who works with the New York City Fire Fighters Counseling Services, and others who were interested in this application for acupuncture. Wendy had a wealth of information and experience, which she shared with enthusiasm and an infectious, can-do attitude. When Hurricane Katrina blew into Louisiana, Wendy called and put me in touch with people I could work with in New Orleans. Wendy's contacts, along with those of Laura Cooley, LAc, were instrumental in initiating bodywork and acupuncture for exhausted firefighters, police, and military service personnel who worked tirelessly while their own homes were destroyed and their families displaced. Wendy and Laura opened the doors for other acupuncturists to enter and work in New Orleans, which was still closed to most civilians. Their example, expertise, and successes were noted by mental health care workers and physicians on site, some of whom were later trained as acupuncture detoxification specialists (ADSs).

While working in New Orleans, I met a fellow volunteer, Todd Shea. Our friendship was instantaneous, and respect grew as we saw each other operate. Todd had a natural ability to think outside the box, acquire supplies and equipment for anyone who asked, and did good work with a smile, no matter how difficult the task. Todd spent 45 days in the New Orleans area; when the earthquake hit Pakistan, he was quick to respond to that emergency. Todd and I kept in touch, and he was instrumental in getting me to Pakistan.

Operation Heartbeat, a non-governmental organization (NGO) started by two physicians from George Washington University in the USA, had a medical team in Pakistan by 16th October. They recruited 20 physicians with different kinds of medical experience. Their team was headed by Todd, who was responsible for all the logistics, getting new teams in the country, and supplying them and other NGOs such as the Pakistan Red Crescent Society and Doctors Without Borders with medicine when needed. The operation was divided into four phases:

1. Acute phase—emergency care of survivors.
2. Subacute phase—emergency outreach into remote, newly accessible, and newly identified areas.
3. Rehabilitative phase—staffing the main field hospital, satellite health units, and outreach teams with local qualified doctors, medical students, and other health care professionals.
4. Reconstructive phase—construction of a permanent hospital at Garhi Dupatta to serve the greater Jhelum Valley.

I arrived in Islamabad and met up with Todd. As our transport hurtled up the bumpy roads, we discussed the current situation and the needs of the local populace. With a new team, we headed to Garhi Dupatta, located in the Jhelum River valley and with mountains on both sides reaching heights of 7000 to 8000 ft (approx. 2100 to 2400 m). As it stood, upon my arrival, Operation Heartbeat's field hospital was only seeing 150 people a day: a marked reduction from the first two weeks, where 450 to 600 patients a day was the norm. The amount of critical injuries had also dropped dramatically, but what was considered necessary were teams to go into the mountains where people were still in need of medical assistance.

On arriving in Garhi Dupatta I started getting medical packs together. Along with the antibiotics, surgical equipment, IV solutions, antidiarrheals, antifungals, and antiparasitics went 3000 acupuncture needles donated by Helio. (Helio was very generous and supplied the project with much-needed supplies.) I was in charge of the medical teams on nine separate operations into the mountains during my stay, with each trip lasting two to three days. Teams consisted of physicians, medical students, an investment banker (who spoke Urdu), surgical technicians, and emergency medical technicians (EMTs), paramedics, midwives, and a naturopath.

Sorties going into the mountains began by first conferring with the Pakistani Army, which supplied helicopters, ground transportation, and, more importantly, had real-time intelligence of what was needed and where medical help was needed. The Pakistani Army had troops in forward bases where they were supplied with tents, food, and bedding brought in by helicopters to distribute to earthquake victims to prepare them for the coming winter.

Our first stop was Nardijean, a small village that had lost 289 people in the quake. Five men were still in the landslide easily visible from the village; they were cutting grass for their cows at the time the earth shook. We treated everything from pneumonia and abdominal pain to infected wounds that had not been cleaned or bandaged for up to three weeks. People who showed overt signs of anxiety or were known to have psychological problems since the earthquake were also asked to come. Our translators did a great job; as people came and were able to get comfortable with us, they began to open up. I spoke to Captain Hammad, who was in charge of the village, and asked his permission to do acupuncture. I also asked the patients. He had no problem with it and showed great interest in the NADA protocol. In fact, as he could see the effect of acupuncture changing people before his eyes, he asked me to teach him how to do it so he could use it on his men. Captain Hammad became the first of four officers and six enlisted men, three medical students from the USA, and two psychologists that I trained in the NADA procedure. After three days and worsening weather, we had to put on our packs and hike out to the nearest army camp that could get transport for us back to Garhi Dupatta. Our supplies were all but gone and Todd asked me to get back so we could redeploy to another area.

Once back in base camp, I would get the medical box ready for our next trip. News of the acupuncture got back to base via the grapevine. I was asked by a major to show

him the NADA protocol. I asked him to sit on a bunk bed and start a natural breathing cycle. As he did this, I inserted the needles and let him "chill" for 40 minutes. When I pulled out the needles, he looked at me with glazed eyes and asked me to teach him the protocol also. The word was starting to spread among the officers of 212th Brigade that someone was putting needles in people's ears and they were starting to feel more relaxed and some of their body pains were going away. All this came from men who climbed over landslides to get into this valley, who were greeted by total destruction, death, and severely injured people. Brigadier General Sherier told me of the suffering he and his men witnessed in the first days as injured people poured out of the mountains into the valleys. The general said it was so painful to see all of the children and women injured, that as he helped the wounded, he would sporadically have to walk away from the scene, cry, and come back to do more work. All of the men I spoke with said the same thing.

While in New Orleans, I had done bodywork on Todd, so he immediately went off and told Brigadier General Amjad of the 10th Brigade that he should come for some bodywork. I took out some essential oils I had brought for such an occasion and worked on the General. He encouraged me to keep doing this kind of work and said that if he could help us in any way, he would. So, we started coming up with Christmas lists of things the camp needed and a list of villages further out that we might try to get to. This is known as the "back-scratching" principle!

After a month of moving about the mountains of Kashmir, I started reflecting on the work accomplished and the work needed to be done. The number of patients started to drop in the villages, although we would easily see 100 a day; though this sounds like a lot, the critical nature of the problems changed. Occasionally, people were still being carried out of the mountains with injuries they sustained during the earthquake. Simple cuts turned into cellulitis and osteomylitis. An example was an old man who came to me clinging onto a friend's back; he could not walk and one glance at his left foot showed me why. The foot, damaged in the quake, was five times larger than the right; it also had two infected wounds that smelled terrible. He asked me not to cut off his foot. I told him we would do everything to save his life first, then save his foot. We dealt with pain and hemorrhaging during childbirth, colds and flu, constipation, diarrhea, fever in infants, adolescents, and adults, plus one man who said his urine was yellow; when I told him to drink more water, he replied that "the water was too cold" and walked out of the tent.

I have been privileged to teach the NADA protocol to Pakistani Army personnel, medical students from the USA, two psychologists, and a few Pakistani nationals. It is funny to see a man doing auricular acupuncture with a machine gun strapped to his back, but I saw it often and the results were good. This was a beginning. I reminded all I worked with that psychological issues take time to heal, and the NADA protocol—with counseling and family and community support—was a great way to help start the healing process. I was able to leave everyone I worked with a few cartons of needles, and I have more to take back with me upon my return.

The job in Pakistan is far from over. I have spoken with acupuncturists in California who want to go to Kashmir to assist in this cause. We are looking for people who not only have an LAc or DOM degree, but people who, like myself, have a Western medical background, be it as an EMT, paramedic, nurse, etc. There is a need for people who believe in a holistic approach to medicine, especially during the acute and subacute phases of this project. Combining Eastern medicine to help Western medicine work better is a beneficial and exciting approach to patient care; one that not only benefits the body, but also the soul. This has been a very positive way to expose Eastern medical science to physicians who have never been exposed to Oriental medicine as they rotate through the camp. I have had the chance to show many doubting physicians, health care workers, and reporters that acupuncture can make a difference to the outcome of many problems. The best part was that when they saw it work, they would then ask if I would train them in the NADA protocol.

I believe there is a window of opportunity in every disaster—an opportunity for change even in old, fixed systems. Action needs to be taken right away and followed up. We, as acupuncturists, can teach others how cooperation and mutual respect for each other's skills benefits not just one group, but our medical community as a whole.

There is another reason for wanting people to have a hand in both camps. The day we left for Islamabad, we learned that a bus went over the side of a high road. The army asked for and transported our medical team to the scene of this terrible accident. Twenty-two people were killed; others were severely injured. You'd think that with the trauma these people had gone through, they should get some kind of break. The news sent my heart plummeting into its own abyss.

Phases two and three are now running into each other and will continue to do so for a short time. As teams go into the field and treat patients, those in the base camp continue making improvements in the field hospital clinic, ER and pediatric units. The army is opening more roads and allowing more villages to be accessed. There is a wonderful commitment by the founders of Operation Heartbeat to see this project through, and I am happy to have been a part of it. My commitment to service in relief efforts runs deep. I hope that people who want to work for the betterment of others, and those who are willing to challenge themselves, will contact me and leave me their contact information so I can begin a database of LAcs who would go to the frontlines of disaster relief work.

Contact Details

Operation Heartbeat
www.operationheartbeat.org

This article originally featured in *Acupuncture Today*, Volume 7, Issue 3, March 2006. It is reproduced here by kind permission.
editorial@acupuncturetoday.com,
www.AcupunctureToday.com

Community Acupuncture

Cynthia Neipris, LAc, New York, New York, USA

Community healing work in a community environment is especially beneficial when a disaster, trauma, or conflict has affected the whole community. Acupuncture in a group setting allows the community as well as the individuals receiving treatment to experience healing.

What is Community Acupuncture?

Community acupuncture is a highly effective and efficient way of treating a variety of individual and community conditions in areas of conflict, disaster, or devastation. Clients are treated in a group, sitting up in chairs, fully clothed. Needles are inserted in the ears based on a protocol developed by the National Acupuncture Detoxification Association (NADA). Other needles may be used on accessible body points as needed.

Much of the conventional treatment for anxiety, depression, and post-traumatic stress disorder (PTSD) in areas of disaster or conflict has been verbal (various forms of counseling) or has required medication. Acupuncture in a group setting has some advantages over these conventional treatments, and it can also be used along with more conventional talking and medication therapies to enhance their effectiveness. I have outlined some of these below.

Effective Treatment

Acupuncture addresses physical and mental health conditions simultaneously in the following ways:

- Immediate effects include a sense of well-being and relaxation, reduced anxiety and depression, and improved sleep.
- General improvements in health (headaches and other pain, digestive complaints, etc.) make it easier for patients to receive other services (like counseling).
- Treatment outcomes improve when patients feel better.
- Effects are immediate, but can also be long lasting, beyond the time the treatment is being given.
- While the treatment alleviates symptoms, it is also a general balancing treatment, which treats not only symptoms, but also the root cause of the symptoms.
- It addresses the whole person and has a comprehensive effect.

Immediate Effects

Few other modalities, except medication, offer immediate relief. This makes community acupuncture ideal while clients are waiting for other services that may take longer to provide.

Simple and Accessible
- No long intake or paperwork is required.
- No complicated equipment is necessary. Clients receive treatments sitting in a group

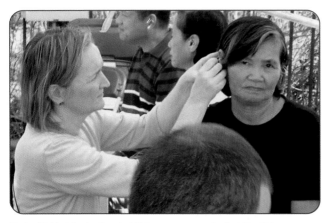

Regina Walsh doing treatment at Vietnamese community, East New Orleans.

so private offices or treatment tables are not required.

- Clients do not need to undress.

Versatile—Effective in a Wide Variety of Settings

- Acupuncture can be integrated successfully into a wide range of programs already in existence, including medical programs that utilize medication, mental health facilities, and social service agencies.
- It can be done anywhere. We treat in parks, churches, and waiting rooms, as well as health clinics.
- Patients with varying needs (trauma survivors, staff, emergency workers, etc.) can be treated in the same group.

Safe

There are almost no side-effects or contra-indications. It is non-addictive.

Cost-effective

Treatments are done in groups, so that many people can be treated at once.

Non-verbal and Non-performance-dependent

- Acupuncture does not require any talking. Patients can relax without fear of exposing themselves or losing control.
- Talking is hard when patients feel scared, tired, sick, hopeless, or embarrassed about feelings. It's hard for patients to articulate clearly what the problem is when they can't think clearly.
- Clients don't have to be able to understand intellectually or express their feelings to get relief.
- Equally effective even when there are language or cultural barriers.

Community-based

The effect of being treated in a group is that the benefit to the group is larger than the benefit would be if each client were treated individually. "Our bodies contain an autonomic mechanism to mimic or unite with a pulse greater than our own—speeding up or slowing

down to sync up with a stronger external rhythm. This concept is called 'entrainment'," explains Frank Lipman, MD, one of the foremost practitioners of integrative medicine in the USA [1]. We entrain to rhythms around us all the time, when we sing in unison with a large group, for example, and the effect is different from just singing the same words alone. Healing work in a community environment is especially beneficial when a disaster, trauma, or conflict has affected the whole community. Acupuncture in a group setting allows the community as well as the individuals to experience healing.

In addition to the current work in New Orleans, according to *Laura Cooley*, licensed acupuncturist and registered NADA trainer, there are "hundreds of international programs using ear acupuncture." Among these are:

- Dakota reservations in the aftermath of a series of tornadoes
- Search and rescue personnel as a de-stressing, revitalizing, and coping tool
- Brigades to Honduras after a hurricane displaced two million people
- Refugee camps in Burma
- Refugees in the USA suffering from PTSD.

Cynthia Neipris, LAc, is the Outreach and Community Education Coordinator for the New York campus of Pacific College of Oriental Medicine. This article may also be viewed on the Acupuncturists Without Borders website at: www.acuwithoutborders.org/community_acupuncture.php.

Reference

1. Lipman F. *Total Renewal: Seven Keysteps to Resilience, Vitality and Long-term Health.* New York: Tarcher/Penguin; 2003.

Contact Details

Cynthia Neipris, LAc
Pacific College of Oriental Medicine
New York, NY, USA
www.pacificcollege.edu

Acupuncturists Without Borders

Diana Fried, MAc, MA, Sandia Park, New Mexico, USA

Acupuncturists Without Borders (AWB) was established to develop and implement acupuncture-based programs that help facilitate community and personal healing in the face of large-scale traumatic events and their aftermath. When left untreated, the emotional and psychological consequences of trauma have the potential to compound the damage, further unraveling lives.

Historically it has been very difficult, if not impossible, to provide timely and cost-effective treatment to the large numbers of people who could benefit from such intervention. The beauty of acupuncture lies in that it is a low capital-intensive modality offering immediate, effective, and easily accessible treatment for large numbers of people, and is easily adaptable for administration under a wide array of circumstances. Acupuncture has proved highly successful in helping to heal the psychological consequences of trauma, with studies showing outcomes comparable to cognitive behavioral therapy.

We are currently working on making community acupuncture part of the standard of care in the immediate aftermath of disasters, alongside traditional medical interventions. We are also developing programs in communities in the global South to facilitate training of local health promoters in basic acupuncture.

Most of our work is done by volunteers. All treatments are given free of charge. AWB members are currently on the ground in Louisiana in the aftermath of Hurricane Katrina, treating evacuees and rescue workers.

The mission of AWB is to help alleviate suffering of people worldwide in urban and rural communities in need, and to support self-empowerment, through community acupuncture treatment and training. Your support for AWB helps establish and maintain our programs so that the benefits of this beautifully simple and effective treatment can be brought to these communities.

N.B.: We are not affiliated with Acupuncture Sans Frontières or Acupuncture Without Borders.

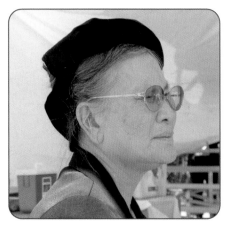

Vietnamese woman receiving acupuncture treatment in East New Orleans.

A Personal Story about Starting AWB, from the Director

I had long had a dream of starting an organization that would offer the extraordinary healing of acupuncture on a global scale. The idea was to serve communities in need around the world, both in the aftermath of disasters, and also with long-term training programs in poor and underserved communities. We would train local professionals in basic acupuncture that they could use for their own communities. This is already being done on an individual basis by several groups internationally. Our plan is still to do this in the longer term, but our commitment right now is to

Louisiana (we are not in Mississippi as well as Louisiana, because the Medical Board will not allow us to serve there).

I was watching the news on TV after Katrina hit. Something struck deep in my heart, and even though I was not planning on starting this organization at that moment, I knew it was time. I knew that I could help make something happen that was unique, and that no one else was doing. I knew that there had to be acupuncturists around the country who would want to help, many of whom understood the power of, and had training in, community acupuncture.

I also felt that it was very important to address needs in the USA, if at all possible. Normally, we would not be able to do this because of licensing issues that prevent out-of-state practitioners from practicing in another state. But in a disaster, those rules are sometimes overidden, as they have been in Louisiana.

Once I put the word out, we had an extraordinary response. I had hundreds of emails from acupuncturists who wanted to help. We had two big challenges: money, of course. But, more importantly, there were the legal questions. It is hard to put this in simple terms, because it has been so complicated.

We spent a great deal of time trying to get answers to whether we could legally do such volunteer work in Louisiana. Due to the confusion and disarray after the disaster we had difficulty even finding the right officials to contact. We did not get responses to numerous phone calls we made.

It turned out that eventually the Governor instituted an Executive Order that suspended state licensing requirements, allowing out-of-state medical and health practitioners to practice in Louisiana within the scope of their out-of-state license until 31st December.

We pushed hard for an extension after December, and had to pull back our teams until the next phase was clear (it takes a while to make plans). Then, on 30th December, the Department of Health and Hospitals announced that out-of-state practitioners could continue to serve until the end of February. There has been no further information about any extension after February, as far as we know.

We continue to have trouble getting clear answers to our questions about legal status. We have been in touch with the Louisiana Recovery Authority, the Louisiana Board of Medical Examiners, and the Department of Health and Hospitals.

We wrote to the Medical Board before the end of the last extension to try to get clarity, and to ask for special exemption for acupuncture because of the unique status of acupuncturists in Louisiana (unlike in most states where acupuncture is its own profession, in Louisiana acupuncturists are considered assistants unless they are a medical doctor). AWB volunteers are all fully licensed in their home states.

At present the future legal status is uncertain. Our commitment, if legally permitted, is to serve the people in need in Louisiana for as long as we can. We believe that the work we do makes a big difference in easing the post-traumatic stress that will continue for a long time to come. We are still getting daily requests to continue the services we are providing.

Contact Details

Diana Fried, MAc, MA
Executive Director,
Acupuncturists Without Borders
www.acuwithoutborders.org

Complementary and TCM Clinic Launched in Essen

Professor Gustav J. Dobos, MD, Essen, Germany

A Bridge between East and West

The first professorial department in Germany devoted to complementary and integrative medicine (or integrated medicine as it is called in Great Britain) was set up at the University of Duisburg–Essen (Germany) in 2004. This University Chair was endowed by the Alfried Krupp von Bohlen und Halbach Foundation and is similar to the Centre for Community Care and Primary Health (CCCPH) set up under Professor Patrick Pietroni at the University of Westminster in London. "In supporting this Chair," said Professor Berthold Beitz, Chairman of the Foundation, "the Krupp Foundation seeks to build a bridge between mainstream medicine and evidence-based complementary medicine." The Chair comprises a department for internal and integrative medicine with 54 beds and an outpatients' clinic for complementary and Traditional Chinese Medicine (TCM) at the Teaching Hospital, Kliniken Essen-Mitte. The table opposite lists the main features of the new Faculty.

The Chair is held by Gustav J. Dobos, MD, Professor for Internal Medicine, who, since 1999, has been conducting research into these fields in his capacity as Chief Physician of the Model Hospital of North Rhine-Westphalia (Internal and Integrative Medicine, Kliniken Essen-Mitte). Professor Dobos studied medicine in Freiburg (Germany), San Diego (USA), and Beijing (China).

In Essen, rapid progress has been made in the transfer of complementary medicine into a verifiable, scientific form and its integration into clinical care. New standards have been set and the basis formed for a kind of medicine that can meet the demands of a society whose population is aging and marked by chronic illness.

Integrative Medicine— "The Best of Both Worlds Combined"

The Department in Essen is preparing the ground for integrative medicine—a combination of mainstream medicine, scientifically verifiable complementary medicines, and TCM. This allows the development of better forms of therapy with fewer side-effects. Alongside TCM, studies are also being made into classical naturopathy and mind/body medicine.

The Chair has two lines of approach: the effectiveness of these forms of treatment has to be verified and valid criteria for quality control have to be established to make treatment transparent and safe. Its research seeks to build on the results of previous studies conducted at the National Center for Complementary and Alternative Medicine (NCCAM) at the National Institutes of Health (NIH) in the USA.

Traditional Chinese Medicine (TCM)

The Department has an outpatients' clinic for complementary medicine and TCM, providing not only acupuncture, Chinese herbal therapy, and *qi gong*, but also *tui na* massage therapy and TCM diet counseling.
An individual therapy plan is drawn up for each patient.

In a project commissioned by the state of North Rhine-Westphalia, quality control criteria have been developed to create a certification system for TCM centers. The Chair is offering lectures and workshops in TCM, and doctoral theses are supervised in current fields of basic and clinical science. Chinese physicians of TCM can apply for a two-year scholarship to pursue a doctoral thesis at the University of Duisburg–Essen. Applicants are required to have completed seven years of study in TCM and have eight years of experience working in the field, as well as proficiency in English.

Classical Naturopathy
One important component of classical naturopathy is therapeutic fasting. Research into the effectiveness and the modalities of therapeutic fasting considers both the basic (fasting and sleep, fasting and neuroendocrine regulation) and clinical aspects (fasting and migraine). In addition, hydrotherapy in the treatment of heart disease and cardiovascular complaints is studied. A special interest lies in the therapy with medical leeches, a centuries-old practice in a wide variety of cultures that has been successfully applied in the treatment of osteoarthritis of the knee, the thumb, and in tennis elbow.

Mind/Body Medicine
Studies reveal that 60–90% of all visits to the doctor in Western countries are due to stress-induced illnesses. Mind/body medicine aims at incorporating stress-alleviation procedures

and new forms of lifestyle-changing methods into people's everyday lives and works on the principle that a health-oriented lifestyle mobilizes self-healing capacities. Mind/body therapy embraces nutrition, exercise, relaxation response, cognitive restructuring, and stress management. Some of the fundamental principles of mind/body medicine were elaborated at the mind/body Medical Institute of Harvard Medical School, Boston (USA) and at the University of Massachusetts, Worcester (USA). Professor Dobos has been collaborating with both institutions for a number of years. The new Chair in Essen focuses on the application of mind/body therapy in cases of coronary artery disease, chronic inflammatory bowel disease, migraine, and cancers such as breast cancer.

Contact Details
Faculty of Integrative Medicine
Clinic Essen-Mitte
Essen, Germany
www.uni-essen.de/naturheilkunde

Structure of the Faculty of Complementary and Integrative Medicine at the University of Duisburg–Essen

Teaching	Research	Hospital
Required to lecture at university	TCM: basic and clinical science	Ward 54 beds
Supervision of doctoral theses	Quality assurance	Institute of CAM and TCM
Postgraduate training in CAM and TCM	Classical naturopathy	Breast cancer outpatients' clinic at university
	Mind/body medicine	

Acupuncture in France—
An Interview with Yves Réquéna

Patrick Rudolph, Physician, Heilpraktiker, LAc, Berlin, Germany

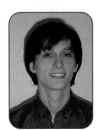

Patrick Rudolph

Introduction

Acupuncture has a long history in France. At the end of the 17th century, Jesuit monks brought the first texts on Chinese medicine to France. In 1671, the first book on this "exotic" medicine was published by Father Harvieu (*Les Secrets de la Medicine des Chinois*). Chinese medicine found its way into practice in France as early as the beginning of the 19th century. But it wasn't until Georges Soulié de Morant, a French consul in China for over 12 years, that acupuncture became known to a broader public and was practiced on a larger scale. His story stands as a model for the situation we still find in France. Being a diplomat, poet, and sinologist, he developed a special interest in Chinese medicine and studied this healing art in China from 1905 on. He practiced acupuncture in hospitals and with important teachers in China and became the first Westerner to be recognized as a Doctor of Chinese Medicine in China.

Returning to France in 1917, he practiced and taught acupuncture in four different hospitals in Paris for more than three decades. His lectures were open to MDs and non-MDs alike. He published various books on acupuncture and gave this method an enormous impetus in France and throughout Europe, making France the center of Chinese medicine in the West for a long time. In the early 1950s he then became accused by medical doctors of illegal practice of medicine. The persecution ruined his health and stopped him from teaching and practicing.

To this day, medical doctors hold a monopoly over the practice of medicine in France. Anyone not holding a French or equivalent medical diploma from a university and practicing acupuncture is doing so illegally. Whether one studied Chinese medicine in China for eight years, studied at an acupuncture school in the West for three years, or moved to France after having practiced in England for many years, it is illegal to practice acupuncture without being an MD.

However, this doesn't stop people from practicing , nor does it stop patients from seeking treatment by specialized acupuncturists outside of the official system. The non-MD community of acupuncturists found its way of establishing their profession through the back door. Nowadays non-MD-acupuncturists have a professional insurance and are being integrated into the social welfare system. They pay taxes and social security contributions from an income they aren't allowed to earn. They obtain professional malpractice insurance cover from insurance companies for treatments they aren't allowed to apply. There are schools teaching Chinese medicine (mostly three-year programs) and professional associations organizing the profession.

Well, everything is alright then, one is tempted to say. No, because this paradoxical situation brings with it a whole lot of problems.

Interview with Yves Réquéna

Mr. Réquéna, how does a patient find his non-MD acupuncturist? Being illegal, it's no doubt difficult to put a sign outside the door saying "Private Acupuncture Clinic."
Only some non-MD acupuncturists dare to put a sign in front of their private practice. But, after all, the sign is not so important anyway. I mean, how many patients come to my clinic because of the sign outside? The patients come because of recommendations. This is the same for MDs and non-MDs.

Can acupuncturists make a living from working undercover?
Not many acupuncturists can live only from their private clinic. But still, there are a grow-

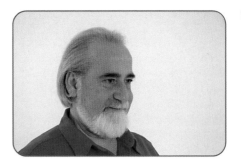

Yves Réquéna

ing number of non-MD acupuncturists who obviously find a way to survive. And they get organized in syndicates/associations that provide them with professional insurance cover. They pay for their taxes and the social security system.

That's difficult to understand, at least for Germans. You get professional negligence insurance for something you're not allowed to do. You fill in an official form, stating that you're doing a job that's being punished by law. Do they really call themselves "acupuncturist?"
I guess so, they can't write "acrobat" if they aren't. The state doesn't really care as long as there's money to be earned. Whether you write "prostitute" or "acupuncturist," they just take the money where they find it.

How dangerous is it to work illegally?
That depends on the situation. The non-MDs aren't constantly being harassed, unless they're advertising or getting too much publicity. From time to time there are cases of prosecution, which regularly end with a fine, and of course the closing of the private clinic. But the bigger problem is that because of the illegal status, professional structures are difficult to establish. For example, the schools of Chinese medicine cannot do practical teaching on patients because they just simply aren't allowed to treat. Problems like this one hinder the development of Chinese medicine in France.

How is the situation for MDs practicing acupuncture?
It's getting worse. I still have the possibility of working under an old regulation, which allows refunding by the health insurance companies with the balance of the fee paid privately by the patient. But the young colleagues have to decide. Either they work with the state health insurance, which pays miserably for acupuncture (about €14/per session), or they generally work privately, earning barely enough to survive. In some big cities it's possible to work privately but in smaller places there are just not enough patients for that. There used to be more MDs working with acupuncture some 15 years ago. Maybe this development will

provide some free space for the non-MDs to find their niche.

The next problem is that the cost of an acupuncture treatment is only reimbursed for a few indications, mainly pain. The benefit must be proven and it should not be the main treatment; it has to be an adjunctive therapy. The situation is becoming increasingly difficult for acupuncture in France. You start to think about emigrating.

Is any research being done on acupuncture at university level?
Very little. Right now there's a study being done in Paris on acupuncture as adjunctive therapy during chemotherapy.

What do you think about the quality of acupuncture treatment by MDs as compared to non-MDs?
Oh, that's difficult to say. In both groups you have people with a sound knowledge who are very skilled and, on the other hand, people I wouldn't recommend. The non-MDs mostly have a very good theoretical knowledge, even Chinese language skills, but they often don't have enough practical training. As I said, the schools have problems providing "bedside teaching" so they often try to compensate this by doing practical training in China. In the end, it depends on the individual acupuncturist and on his/her commitment and ability.

How is the relationship between the two acupuncture communities of MDs and non-MDs? Is there a discussion on common topics, for example, on treatment strategies for certain diseases? Are there common events, like conferences?

The relationship is pretty bad. There's virtually no professional exchange on topics of Chinese medicine between these two groups. But actually it mostly depends on whether the acupuncturist comes from a traditionalist or a scientific faction. You sometimes see MDs who are more traditionalist at conferences with non-MDs.

How is the communication between these two groups with regard to a common patient? Does the MD know that there is a parallel treatment by a non-MD?

Oh no. That would mean war. It only happens in a case where the two therapists know each other already. Like sometimes you have a couple that work together, or when there is a personal friendship between them they can talk to each other. But it doesn't happen that a non-MD calls up some MD he doesn't know and says: "Hi, I wanted to talk to you about our mutual patient."

And the patients keep quiet as well?

Well, often the patients just think: "My little doc doesn't need to know everything."

The patient could threaten to accuse the practitioner. Does the fact of illegal practice influence the relationship between acupuncturist and patient?

No, if the patient chooses a non-MD, he or she takes responsibility and is aware of the situation.

How do you see the prospects for Chinese medicine in France?

Rather difficult, after all it depends on the political aims. If you look around you see Germany with the *Heilpraktiker* (alternative healing practitioner), the UK we don't need to talk about; everyone is free to do what they like. Then in Belgium, Portugal, and Spain a lot changed recently. Worldwide there are attempts by the UN to integrate traditional medicine. Cuba is very much ahead concerning the integration of acupuncture, also because of the embargo, which led to an insufficient supply of medical drugs. In Mexico there are "barefoot doctors" who have been trained in acupuncture, a bit like in Mao's era, to ensure public health. The dialogue between MDs and non-MDs is promoted, or at least the mutual respect and recognition is attempted. Furthermore there is China, interested in spreading its culture to the world and trying to increase the export of Chinese herbs. We can be curious about the further development of Chinese medicine.

Patrick Rudolph, currently practicing in Berlin, Germany, is a course instructor in Chinese Herbs, Pulse and Tongue Diagnosis.

Yves Réquéna, MD, specialized in acupuncture, practicing in Aix-en-Provence and in Paris, France, teaches acupuncture and *qi gong*.

Contact Details

www.yves-requena.com
pat@chinadoc.de

Acupuncture in Western Europe

Professor Gunnar Stollberg[1], PhD, Bielefeld, Germany

While the term "hybridization" is particularly well suited to describing innovations consisting of (literally) existing ingredients, the term is problematic in that it implies the existence of non-hybridized culture. However, societies without processes of transfer, exchange, and transformation are rare. When Elwert [1] described culture as the social organization of syncretism, he strengthened the idea of culture as open and dynamic structures instead of static and isolated formations. Nederveen Pieterse [2] talked of the "hybridization of hybrid cultures." If every culture is hybridized, the term loses its significance. It may only still be relevant for challenging essentialist discourses [3]. Is it obsolete for other research topics?

I will first look for an original version of Chinese medicine in China. Having outlined various forms of Chinese medicine in the West, and after a short history of acupuncture in Europe, I will describe hybridized forms of Chinese medicine in Germany and in the UK. I will then look for hybridization in acupuncture education and present a British medical conception of minimal acupuncture. Finally I will outline recent results of German acupuncture randomized controlled trials (RCTs) and their potential consequences.

Is There an Original Chinese Medicine in China?

Anthropologists often know about the original versions of, say Asian, cultures and their elements, and they often have contempt for their Western imitations. This is especially true for versions that became popular in the West, with the contempt arising for the milieu that is popular Western culture. The thesis of the McDonaldization of the world [4] does not derive from a deep admiration of McDonald's,

but from its contempt. On the other hand, non-European cultural elements are admired for their originality and for being adapted to local circumstances and requirements. They are embedded, and on their way to Europe they become dis-embedded. A nod to economy de-legitimizes this process and its results.[2]

If we relate this criticism to the Westernization of Chinese medicine, we could state that there is a broad tradition of medical knowledge in China, well embedded in Daoist and Confucian philosophy. Some elements of this rich tradition migrated to Europe and to the USA, where they became dis-embedded from their philosophical background, and decayed to mere technologies, adapted to biomedical conceptions—a poor shadow of the originals, minimized for economic reasons.

But if we look at recent descriptions of Chinese medical knowledge [8, 9], there is not a mere original, rather there are many faces of Chinese medicine in China.[3] Parts of the broader tradition were transformed into the curricula of Traditional Chinese Medicine (TCM) that are taught at Chinese colleges. TCM and a few other elements of Chinese medicine migrated to Europe. In the cities of mainland China, Hsu [8] observed different ways and social settings of the transmission of traditional medical knowledge:

- First there are popular and folk practitioners. Herbalists and *qi gong* masters practice folk medicine outside the clinics. They established an oral tradition of secret knowledge, Daoist verses, which accompany the breathing techniques of *qi gong* in their pronunciation and emphasis.
- Chinese medical doctors work in or outside clinics, and pass on personal knowledge, consisting of long classical Chinese texts, which are reproduced by heart. These texts remain polysemic; the practices are virtuous.

- Traditional Chinese medicine doctors work in clinics and reproduce a standardized body of knowledge consisting of shorter passages from medical textbooks. These texts aim at reducing the polysemic character of the classics. Theory and practice are clearly separated, as they are in biomedicine.

These three knowledge styles may be illustrated by three conceptions of *qi*.[4] In the secret knowledge of *qi gong*, *qi* can be felt by touching the body surface. In personal knowledge, its movement can be realized by pulse diagnosis. Standardized knowledge stresses the permanent fluctuation of *qi*, and contrasts that to blood and other bodily fluids [11]. Thus, we cannot simply state that a Chinese original became polluted by migrating to the West.

Various Forms of Chinese Medicine in the West

In the USA, a medical counter-culture developed in the 1960s. It comprised European-American acupuncturists. Some of them had learned TCM in mainland China. Barnes [12] lists two other groups of acupuncturists in the USA: older Chinese-Americans who had learnt acupuncture through lineage systems, often from older generations, and/or in pre-war educational programs who practice in the American-Chinese community; Chinese-American practitioners from mainland China who had gained various biomedical qualifications in China, and had additionally achieved some acupuncture knowledge. "Most European-American practitioners neither speak nor read Chinese ..." They "define themselves ... as holders of a working knowledge that approximates aspects of the curriculum in Chinese medical schools." [13]

Authors differ in their interpretation of whether the counter-culture changed into a complementary culture or not. Baer [14] keeps the flag of the social movement flying: "An authentically holistic and pluralistic medical system would not simply provide working-

class people, peasants, and indigenous people with traditional medicine as a cheap alternative but would need to be part and parcel of a democratic socialist global system that would provide all with the benefits of both biomedicine and heterodox healing systems."[5] But Barnes [16] remains skeptical: "There continues to be a large number of acupuncturists who, while they may no longer see themselves as 'alternative' practitioners working in opposition to biomedicine, still define themselves as 'complementary'; that is, as distinct from biomedical practice but able to work as partners."

In Western Europe, we find various forms of Chinese medicine. In a traditional immigration country like the UK there exists a Chinese folk medicine sector, but its use seems not to be widespread in the Chinese community.[6] In the German and British indigenous population, *qi gong* and *shiatsu* became popular in the wellness and massage areas; Chinese herbal teas are served in expensive wellness hotels; Chinese herbal medicine is spreading over the UK; and acupuncture is practiced by many biomedically oriented physicians as well as by non-medically qualified personnel. China is no more than a frame of reference for all of them. In this article, I will especially look at acupuncture.

An Historical Overview of Acupuncture in the West

Chinese medical tradition includes many therapeutic forms like drugs, movement, and respiration (*qi gong*, etc.), massage and so on. Acupuncture is one aspect of the Chinese medical sub-discipline "acupuncture and moxibustion" (*zhen jiu*) in China. It is distinctive for two reasons: first, it is based on a theory of the body that views the body as permeated with channels (or "meridians"), *jing luo*, which reach from the extremities to internal body parts. Second, it makes use of particular instruments, needles. According to Chinese medical theory, the manipulation of the needles in particular points on the channels regulates the balance of *qi*, *yin*, *yang*, and the so-called Five Elements (*wu xing*) in the body. These ideas can be traced to the earliest canonical writings on acupuncture and moxibustion in China, the *Huang Di Nei Jing* (The Yellow Emperor's Classic of Medicine) written about 2000 years ago.

The European history of acupuncture is marked by different attitudes toward the needling therapies that their promoters called "acupuncture."[7] Well-known are the publications of physicians of the East India Company, like that of the Dutch Willem ten Rhyne in 1683 and of the German Engelbert Kämpfer in 1712, who reported with admiration on these techniques—based on information from Jesuit missionaries (ten Rhyne reported on needling only, but Kämpfer also reported on moxa). However, just as physicians who wrote with admiration on Chinese pulse diagnostics (Floyer in 1707), faced hostility among the emerging university-based medical colleagues, those advocating needling were severely criticized throughout the 18th century in Germany and Britain.

This changed drastically in the early years of the rise of clinical medicine in France, when there was an upsurge of experimentation with needling techniques.[8] However, by the beginning of the 20th century, acupuncture had vanished from medical practice in Europe.

The recent spread of acupuncture in the West started before World War II with Soulié de Morant (1934) in France. From there it spread after the War, to Western Germany in the 1950s [25]. The founding father of the German Medical Association of Acupuncture (DÄGfA), Dr Gerhard Bachmann (1895–1967), adopted the conceptions of Dr Roger de la Fuye (1890–?) who had worked as a military physician in Indochina, and had published textbooks on acupuncture and on "homeosiniatry," a combination of homeopathy and acupuncture.[9] Dr Heribert Schmidt, who chaired the DÄGfA from 1967 to 1970, had learned *kanpo*, the Japanese form of Chinese medicine, in Japan. Thus, non-Chinese forms of acupuncture were prevalent in these years. The Chinese form disseminated in the 1970s, when American journalists reported about acupuncturist analgesia. Today, the professio-

nal organizations mostly teach Chinese forms of acupuncture.

In the then Eastern Germany (GDR), acupuncture met the hostility of powerful persons and institutions. In the 1970s, a set of needles was officially destroyed in Ichtershausen (close to Arnstadt and Erfurt). Otto Prokop, Head of the Berlin Institute for Forensic Medicine, published many articles against heterodox medicine and especially acupuncture, which he declared to be a form of magic [27]. Thus, there were only few physicians practicing and training in acupuncture in their personal networks. In the 1980s, some of them had the opportunity to study acupuncture in Austria and even in China [28]. Since that time, this therapy has become established within the framework of the Working Group for Neural Therapy (Arbeitsgemeinschaft für Neuraltherapie), which had a membership base of some 900 physicians in the late 1980s [29]. In 1990, the name changed to DGfAN, which was divided into sections for acupuncture and neural therapy[10] [30].

Acupuncture in Germany

It is currently impossible to gauge the number of acupuncturists as well as the extent of acupuncture use. Table **1** shows that many German physicians and fewer non-medical practitioners are members of acupuncture organizations.

The extent of treatment through acupuncture is thus difficult to gauge. Holding an acupuncture qualification neither necessarily means practicing acupuncture on all patients, nor necessarily on any patient. Acupuncture will usually be one of several treatments carried out by any one practitioner. Robert Frank and I [31, 32] found different types of the hybridization of Asian and biomedicine in German medical practice. From interviews with medical acupuncturists we constructed the following types of hybridization, shown in Table **2**.

In the introduction I asked whether the term "hybridization" is obsolete in cultural studies because every "original" culture is hybridized. As may be seen from Table **2**, we tried to escape this terminological dilemma by pursuing an empirical path. We break down this rather vague concept into different modes of hybridization. We first differentiated for the gravitational center of the process: was it biomedicine or heterodox medicine? Second, we looked for weak and strong degrees of hybridization. The combination of these criteria produced a matrix containing four fields:

- The first one shows a biomedically dominated coexistence of biomedicine and heterodox medicine. I give an example for this mode of hybridization from our interviews with medical acupuncturists: "I believe that Western and Eastern medicine should complement each other. Both have their areas of application" (acupuncturist no. 3). Most of "our" medical acupuncturists practiced acupuncture in this way.
- The second field shows a coexistence of biomedicine and heterodox medicine subject to heterodox dominance. Here is an example again: "For me, decent diagnostics have to precede acupuncture. I never insert needles in anyone who comes in here saying, 'I've got this and that—what are you waiting for?'" (acupuncturist no. 12). This heterodoxically dominated coexistence was practiced by a few acupuncturists working in private practice.
- The third field shows a biomedical incorporation of Asian medicine. For example: "There is feedback in the brain, which triggers the selective distribution of opiates. Reflexes are triggered and a selective relaxation takes place—particularly in muscular and orthopedic conditions. I don't think it would be too difficult to prove that scientifically" (acupuncturist no. 2). This pattern is widely represented in teaching Asian medicine, but we could rarely find it in medical practice.
- The fourth field shows a great melting pot. A last example: "I combine acupuncture with other modes of treatment—homeopathy or bioresonance—in 80% of my cases. I use Chinese concepts—like the Five Elements or touching the meridians—for everyone. I decide later whether to insert needles or proceed differently. Right now, I avoid it whenever possible" (acupuncturist no. 9). Few of "our" acupuncturists came close to this pattern.

Table 1 Membership of acupuncturist associations in Germany, 2003

Organization	Membership
German Academy for Acupuncture and Auriculomedicine (Deutsche Akademie für Akupunktur und Aurikulomedizin; DAAAM; established 1974)	13 600[1]
German Medical Association of Acupuncture (Deutsche Ärztegesellschaft für Akupunktur; DÄGfA, established 1951)	11 000[2]
German Society for Acupuncture and Neural Therapy (Deutsche Gesellschaft für Akupunktur und Neuraltherapie; DGfAN; in the former GDR, established 1971)	3200[3]
German Acupuncture Society Düsseldorf (Deutsche Akupunktur Gesellschaft Düsseldorf; DAGD, established 1978)	1600[4]
Association for Classical Acupuncture and TCM (Arbeitsgemeinschaft für klassische Akupunktur und Traditionelle Chinesische Medizin; AGTCM; non-medically qualified *Heilpraktiker*; established 1954)	1050[5]

[1] Personal information provided by Dr Frank Bahr, Munich, September 2003; see also the website www.akupunktur-arzt.de.
[2] Personal information provided by Dr Wolfram Stöhr, Munich; see also the website www.daegfa.de.
[3] The majority of the members of the DGfAN practice acupuncture, and not neural therapeutics. Personal information by Dr Reinhart Wagner, Ebersdorf/Thüringen; see also the website www.dgfan.de.
[4] Personal information provided by Dr Gabriel Stux, Düsseldorf; see also the website www.acupunctureworld.com/ge/deakdu.
[5] Personal information provided by Andreas A. Noll, Berlin; see also the website www.agtcm.de.

The prevalence of the biomedically dominated coexistence of biomedicine and acupuncture shows that acupuncture is widely used in a complementary, and not in an alternative manner. Acupuncture is not taught at universities or medical schools. There is but one German professorship officially entitled to teach Chinese medicine.[11] Acupuncture, rather, is taught within the framework of further medical education. The German Medical Association has published guidelines for this education in general. In the 1980s, the professional acupuncturist organizations adapted their education schemes to these guidelines, and the regional medical chambers accepted these schemes within the framework of natural curing procedures.

Official medical organizations moved from skepticism against acupuncture to a series of trials and regulatory models. The older skepticism is represented by memoranda of the Scientific Advisory Council of the German Medical Association (Wissenschaftlicher Beirat der Bundesärztekammer) in 1957 [33] and 1992, and by the German Physicians' Drug Commission (Arzneimittelkommission der deutschen Ärzteschaft), which in 1998 recommended not including complementary and alternative medicine (CAM) in the public health insurance schemes. As late as 2001, the Federal Joint Committee (Bundesausschuss der Ärzte und Krankenkassen)[12] published a skeptical report about acupuncture: its efficacy was said to result for the most part from the care given by the healer, and such efficacy was not considered to depend on the healer's training or on a specific medical conception. Thus acupuncture is situated on the level of many other therapies that have not been tested in RCTs [34]. However, in 1999 a group of German public insurance companies have embarked on a huge trial regarding the efficacy and efficiency of acupuncture and other heterodox therapies. I will comment on these RCTs later on. They will not only change the status of reimbursement for acupuncture treatment, but will also be relevant for the regulation and further spreading of acupuncture knowledge among German physicians.

In 2003 the German Medical Association published special rules for further education in acupuncture, which will become a model for respective rules to be published by the medical chambers of the German states. These rules establish an additional title (*Zusatzbezeichnung*) "Medical Acupuncturist."

Acupuncture in the UK

The 20th-century history of acupuncture in the UK[13] is fairly distinct from that on the continent, though in the UK, as in Germany, Japanese, South-East Asian, and other non-Chinese forms of acupuncture were widespread until the 1970s [35]. In the UK, one particular per-

Table 2 Types of hybridization

Degree of Hybridization	Gravitational Center	
	Biomedicine	Heterodox Medicine
Weak	Complementing biomedical practice with Asian medicine	Complementing heterodox medical practice with biomedical procedures (at least diagnostics)
	Criteria: biomedical disease category; patients' demands	No further meta-theory
		Loose combination
	No further meta-theory	
Strong	Inclusion of Asian medicine in biomedical paradigms	Fusion of all conceptual ingredients into universal model of medical theory and practice
	Use of Asian medicine in predominantly biomedical practice	

son, Jack R. Worsley (1923–2003), has been extremely influential.[14] Not that he was the first to practice acupuncture in 20th-century Britain,[15] but he trained many non-medically schooled practitioners in Five Element theory.[16] Those practitioners later educated themselves further—some started to practice acupuncture and Chinese herbal medicine according to entirely different medical paradigms from Five Element theory—and several founded acupuncture colleges in the 1980s.

These mainly British acupuncturists have more recently made efforts to re-unite themselves under the auspices of the British Acupuncture Council (BAcC), and after a meeting in October 2001, decided to set up standards for self-regulation. Quite apart from those, exponents of the British medical profession have continuously made use of acupuncture as a technique, and have trained physicians in these techniques. At last, there is a third current of practitioners to consider: after the economic reforms in the People's Republic of China, the UK has seen an unprecedented influx of Chinese who practice Chinese herbal medicine, acupuncture, *qi gong*, and other skills.

In the UK, acupuncture is taught at acupuncture colleges, at universities (in departments of primary health care or community health care, for instance), and within professional societies who offer short- and long-term courses. There is also a plurality of acupuncture organizations, medical and non-medical (Table **3**). Furthermore, there is a substantial body of Chinese medical doctors of Chinese origin who offer mostly Chinese herbal medicine. But medical doctors of Chinese origin only seldom offer training.[17]

Acupuncture is taught at specialized colleges of acupuncture, at universities, and within professional acupuncture associations. The British Medical Acupuncture Society (BMAS) offers basic and advanced courses to health care professionals who are registered by statute in the UK. This includes nurses, midwives, health visitors, physiotherapists, osteopaths, chiropractors, and podiatrists.

Table 3 Membership of acupuncturist associations in the UK, 2004[1]

	Relevant Acupuncture Organization	Estimated Number
Medical practitioners	British Medical Acupuncture Society (BMAS)	2300
Traditional acupuncturists	British Acupuncture Council (BAcC)	2500
Traditional Chinese medical doctors, including acupuncturists	Legislative Association for Chinese Medicine Practitioners: Association of Traditional Chinese Medicine (ATCM), (since 23rd November, 2003 includes British Society of Chinese Medicine)	1200
	General Council of TCM, which includes the following three: ▪ Association of Chinese Medicine Practitioners (ACMP) ▪ Chinese Medical Institute and Register ▪ Chinese Healthcare Institute Register	
Auricular acupuncturists/ substance abuse	SMART (Self Management and Recovery Training) NADA (National Acupuncture Detoxification Association) Society of Auricular Acupuncturists	2500
Physiotherapists	Acupuncture Association of Chartered Physiotherapists	2650
Dentists	British Dental Acupuncture Society	100
Nurses	British Academy of Western Acupuncture	250

[1] Acupuncture Regulatory Working Group [40] Appendix 3.

The BAcC offers education for non-medical acupuncturists.[18] The British Acupuncture Accreditation Board (BAAB)[19] has accredited seven colleges in the UK, and another four are currently Stage One accredited and committed to ongoing development of the course to reach full accreditation.

The British Medical Association (BMA) has made a turn in its policy towards acupuncture. In 1986, it presented complementary therapies as ineffective, not evaluated, and sometimes harmful to patients [41]. In 1993, it stressed the necessity of regulating education in heterodox practices, and of establishing codes of medical ethics for all forms of medicine [42, 43]. In 2000, it recommended formalizing education in acupuncture and integrating this treatment into the National Health Service (NHS) [44].

The Department of Health (DH) took up official purposes for a statutory regulation of the acupuncture profession. They had been raised by a committee of the House of Lords in 2000, followed by an Acupuncture Regulatory Working Group (ACRWG) in 2003. The ACRWG suggested establishing a General Acupuncture Council to govern an official register of acupuncturists: "Registration should confer the title 'Registered Acupuncturist.' Certain subsidiary designations might be considered in the interests of informed patient choice." [45] The DH took this proposal up, widened the council proposed to a CAM Council, and suggested the following subsidiary designations for acupuncturists: "Traditional acupuncture; Western medical acupuncture; auricular acupuncture." In addition, the title of a "Traditional Chinese Medicine Practitioner" might be supplemented by "(herbal medicine and acupuncture), or (herbal medicine), or (acupuncture)." [46]

The DH consulted many professional organizations for their response to its proposals. While the majority of responses indicated support for the introduction of statutory regulation of CAM, the BacC raised a number of concerns [47]. In our context, the criticism of the proposed titles is of special interest: "It was suggested that there was no commonly agreed definition of Traditional Chinese Medi-

cine and that the public may not therefore understand the title's meaning." [48]. The BAAB [49] clearly stated: "The Board considers that the titles 'acupuncturist' and 'herbal medicine practitioner' are clear to the public and that these two titles should be the basis for registration." Though there is no explicit criticism of the proposed subsidiary "Western medical acupuncture," this was not welcomed by any of the professional organizations.

Hybridization in Acupuncture Education

Is it appropriate to interpret acupuncture education as minimizing acupuncture? In her observations of the New York acupuncture scene, Hare [50] presented a hybridization of a Confucian and Daoist model of order and moderation and US individualism that may be forming a US type of Chinese medicine. She reported about a dentist who had been trained in New York, and later on studied acupuncture in the UK, and commented on Chinese philosophy and acupuncture: "Lao Tze is also the basis of Chinese acupuncture—'affect without enforcing.' ... The foreword of the *I Ching*[20] is all about Five Element acupuncture." [51]

But we would hardly meet a German (medical or non-medical) acupuncturist, who would be able to comment on classical Chinese texts. Acupuncture education is framed by the rules of *further* medical education, not as learning a totally new medical system. To obtain the additional title "acupuncturist" a German physician must be recognized as a medical specialist and undergo 200 hours of acupuncture training consisting of 120 hours of theory lessons, 60 hours of acupuncture treatment practice, and 20 hours of seminar courses debating treatment cases. These requirements are quantitatively the same for all additional titles, and there is neither a special reduction nor a special extension for acupuncturists.

University education in Chinese medicine or acupuncture is in its very beginning. The well-established professional organizations offer a lesser and a greater diploma. The DAAAM (see Table **1** for an overview of organizations) offers a basic course of 140 units, which leads to the Diplom A qualification. A further 210 units are required for Diplom B. In the DÄGfA the basic course (Diplom A of 144 hours) previously offered has now been adapted to the new guidelines for qualification as a "medical acupuncturist" mentioned above. A higher qualification (Diplom B of 200 hours), which can be achieved in one of three different course structures, is also offered. The B diplomas include much more medical and philosophical Chinese background, than the A diplomas do, and sometimes offer a small special education in a special medical branch.

The largest non-medical acupuncture association, the Association for Classical Acupuncture and TCM (AGTCM), offers basic courses that last three years and consist of at least 750 hours, as well as a wide variety of specialist courses of varying durations, underlying a credit system. A certain degree of attendance is compulsory to continue membership.

The British BMAS offers basic and advanced courses to physicians and to other medical professionals. A four-day course and a record of 30 treated cases lead to the Certificate of Basic Competence (COBC). After another 100 hours' training and more than 100 case records candidates may apply for the Certificate of Accreditation (COA).

The BAcC offers education to non-professionals. The required training was 2400 hours since 1989, and it increased to 3600 hours in 2002. About one-third of this training covers anatomy and physiology, pathology, and other related medical topics.[21] (See also "Chinese Medicine Education in the UK," p. 213, Education.)

If you look at the number of lessons required for formal registration in Britain, those for medical professionals hardly differ from the German figures. Those for non-professionals are very high, but include a basic medical education. In this respect, it is impossible to compare the German situation directly, because the education of the non-medically qualified *Heilpraktiker* has not been regulated.[22]

So far, we have not discussed minimal acupuncture, but there are two developments that directly relate to this topic. The first is a medical conception minimizing acupuncture for standard therapies. The second is an unexpected outcome of acupuncture RCTs in Germany.

Minimal Acupuncture as a British Medical Conception

Dr Felix Mann had trained many physicians in acupuncture. As a junior doctor, he had gone to France and Germany in the mid-1950s, where he was introduced into acupuncture. He completed his studies in Peking, Nanking, and Shanghai. After his return to London in 1958, he started to teach acupuncture in his house in London West End [52]. Though Mann had started as a traditional Chinese-style acupuncturist, he developed his own methods later. Dr Anthony Campbell, a homoeopathic physician, who became trained in acupuncture by Mann in 1977, recalled: "The first thing Felix told us was that he did not believe in the traditional apparatus of Yin and Yang, meridians, acupuncture points and so on." [53]

In 1992, Mann published the thesis that acupuncture does work, but its efficacy is not limited to needling the classical points. Campbell propagated the credo of a "modern, non-traditionalist acupuncturist." He explained the efficacy of acupuncture via the nervous system, via endogenous opioids, etc., and he taught his practice to doctors and physiotherapists in two-day courses [54]. The development of non-classical forms of acupuncture was, on the other hand, due to conceptualizing randomized clinical trials in acupuncture. For superficial acupuncture, special needles were invented. They did not penetrate the skin, but sprang back into their holder. For sham acupuncture, the needle is inserted at a different site from that of the traditional treatment points.[23] In some of the studies that sham acupuncture had been developed for it proved to be more efficient than a "normal" placebo.[24] This result was taken up by some researchers and doctors[25] for therapeutic means, because it "can be learnt by medical practitioners in short courses of between 2 and 5 days, which aim to teach knowledge and skills sufficient to treat conditions that are commonly seen in primary care." [58]

Ballegard [59] found "no significant difference between the effect of the traditional and non-standard acupuncture on angina pectoris, both effecting a reduction in nitroglycerin consumption and in anginal attacks. Thus, it was concluded that the clinical improvement was due either to a specific effect of both methods or a placebo effect."

Davies [60] could not report statistically significant results from his study on minimal and traditional acupuncture in minimizing hot flushes following breast cancer treatment.

Ross, White, and Ernst [58] give an account of the use of "minimal acupuncture" for neck pain: "Doctors were free to decide what areas or acupuncture points to treat ... This ... study has found the majority of patients ... were apparently successfully treated with between one and six brief sessions of minimal acupuncture."

This form of acupuncture is dis-embedded from the Chinese philosophical background. Indeed, it is intentionally dis-embedded. But this medical conception is in the minority.

German Randomized Trials on Acupuncture

There has been a debate about how to prove the efficacy and efficiency of CAM therapies since the 1990s. Authors often aimed at better recognition of these therapies by medical science, at reimbursement of the patients by insurance schemes, and at separating the wheat from the chaff. While RCTs were criticized as scarcely viable for CAM therapies, and even for ethical aspects [61], RCTs became increasingly accepted in the CAM scene, as may be seen from the foundation of the journal *Forschende Komplementärmedizin*. In 1999, a group of German health insurance companies initiated acupuncture RCTs.

Patients who had been treated for chronic diseases like low back pain, arthrosis, and mi-

graine for a longer time were offered acupuncture treatment. In a first stage of the tests, the patients were interviewed by scientific institutes to ascertain whether they were feeling better or not. The second stage of the tests was formed by one-side blinded[26] randomized studies, which were performed at the physicians' offices, and supervised by university institutes. The physicians had to hold the (lesser) Diplom A at least, and they received special training for the tests. The patients who were willing to take part in the trials were divided into groups according to the respective disease, and then subdivided into three groups. Again:[27]

- The first group received a series of 12 semi-standardized acupuncture sessions. They were needled at certain basic points according to a common acupuncture textbook; some other points could be needled in addition. The physicians aimed at producing a *de qi* sensation.[28]
- The second group was supposed to be the control group. These patients received sham acupuncture, which was called minimal acupuncture in the directory. Physicians were told not to talk of a placebo. They should neither manipulate the needles, nor produce a *de qi* sensation. The needles should be inserted into at least five out of ten points, which varied for the three diseases treated, and which were not common acupuncture points. Three experienced acupuncturists and two associations[29] had agreed upon the localization of these points [64].
- The third group received verum acupuncture, but only after six months on a waiting list.

The most astonishing results were those of the minimal (sham) acupuncture groups.[30] The researchers had presented the first results at a conference in Berlin in May 2004. The results were almost the same for all diseases tested. First published were those on patients with tension headache [63] and with migraine [62]. Two hundred and ninety-six headache patients were randomized in the way described above. In the end, 132 received verum acupuncture, 63 minimal acupuncture,[31] and 75 were on the waiting list. The number of days with headache decreased by 7.2 days in the verum, by 6.6 days in the 'minimal,' and by 1.5 days in the waiting list groups. The response rates[32] were 46% in the verum, 35% in the minimal acupuncture, and 4% in the waiting list groups.[33]

As for the migraine patients, 304 were randomly assigned, and finally valid data were available for 132 patients in the verum acupuncture, for 76 in the sham acupuncture groups, and for 64 patients on the waiting list. The days with headache of moderate or severe intensity decreased by a mean of 2.2 days in the verum, of 2.2 days in the sham acupuncture, and of 0.8 days in the waiting list groups. The response rates to the treatment were 51% in the verum, 53% in the sham acupuncture, and 15% in the waiting list groups.

"Results in the sham acupuncture tended to be slightly better than those in the acupuncture group, but the differences were not significant." [67] Indeed, the results for the sham (or minimal) acupuncture group are most astonishing. How is the phenomenon explained by the authors? First, they stress that the data are valid, and that the sham results are above those expected from a mere placebo: "An interesting finding of our trial is the strong response to sham acupuncture. The improvement over and the differences compared with the waiting list group are clearly clinically relevant. ... response rates in placebo groups are typically around 30%. ... The strong response to sham acupuncture in our trial could be a chance finding. It could also be that the study patients with high expectations of acupuncture treatment reported positively biased data. However, the validity of our results is supported by the consistency of findings as judged by a variety of instruments including a headache diary and validated questionnaires on quality of life, disability, and emotional aspects of pain." [68]

The authors offer two explanations. The first one is that of an active placebo:[34] "... we cannot rule out that this [sham] intervention may have had some physiological effects. The non-specific physiological effects of needling

may include local alteration in circulation and immune function as well as neurophysiological and neurochemical responses. ... our minimal acupuncture intervention was clearly an appropriate sham control although it might not be an inert placebo." [68]

The second explanation offered is that of potent placebo effects: "Another explanation for the improvements that we observed could be that acupuncture and sham acupuncture are associated with particularly potent placebo effects. There is some evidence that complex medical interventions or medical devices have higher placebo effects than medication. Furthermore, acupuncture treatment has characteristics that are considered relevant in the context of placebo effects, including exotic conceptual framework, emphasis on the 'individual as a whole,' frequent patient–practitioner contacts, and the repeated 'ritual' of needling." [68][35]

While the first explanation is situated on a physiological level, the second is a cultural one: ritual and holism, associated with alternative medicine, might produce health effects in their respective believers. I do not aim to search for the correct answer. But which consequences might these results have? If the classical "very" acupuncture points are less relevant than the needling process itself, this may first strengthen the tendency to disembed acupuncture from its philosophical and cultural background, and second, weaken the motivations of Western physicians to achieve the higher diplomas offered by the acupuncturist organizations. Trigger or acupuncture points, Indian chakras or Chinese meridians:[36] a great melting pot of medical conceptions is offered behind a number of convergent practices. (See also "Acupuncture Quo Vadis?—On the Current Discussion Around its Effectiveness and 'Point Specificity'," p. 29; "Comments on the German Acupuncture Studies," p. 37, Research; and "Acupuncture in Germany in 2006," p. 191, Professional Developments, Legislation, and Regulation.)

Conclusion

Arriving in the West, acupuncture has certainly been dis-embedded from its original philosophical and theoretical background. But this is at least partly true for TCM in China itself already, as previously stated. In Western practice, acupuncture has become isolated from other forms of Chinese medical practices. It has become hybridized with various forms of biomedicine, and also with other CAM therapies, especially with homeopathy. But this does not necessarily imply that acupuncture has become minimized. Some medical professional organizations and a few universities take heed of acupuncture in the same way as other medical specialties are heeded. Minimal acupuncture as a medical conception remains marginal. But the extension of Chinese medical philosophy and a re-embedding of acupuncture to its original background cannot be expected. With regard to hybridization, it has opened paths for empirical research. Though you will look in vain for non-hybridized cultural forms, it makes sense to look for different modes of hybridization. In Western Europe, I could present some forms of acupuncture hybridized with biomedicine, but that does not necessarily imply that they represent minimized shadows of an Eastern original.

Notes

1. A special thanks to Robert Frank, Berlin, who commented on earlier versions of this article.
2. In the field of medicine, the Asian original admired is less Chinese than Indian medicine. See, for instance, Bode [5] for the industrial production of Indian pharmaceuticals, or Zimmermann's criticism [6] of the Maharishi Ayurveda. For a history of yoga that shows its spiritualization before its way to the West, see De Michelis [7].
3. See Nordstrom [10], who found many faces of Ayurveda in modern India.
4. *Qi* can be described as similar to an immaterial force/energy. Its paths through the human body can be localized on 12 routes, called channels or meridians, most of them connected

to an organ, even though these organs differ strongly from their biomedical equivalents.
5. See in a similar way, but less enthusiastically, Brown and Zavestoski [15] on social movements in health.
6. Some 71% of the Chinese population never visited a traditional Chinese doctor, though 54% agreed that for some health problems traditional might be better than Western medicine. Some 59% agreed that traditional medicine is too expensive to be used regularly [17].
7. Researchers who have written on the subject distinguish between various stages; see [18–24].
8. In France, e.g., Berlioz in 1816, Haime in 1819, Beclard in 1821, Sarlandière in 1825; in Britain, e.g., Churchill in 1822; in Germany, e.g., Kerber in 1832; in Italy, e.g., Da Camino since 1834.
9. For a modern form see Ebert [26].
10. Neural therapy following Huneke is a medical concept eliminating disruptive fields by injecting local anesthetics.
11. The Chair for Natural Healing Science at the University of Essen, established in 2004. Professor Gustav J. Dobos is holding this Chair.
12. Its members come from a federal organization of physicians practicing within statutory sickness funds, and from these funds themselves. It admits new diagnostic and therapeutic methods, etc.
13. The information on the UK owes many details to Elisabeth Hsu and Verena Timbul, Oxford.
14. "...the so called Worsley style ... is very 'personality' based and has a strong emphasis on emotional manifestations of the 5 phases" (www.medicinechinese.com/A55800/tcmforum.nsf; 9/15/2002) [36].
15. Felix Mann, for instance, was another early proponent [37].
16. There are Five Element acupuncture traditions, mostly in Taiwan, Japan, and Vietnam. They derive Chinese Tang dynasty (7th to 10th centuries AD). See Adam Atman [38].
17. According to some authors [17, 39], they practice Chinese medicine outside the formal professional system.
18. Personal information provided by John Wheeler, London, February 2002.
19. This board was set up in 1989 by the precursor of the BAcC as an independent body that was intended to set the standards of accreditation for courses offering training in acupuncture.
20. A classical Chinese text, edited and translated by R. Wilhelm and C.F. Baynes in 1950.

21. Personal information provided by John Wheeler, London, February 2002.
22. They must pass an examination, whose regulations vary for the single German states, and even municipalities. The examination requires no special education.
23. Ballegard [55].
24. For an overview of studies using acupuncture and sham acupuncture in RCTs see Cummings [56].
25. There is a stream in the BMAS advocating this "modern, Western-orientated form" of acupuncture [57].
26. Blinding has been introduced into clinical trials (originally of drugs) in order to correct personal influences. One-side blinding means that the physician knows whether he/she gives a verum or a placebo, while the patient does not. In double blinding neither the physician nor the patient knows.
27. For the trials see Linde et al [62] and Melchart et al [63].
28. An itching feeling of the circulation of *qi*, starting from the needled point, and caused by manipulating the needle.
29. The DÄGfA and the International Society for Chinese Medicine, both situated in Munich.
30. A Norwegian study on sinusitis patients produced no clear results [65].
31. The authors of the ART-Studies sometimes call the control group minimal [63] and at other times the sham acupuncture group [62].
32. Defined by a reduction of at least 50 % in headache days.
33. For a smaller study on acupuncture for chronic headache see Coeytaux et al. [66].
34. This explanation has been used by Ezzo et al. in: Stux and Hammerschlag [69] before, as a result of acupuncture systematic reviews.
35. See also the debate on the results of sham acupuncture; National Center for Complementary and Alternative Medicine: odp.od.nih.gov/consensus/cons/107/107_statement.htm.
36. See Shang in Stux and Hammerschlag [69] for a comparison.

References

1. Elwert G. Kulturbegriffe und Entwicklungspolitik—über "soziokulturelle Bedingungen der Entwicklung." In: *Kulturen und Innovationen: Festschrift für Wolfgang Rudolph*. Berlin; 1996: 51–88.
2. Nederveen PJ. Globalisation as hybridisation. *Int Soc* 1994;9:180.
3. Rosaldo R. Foreword. In: Garcia Canclini N. *Hybrid Cultures: Strategies for Entering and Leaving Modernity*. Minneapolis: Pine Forge Press; 1995: xi–xvii.
4. Ritzer G. *The McDonaldization of Society.* Thousand Oaks: University of Minnesota Press; 1993.
5. Bode M. *Ayurvedic and Unani Health and Beauty Products: Reworking India's Medical Tradition.* Amsterdam: Amsterdam University; 2004.
6. Zimmermann F. Gentle purge: the flower power of Ayurveda. In: Leslie C, Young A, editors. *Paths to Asian Medical Knowledge.* Berkeley: University of California Press; 1992: 209–223.
7. De Michelis E. *A History of Modern Yoga: Patañjali and Western Esotericism.* London: Continuum, International Publishing Group; 2004.
8. Hsu E. *The Transmission of Chinese Medicine.* Cambridge: Cambridge University Press; 1999.
9. Scheid V. *Chinese Medicine in Contemporary China.* Durham: Churchill Livingstone; 2002.
10. Nordstrom CR. Exploring pluralism—the many faces of Ayurveda. In: *Soc Sci Med* 1988;27(5): 479–489.
11. Hsu op.cit.:235ff.
12. Barnes LL. The acupuncture wars: the professionalizing of American acupuncture—a view from Massachusetts. *Med Anthropol* 2003;22:261–301.
13. Ibid.:268.
14. Baer HA. The growing interest of biomedicine in complementary and alternative medicine: a critical perspective. *Med Anthropol Q* 2002; 16:405.
15. Brown P and Zavestoski S. Social movements in health: an introduction. *Sociol Health Illn* 2004; 26:679–694.
16. Barnes op.cit.:291.
17. Sproston K et al. *Health and Lifestyles of the Chinese Population in England.* London: Health Education Authority; 1999.
18. Arnold H-J. *Die Geschichte der Akupunktur in Deutschland.* Heidelberg: Verlag Karl F Haug; 1976.
19. Lu, Gwei-Djen and Needham J. *Celestial Lancets. A History and Rationale of Acupuncture and Moxa.* Cambridge: Cambridge University Press; 1980.
20. Unschuld PU. *Medicine in China. A History of Ideas.* Berkeley; 1985.
21. Hsu E. Outline of the history of acupuncture in Europe. *J Chin Med* 1989;29:28–32.

22. Saks M. *Profession and the Public Interest. Medical Power, Altruism, and Alternative Medicine.* London/New York: Routledge; 1995.
23. Jütte R. *Geschichte der Alternativen Medizin.* Munich: Verlag CH Beck; 1996.
24. Bivins R. *Acupuncture, Expertise and Cross-cultural Medicine.* New York: Palgrave Macmillan; 2000.
25. Gleditsch J. 50 Jahre DÄGfA. Zur Geschichte der deutschen Ärztegesellschaft für Akupunktur. *Deutsche Zeitschrift für Akupunktur* 2001; Special Issue 2a:176–191.
26. Ebert H. *Homöosiniatrie. Die Komplementarität von Homöopathie und Akupunktur in neuer und erweiterter Form.* Heidelberg: Verlag Karl F Haug; 1992.
27. Hahn RE. *Die Diskussion um die Akupunktur in der DDR.* Med. Diss. Leipzig (MS); 2002: 50ff, 70ff.
28. Ibid.:44.
29. Ibid.:59ff.
30. Ibid.:64.
31. Frank R, Stollberg G. Cenceptualising Hybridisation—on the Diffusion of Asian Medical Knowledge to Germany. In: *International Sociology* 2004;19:71–88.
32. Frank R, Stollberg G. Medical Acupuncture in Germany: Patterns of Consumerism among Physicians and Patients. In: *Sociology of Health & Illness* 2004;26:351–372.
33. Gleditsch op. cit.:181.
34. Bundesausschuss der Ärzte und Krankenkassen. *Akupunktur. Zusammenfassender Bericht des Arbeitsausschusses „Ärztliche Behandlung" des Bundesausschusses der Ärzte und Krankenkassen über die Beratungen der Jahre 1999 und 2000 zur Bewertung der Akupunktur gemäß § 135 Abs. 1 SGB V.* Cologne, 2001.
35. Eckman P. Tracing the historical transmission of traditional acupuncture to the West: in search of the Five Element transfer lineage and a higher vision. *Am J Acu* 1997;25(1):59–69.
36. Barnes op.cit.
37. Baldry P. The integration of acupuncture within medicine in the UK—the British Medical Acupuncture Society's 25th anniversary. *Acupunct Med* 2005;23:2–12.
38. Acupuncture articles. http://adamatman.com/articles/.shtml. 15th September, 2005.
39. Gervais M-C and Jovchelovitch S. *The Health Beliefs of the Chinese Community in England: A Qualitative Research Study.* London: Health Education Authority; 1998.
40. Acupuncture Regulatory Working Group (ACRWG). *The Statutory Regulation of the Acupuncture Profession.* London: The Prince of Wales' Foundation for Integrated Health; 2003.
41. Fulder, Stephen 1988: *The Handbook of Complementary Medicine,* 2nd ed. Oxford: Oxford University Press (1st ed. 1984).
42. Sharma UM. Using alternative therapies: marginal medicine and central concerns. In: Davey B, Gray A, Seale C, editors. *Health and Disease. A Reader,* 2nd edition. Buckingham/Philadelphia: Open University Press; 1995:38–44.
43. Tovey P. Contingent legitimacy: UK alternative practitioners and inter-sectoral acceptance. *Soc Sci Med* 1997;45:1129–1133.
44. British Medical Association. *Acupuncture: efficiency, safety and practice.* London: BMJ Bookshop; 2000.
45. ACRWG op. cit.:20.
46. Department of Health (DH). *Regulation of Herbal Medicine and Acupuncture.* www.dh.gov.uk; 2004:20.
47. Department of Health (DH). *Statutory Regulation of Herbal Medicine and Acupuncture. Report on the Consultation.* www.dh.gov.uk; 2005:4.
48. Ibid.:6.
49. British Acupuncture Accreditation Board (BAAB). *Response to the Department of Health Consultation Document on the Regulation of Herbal Medicine and Acupuncture.* www.acupuncture.org.uk/content/baab; 2004:4.
50. Hare ML. The emergence of an urban US Chinese medicine. *Med Anthropol Q* 1993;7:31.
51. Ibid.:42.
52. Baldry op.cit.
53. Campbell A. A doctor's view of acupuncture: traditional Chinese theories are unnecessary. *Complement Ther Med* 1998;6:152.
54. Ibid.:152–155.
55. Ballegard S. Acupuncture and the cardiovascular system: a scientific challenge. *Acu Med* 1998;16:5ff. www.medical-acupuncture.co.uk/journal/may1998/one.shtml.
56. Cummings M. Research review. *Acu Med* 2004; 22:22–225.
57. Baldry op.cit.:10.
58. Ross J, White A, Ernst E. Western, minimal acupuncture for neck pain: a cohort study. *Acu Med* 1999;17:5.
59. Ballegard op.cit.:11ff.
60. Davies FM. The effect of acupuncture treatment on the incidence and severity of hot flushes experienced by women following treatment for breast cancer: a comparison of traditional and

minimal acupuncture. In: *The European Journal of cancer* 2001;37:S438.

61. Kiene H. *Der Wissenschaftsstreit am Ende des 20 Jahrhunderts.* Stuttgart–New York: Schattauer Verlag; 1994.

62. Linde K, Streng A, Jürgens S, et al. Acupuncture for patients with migraine: a randomized controlled trial. *JAMA* 2005;293;(17):2118–2125.

63. Melchart D, Linde K, Streng A, et al. Acupuncture Randomized Trials (ART) in Patients with Migraine or Tension-type Headache—Design and Protocols. In: *Forschende Komplementärmedizin und Klassische Naturheilkunde* 2003;10:179–184.

64. Linde op.cit.:187.

65. Rössberg E, Larsson PG, Birkeflet O, Söholt L-E, Stavem K. Comparison of traditional Chinese acupuncture, minimal acupuncture at non-acupoints and conventional treatment for chronic sinusitis. *Complement Ther Med* 2005;13:4–10.

66. Coeytaux RR, Kaufman JS, Kaptchuk TJ, et al. A randomized, controlled trial of acupuncture for chronic daily headache. *Headache* 2005;45:1113–1123.

67. Linde op.cit.:2122.

68. Linde op.cit.:2124.

69. Stux G. and Hammerschlag R, editors. *Clinical Acupuncture: Scientific Basis.* Berlin: Springer Verlag; 2001:29.

The original version of this article will be published in: Dominique Schirmer, Gernot Saalmann, Christl Kessler (Eds.), *Hybridising East and West. Tales Beyond Westernisation: Empirical Contributions to the Debates on Hybridity,* Münster, LIT-Verlag (in print).

Education and Practice of Chinese Medicine in Taiwan

Nigel Wiseman, PhD, Guishan, Taiwan

Introduction

Although in the 1920s the Nationalist government of the newly founded Republic of China almost abolished Chinese medicine, it nevertheless allowed it to coexist with Western medicine after its withdrawal to Taiwan. In the country today, the number of physicians practicing Chinese medicine is only one-tenth of those practicing Western medicine, and currently acupuncture plays a much smaller role than medicinal therapy. The widespread use of Chinese medicine, not least as a result of the interest of Western industrial countries, has contributed to its incorporation into the health service, which three years ago was extended to the whole population. The education of Chinese medical education in Taiwan is gradually being absorbed into the university education system. Nevertheless, attempts to integrate its practice with that of Western medicine have so far achieved limited success.

Western interest in Chinese medicine has undergone a huge growth in popularity since the early 1970s. Nixon's historical visit to the People's Republic of China (PRC) brought news that the Chinese were experimenting in the use of the country's ancient needle therapy to provide analgesia to permit the performance of surgical operations. Mao Zedong's government promoted the use of Chinese medicine, including acupuncture, as part of national health care, and government support on the mainland has encouraged Westerners to associate Chinese medicine with the mainland rather than with any other part of the Chinese-speaking world.

History

The development of Chinese medicine in Taiwan is of interest to us if we are to understand how it has progressed in the modern age. Taiwan is the only part of China to have remained under the Republic of China flag since the overthrow of the Qing dynasty in 1911, and the development of Chinese medicine on the island shows how it has fared in a Western capitalist environment of modernization for nearly a hundred years. With the economic failure of socialist policies and increasing liberalization in the PRC, the development of Chinese medicine in Taiwan may in fact provide important indicators for future trends in the Chinese region as a whole.

To understand the general development of Chinese medicine in the modern era, we should go back to the nineteenth century, when China's contacts with the West first began to intensify.

The incursion of European traders in China in the nineteenth century brought the Chinese to the painful realization that their great civilization was a thing of the past, and that they were technologically backward, militarily weak, and economically impoverished. The dominating reaction to this plight was the conviction that China had to acquire Western knowledge if the country were to compete and survive in the world.

The Chinese began to acquire a vast gamut of Western learning, starting with military and technological knowledge. Although China had its own sophisticated healing traditions, the medical field certainly did not escape Western influence. Because missionaries, who followed traders into China, used healing of the sick as a concrete embodiment of Christian love, Western medicine was introduced by foreigners rather more than by Chinese initiative.

Western medicine was accepted because it was the medicine of a civilization accorded high prestige, as it was based on a scientific approach seen to be at the core of Western economic superiority, and not least, perhaps, because Western medicine shared certain similarities with Chinese medicine.

With the fall of Qing imperial rule, the Republic of China was established by the Kuomintang or Nationalist Party, which ushered in a period of intense Westernization. Chinese medicine had its defenders, and support for it was strong enough to prevent attempts within the government to abolish it. Nevertheless, support was not strong enough to allow it to be incorporated into the education system of that time. It became a folk medicine, tolerated but not encouraged. The cultural eclipse is neatly symbolized by a change in terminology. What had been simply been called *yi*—"medicine"—now came to be referred to as *zhong yi*, "Chinese medicine."

At the end of the 1920s, civil war broke out between the ruling Nationalists and insurgent communists. The situation was exacerbated when the Japanese invaded China in 1937. In 1945, Nationalist forces succeeded in winning back Taiwan from the Japanese, who had occupied the island for 60 years. As they found themselves losing the civil war, Taiwan offered a haven free of communists, to which they retreated.

The Japanese invasion and the civil war left the communists in control of the mainland and the Nationalists now only in control of Taiwan. In both the mainland and Taiwan, Western medicine was adopted as the principal form of medicine, and as the main arbiter of all health and hygiene matters. The difference in policy between the two governments is reflected in the development of medicine.

Modern Development of Chinese Medicine in Taiwan

In mainland China, Chinese medicine was actively promoted alongside, though not to the same degree as, Western medicine. Various reasons have been given to explain why this occurred. One is that while resources were insufficient to provide adequate Western health care for the entire population, Chinese doctors were nevertheless available in large numbers.

Another is that Chinese medicine was considered to be the only method the Chinese people experienced in fighting against disease. A third is that it was thought that Chinese medicine could be made into a mouthpiece for communist ideology.

In Taiwan, on the other hand, the Nationalists continued to keep Chinese medicine as a popular feature of health care. In so doing, they were in fact continuing the same basic policy line that the Japanese had applied during their 60-year colonial rule of the island that the Nationalists had ended in 1945.

To provide some idea of the relative importance accorded to Chinese and Western medicine, respectively, in the Chinese area, it is interesting to note that the ratio of Chinese to Western medical doctors is about one in ten in Taiwan, while in the PRC it is about one in three. Despite the huge difference in these figures, it is nevertheless evident that Chinese medicine is accorded a much lower priority than Western medicine in the mainland in comparison to that in Taiwan.

Many people returning to the West after visiting China have the impression that the PRC government accords equal status to Chinese and Western medicine. As a result of nationalist pride encouraged by the PRC government, people receiving foreign students and guests have tended to exaggerate the importance accorded to Traditional Chinese Medicine (TCM) in the PRC. But the propaganda should be understood against hard facts. Resources invested by the mainland government in training physicians are actually a more reliable indicator.

Since antiquity, a wide variety of methods have been available for maintaining and restoring health. Besides the classical forms of medicine, based on traditional literature, acupuncture and medicinal therapy, there have been many others: orthodox drug therapy, acupuncture, herbalism, shamanist practices, prescription pharmacy, patent medicine pharmacy, bone-setting, various forms of *tui na* and hygienic exercises, health-protecting amulets, etc. Here it is interesting to note that although acupuncture is the Chinese healing practice best known in the West, it has not been widely practiced in China for centuries.

In the PRC, where the government tightly controls publications, magical elements have largely been expunged. The modern form of Chinese medicine that has evolved in the PRC, where it is rather misleadingly called Traditional Chinese Medicine (TCM) in English, is a modernized version of various literary traditions. The encouragement of Chinese medicine in the mainland has given rise to the production of a vast amount of literature that has drawn out what is now considered to be the useful elements of TCM. These elements have been presented in a way acceptable to present-day readers, often combined with modern medical perspectives.

In Taiwan, magical and religious practices have been subject to no such restriction. Thus, supernatural healing practices that have been suppressed in the PRC have survived in Taiwan. Although Taiwan is, in many ways, more modernized and Westernized than the mainland, it has been much more conservative in the realm of traditional healing practices.

Arthur Kleinmann, in his classic study on traditional healing practices in Taiwan, describes the large variety of traditional practices designed to maintain and restore health that still survived in Taiwan at the end of the 1970s. Anyone wishing to understand what we call "Chinese medicine" or "Traditional Chinese Medicine" in the traditional context of healing practices and in the context of culture should read Kleinmann's book.

Regulation, Practice, and Education

In spite of its laissez-faire attitude to traditional healing practices, the Nationalist government has nevertheless tried to regulate the practice of Chinese medicine. In the 1940s, provisions for a Special Examination for Chinese Medicine (*zhong yi te kao*) and licensing were introduced for Chinese medical physicians. This has survived to this day, although it is now to be phased out.

According to these provisions, certain texts are prescribed for the examination but no educational framework was established. Although numerous privately run cram-schools have sprung up to get candidates through the examination, no university level course has ever been established with the specific aim of training students to pass this examination. For the past few years, students passing the Special Examination have been required to receive practical instruction, but there has never been any formal instruction prior to the examination. Patently, the aim of the regulations was to institute standards in the field, in which training traditionally followed the master–apprenticeship pattern.

Today, the Special Examination requires students to have a rudimentary knowledge of basic Western medicine and very broad and detailed knowledge of traditional Chinese medical literature, notably the *Huangdi Neijing, Nanjing, Shanghanlun,* and *Yizhong Jinjian,* etc. The examination is notable in that it requires a large amount of memorization and is notoriously hard to pass.

According to government regulations, only those passing the licensing examination are allowed to practice Chinese medicine. Nevertheless, because Chinese pharmacists are allowed to sell Chinese medicines without a physician's prescription, this enables them to advise people on what remedies to buy, or even provide a diagnosis.

In 1958, a group of Chinese medical enthusiasts established China Medical College in Taichung. This was the first ever college in the history of the Republic of China to offer a university-level program in Chinese medicine. The Department of Medicine trained students in both Chinese and Western medicine. The Chinese medicine taught in the School of Chinese Medicine covers more or less the same content as the Special Examination. Emphasis is placed on familiarity with classical literature. The national examination that students of the Department of Chinese Medicine take, however, is different from, and notably easier than, the Special Examination.

After graduation, students were allowed to sit a national examination to obtain a license to practice Chinese medicine. If they passed this, they could then take the national licensing examination for Western medicine.

The dual licensing system for students of the School of Chinese Medicine has continued to the present. Its success has always been hotly debated. It is generally admitted that most students entering the Chinese medical department do so because they previously failed to obtain high enough scores in the national university entrance examination to enter a regular Western medical college. On average, about 60 % of graduates of the Chinese medical department go into Western, rather than Chinese medicine.

Enthusiasm for Chinese medicine in the Department of Medicine was so low that in 1960 it ceased the dual program instruction in Chinese and Western medicine. Chinese medicine was transferred to a newly created Department of Chinese Medicine, while the Department of Medicine henceforth provided instruction only in Western medicine. Since that time, the Department of Medicine has for most of the time had a larger intake of students than the Department of Chinese Medicine. In the meantime, a standard array of medical college departments has sprung up, including pharmacy, nursing, public health, medical technology, etc. In deference to the founding goals of China Medical College, students in most departments learn, or at least have the opportunity to learn, something of Chinese medicine. Nevertheless, as the College has grown, the Chinese medical element has shrunk proportionally.

In reaction to the continual brain drain from Chinese to Western medicine, a Post-Baccalaureate School of Chinese Medicine was established in 1984. Graduates of this school were to be allowed to take only the Chinese medical licensing examination that students of the Department of Chinese medicine sat. The Post-Baccalaureate curriculum includes quite a lot of instruction in basic Western medicine, but not nearly as much as that which is in the curriculum of the School of Chinese Medicine. As the name suggests, the Post-Baccalaureate School only takes in students that have at least a bachelor's degree in some other field.

The Post-Baccalaureate School of Chinese Medicine takes in as many students as the School of Chinese Medicine. The five-year course is particularly attractive to graduates from other schools and departments that have less lucrative career openings.

As mentioned above, the curricula for the Special Examination and for the two Chinese medical departments of the China Medical College are quite traditional. As such, they differ somewhat from the PRCs modernized version of Chinese medicine, which places more emphasis on modern literature synthesizing traditions than on study of the classics. Taiwan has been isolated from the mainland, but nevertheless mainland literature has found its way into the island. Although books in the simplified characters were, until recently, banned in Taiwan, medical literature was smuggled in and reprinted with complex characters. Now, Taiwan's participation in the international copyright convention and relaxation of the ban on simplified characters has increased the availability of PRC TCM literature and allowed it to become popular background reading among students.

In 1980, China Medical College created its own teaching hospital. The hospital provides a full range of Western medical services, but also has a large Chinese medical department that is divided into various sections of internal medicine, traumatology, and acupuncture. All physicians in the Chinese Medical Department are qualified in both Western and Chinese medicine, but generally practice a traditional style of Chinese medicine, basing treatment largely on traditional Chinese medical diagnosis.

Influence of Insurance

In 1992, government health insurance, originally established for certain segments of the population only, was extended to a full national health service. Soon after, coverage for Chinese medical treatment was included. National health insurance covers drug therapy, acupuncture, and *tui na* for outpatients. Provisions to develop inpatient treatment of Chinese medicine generally wait to be accomplished.

The decision to incorporate Chinese medicine into the national insurance system has undoubtedly been encouraged by world interest in Chinese and other alternative medicines, and by Western precedents regarding insurance cover for acupuncture treatment.

The inclusion of Chinese medical treatment within the national insurance system has affected the structure of Chinese medicine. People who previously sought Chinese remedies are given greater encouragement to do so since they no longer have to pay for them. But the insurance system encourages such patients to go to licensed physicians only and not to traditional pharmacists providing advice about a choice of remedies, or any other traditional healing practices. In the future, we can therefore expect a diminishing plurality of traditional healing practices.

The national health insurance system favors industry since it only covers factory-produced powdered medicines; it does not cover crude drugs traditionally used in decoctions. Factory-produced powdered drugs are said to enable more exact control of drug quality and control of quantities in compound formulas. Such arguments have, of course, emanated from the factories producing the powders. Crude drugs are now becoming a luxury that people have to pay for themselves.

The inclusion of Chinese medicine within the national health system has encouraged many larger Western medical hospitals to establish Chinese medical departments. One other medical college, part of Changgung University, has also established a department of Chinese medicine, the students of which take the same examination as those of the China Medical College. Changgung Memorial Hospital has experimented with the integration of Chinese medicine with Western medicine. Unlike China Medical College Hospital, where Chinese medicine is considered a specialty in its own right, Changgung expects all its physicians to gain Western medical specialty qualifications. The result of this approach has been effectively to make Chinese medicine an optional therapy provided by physicians whose

principal training is in Western medicine. This has tended to encourage a lack of respect for Chinese medicine that has made the approach unsuccessful. The hospital's regulations are shortly to undergo revision for China Medical College's model to be adopted.

China Medical College has been slower to develop integration. It was only recently that China Medical College Hospital established a Department of Integrated Chinese Medicine, and the College created an Institute of Integrated Chinese and Western Medicine.

At the present time, the Special Examination physicians are the most numerous licensed Chinese medical physicians. They have their own, highly influential, Association of Chinese Medical Physicians, which is separate from that of medical college graduates. A bill to phase out the Special Examination has recently been passed, so that in future the only licensed physicians practicing Chinese medicine will be those who have graduated from a medical college, and have received as part of their training a greater or lesser amount of Western medicine. The future providers of Chinese health care in Taiwan will be working either in Chinese medical departments of Western medical hospitals or in individual or group practices, but in either case within the framework of the national health system.

Conclusion

Although the education and practice of Chinese medicine will increasingly be brought into the same framework, it remains to be seen to what extent and in what way Chinese medicine will actually be integrated with Western medicine. While on the mainland the government has supported Chinese medicine and imposed a modus vivendi with Western medicine, this cannot be done within the free academic environment of Taiwan. The speculative nature of its concepts makes Chinese medicine unacceptable to Taiwan's Western medical community as much as to that of the West.

Attitudes to Chinese medicine amongst its proponents in Taiwan differ from those of its Western proponents. In the West, supporters of Chinese medicine tend to see it as either an alternative or as complementary to Western medicine. Westerners perceive Chinese medicine to be natural and holistic, and therefore based on a philosophy entirely different from not only Western medicine but also science and technology.

The concerns of the Chinese are entirely different. Of paramount importance in their lives is the economic and scientific edge that the West has over them. They are more aware of the benefits than of the problems science and technology may cause. For the Chinese, Chinese medicine is still popular because it responds to traditional notions of health and sickness. It also retains its popularity because it allows for the traditional freedom of shopping around for cures rather than having to accept the often "single verdict" of Western medicine.

The Chinese medical community in Taiwan, as well as that within the PRC, believes that if Chinese medicine really does have any clinical value, it has to be possible to integrate it with any other clinically valuable medicine. It also believes that if it is to convince the rest of the world of the value of Chinese medicine, it has to prove its worth to the dominant modern medical community.

The problems with this stance are immense. There is no place in Western medicine for any medical practice that does not rest entirely on a scientific footing. Any form of Chinese medicine that is stripped of all of its many speculative concepts (for instance, channels, organ functions, and diagnostic categories of the pattern) would barely be Chinese medicine at all. The road ahead to proving the scientific bases of Chinese medicine is thus fraught with difficulties. Whether or not the challenge can successfully be met, before traditional ideas of health and sickness that currently continue to ensure the popularity of Chinese medicine fade away, remains to be seen.

Bibliography

1. Birch S, Felt RL. *Understanding Acupuncture.* London: Churchill Livingstone; 1999.
2. China Medical College. *Zhongguo Yiyao Xueyuan Ershi Nian* [China Medical College, 20 Years]; 1978.
3. China Medical College Taichung, Taiwan: http://www.cmc.edu.tw/english/indexe.htm.
4. Kleinmann A. *Patients and Healers in the Context of Culture: An Exploration of the Borderland between Anthropology, Medicine, and Psychiatry.* Berkeley: University of California Press; 1980.
5. R.O.C. Health Department. *Taiwan Diqu Gonggong Weisheng Fazhanshi* [History of Public Health in the Taiwan Area]. Taipei: Health Department of the Administrative Yuan; 1995.
6. Sivin N. *Traditional Medicine in Contemporary China.* Ann Arbor: Center for Chinese Studies, University of Michigan; 1987.
7. Unschuld PU. *Medicine in China: A History of Ideas.* Berkeley: University of California Press; 1985.
8. Unschuld PU. *Chinesische Medizin* [Chinese Medicine]. Munich: Verlag CH Beck; 1997.

Contact Details

Nigel Wiseman, PhD
School of Traditional Chinese Medicine,
Chang Gung University, Guishan, Taiwan

The Development, Regulation, and Practice of Traditional East Asian Medicine in Australia

Kylie O'Brien, PhD, Melbourne, Australia

The regulatory context for the practice of traditional East Asian medicine (TEAM), and more particularly Chinese medicine, in Australia is non-uniform across its seven states and territories. Each state/territory has its own legislation and regulations governing healthcare provision, including those relating to the statutory regulation of healthcare practitioners. Victoria became the first state in a Western country to regulate the practice of Chinese medicine comprehensively, with the passing of the Chinese Medicine Registration (CMR) Act in 2000. A form of self-regulation of Chinese medicine practice currently exists in all other states and territories via professional associations, though the states of Western Australia and New South Wales are considering statutory regulation.

Statutory Regulation of Chinese Medicine Practice in Victoria

Several factors provided the initial impetus for consideration of statutory regulation of Chinese medicine in Victoria. These included increasing complaints concerning herbal medicines to the (then) Victorian Health Protection Section's Therapeutic Goods Unit, a perceived increase in demand for, and use of, Chinese medicine in Victoria, and support for regulation from the Chinese medicine professional community [1]. Although statutory regulation of health occupations is the responsibility of individual state governments, rather than the Commonwealth government, the Australian Health Ministers' Advisory Council (AHMAC), established by state and Commonwealth health ministers to advise them on health matters, agreed that states should only proceed with statutory regulation of a new health occupation if the majority of states agree [1]. The AHMAC has agreed on a set of criteria and processes for deciding whether to proceed with statutory regulation of unregistered occupations, in order to develop a uniform approach to the regulation of health professions. The process of regulation of Chinese medicine practice in Victoria was thus guided by the AHMAC, in particular its "Working Group on Criteria and Process for Assessment of Regulatory Requirements for Unregulated Health Occupations," the purpose of which is to assess the application for statutory regulation from occupational groups. Essentially, Victoria became the test case in Australia for statutory regulation of Chinese medicine.

A review of the practice of Chinese medicine in Australia was commissioned in 1995 by the Victorian Department of Human Services, which included potential risks and benefits, workforce data, and analysis of the need for statutory regulation. A report entitled *Towards a Safer Choice: the Practice of Traditional Chinese Medicine in Australia* was produced. Its key recommendation was that: "Traditional Chinese Medicine practitioners be subject to statutory occupational regulation and that the focus of this regulation be the protection of the public by ensuring practitioners have adequate qualifications for safe and competent practice." [1] A series of discussion documents was presented for public comment in 1997 and 1998 by the Victorian Ministerial Advisory Committee on Traditional Chinese Medicine, which canvassed options for regulation and key recommendations in relation to the regulation of Chinese herbs currently restricted under drugs and poisons legislation. The Chinese Medicine Registration Act 2000 [2] was passed in Victorian parliament in May 2000, and the first Chinese Medicine Registration Board of Victoria was subsequently appointed.

Statutory regulation of Chinese medicine practice in Victoria is by "protection of title" rather than by "protection of practice." Essentially this means that, under the Chinese Medicine Registration Act 2000, it is an offence to use titles protected under the Act, including "Registered Acupuncturist," "Registered Chinese Medicine Practitioner," "Registered Chinese Herbal Medicine Practitioner," "Registered Oriental Medicine Practitioner," "Registered Chinese Herbal Dispenser," or any other title "calculated to induce a belief that the person is registered as a practitioner under this Act." [2] It is also an offence under the Act to claim to be registered under the Act or to "carry out any Act which is required to be carried out by or under an Act by a person registered as a practitioner under this Act." [2] It is also an offence to claim to be qualified to practice as a Chinese medicine practitioner.

The Victorian Chinese Medicine Register has three divisions: Acupuncture, Chinese Herbal Medicine, and Chinese Herbal Medicine Dispensing. As of 22nd February, 2006, there were 822 practitioners registered in Victoria: 329 in the division of Acupuncture, 32 in the division of Chinese Herbal Medicine Practitioners, and 459 registered in both. The process of registration in the division of Chinese Herbal Medicine Dispensing began in 2002, though to date only a small number of applications have been received by the Chinese Medicine Registration Board (CMRB) and none have yet been registered.

The CMRB consists of nine members: two non-practitioner members, one lawyer, and six practitioner members (practicing a minimum of five years). The CMRB's functions, outlined in Section 68 of the Chinese Medicine Registration Act 2000, include:

- Registration of practitioners who comply with the requirements of the Act.
- Regulation of the standards of practice of Chinese medicine and the dispensing of Chinese herbs.
- Receipt and investigation of complaints about practitioners.
- Approval of courses that provide qualifications for registration of Chinese medicine practitioners and Chinese herbal dispensers.
- Approval of courses of study or training that provide qualifications for endorsement

of registration to use Schedule 1 Chinese herbs (discussed later).
- Publication of codes for the guidance of registered practitioners about standards recommended by the Board relating to the practice of Chinese medicine, and the prescribing, labeling, storage, dispensing, and supply of Chinese herbs, including Schedule 1 poisons within the meaning of the Victorian Drugs, Poisons, and Controlled Substances Act 1981.

Statutory Regulation of Chinese Medicine Practice in Other Australian States/Territories

New South Wales and Western Australia are currently considering statutory regulation of Chinese medicine practice. The Committee on the Health Care Complaints Commission's *Report into Traditional Chinese Medicine* may be consulted for further information about the New South Wales process [3]. The discussion paper *Regulation of Practitioners of Chinese Medicine in Western Australia* [4] may be consulted for further information about potential regulation of Chinese medicine practice in Western Australia.

Access to Chinese Herbs in Australia

In Australia, access to a number of potentially toxic raw Chinese herbs is subject to state-based drugs and poisons legislation. Several Chinese herbs are listed in the schedules and appendices of the national Standard for the Uniform Prescribing of Drugs and Poisons (SUSDP). The SUSDP is a national classification system for drugs and poisons that is adopted by the individual states/territories to varying degrees into their legislation. Access to items, including Chinese herbs, that are listed in various schedules and appendices of state/territory poisons lists, is limited to certain registered health practitioners (such as registered medical practitioners, pharmacists, dentists, and veterinary surgeons) and excludes Chinese medicine practitioners.

In Victoria, Schedules 2–9 of the SUSDP have been adopted into the Victorian Poisons List, Schedule 1 of the SUSDP remaining unnamed and blank [5]. Under Victorian legislation, specifically the Victorian Drugs Poisons and Controlled Substances Act 1981, it is illegal for a Chinese medicine practitioner or dispenser to "obtain, possess, use, sell, or supply" herbs listed on the Victorian Poisons List, unless they are also a registered medical practitioner, dentist, veterinary surgeon, or pharmacist [5]. However, as a consequence of the passing of the Chinese Medicine Registration Act 2000, there were changes made to the Victorian Drugs Poisons and Controlled Substances Act 1981 that have provided a mechanism by which suitably qualified practitioners of Chinese herbal medicine may have access to Chinese herbs listed on the Victorian Poisons List.

Schedule 1 of the Victorian Poisons List has been renamed: "Poisons of plant, animal, or mineral origin that in the public interest should be available only from a person registered under the Chinese Medicine Registration Act 2000 or authorized under another Act."

The amendments to the Drugs Poisons and Controlled Substances Act 1981 empower the Victorian Minister for Health to directly amend the Victorian Poisons Code to specify substances to be included in Schedule 1 in the Poisons List, and amend, revoke, substitute, or insert substances [2]. Under Section 8 of the Chinese Medicine Registration Act 2000, suitably qualified Chinese herbal medicine practitioners and dispensers may have their registration endorsed to obtain, possess, use, sell, or supply herbs listed in Schedule 1 of the Victorian Poisons List [2]. Practitioners will be required to complete a CMRB-approved course of study to obtain endorsement; registration alone under the Chinese Medicine Registration Act 2000 is not sufficient to have access to Schedule 1 herbs. In addition, it is likely that the endorsement to prescribe or dispense Schedule 1 herbs will be subject to annual renewal [5]. The CMRB is in the process of establishing standards for courses of study for the purposes of endorsement of registration

under Section 8 of the Chinese Medicine Registration Act 2000.

The CMRB set up a Scheduling Committee to provide recommendations for the Board to put to the Victorian Minister for Health that will include a list of Chinese herbs for inclusion into Schedule 1 of the Victorian Poisons List. As part of this process, the Scheduling Committee produced a discussion document entitled "Safe Access to Chinese Herbs," available at: www.cmrb.vic.gov.au. The Committee developed an herb monograph pro forma that will form part of the submission to the minister for health, and is currently formulating guidelines that relate to other issues raised in the discussion document, including standards of training for Schedule 1 endorsement and quality assurance. The Committee proposed that an initial submission to the Minister of Health contain four herbs chosen for their therapeutic importance that are currently illegal for practitioners of Chinese medicine to use, due to inclusion in Schedules of the Victorian Poisons List. These herbs are: *zhi fu zi* (processed *Aconitum carmichaeli Debx.*), *ma huang* (*Ephedra sinica Stapf, Ephedra intermedia Schrenk ex Mey, Ephedra equisetina Bge.*), *bing lang* (*Areca catechu L.*), and *ban bian lian* (*Lobelia chinensis Lour.*) [5].

In contrast to raw Chinese herbs, proprietary Chinese herbal medicines are controlled under Commonwealth legislation. The Therapeutic Goods Administration (TGA) has a two-tiered system of registering and listing medicines, including complementary medicines, on the Australian Register of Therapeutic Goods (ARTG). A listed medicine has been assessed for safety and quality, whereas a registered medicine has in addition been assessed for efficacy. For a therapeutic claim or indication to be made about a proprietary medicine, it must be registered [6]. The majority of Chinese herbal medicines are listed on the ARTG.

Chinese Medicine Education in Australia

Until the 1990s, Chinese medicine education was delivered in privately operated institutions offering predominantly diploma or advanced diploma level training. There are now several Australian universities and privately operated schools offering either four- or five-year degrees in Chinese medicine, including the Academy of Traditional Chinese Medicine, the RMIT University (Royal Melbourne Institute of Technology), the Southern School of Natural Therapies, the University of Western Sydney (UWS), the University of Technology Sydney (UTS), Victoria University, and the Australian College of Natural Medicine. In addition, there are several postgraduate degrees in acupuncture and Chinese medicine offered at universities including UWS (Master of Traditional Chinese Medicine and Master of Acupuncture), RMIT University (including the Master of Applied Science [Acupuncture] and Master of Applied Science [Chinese Herbal Medicine]) and UTS (Master of Health Science in Traditional Chinese Medicine). The masters degrees at UWS and UTS are designed for students who have already completed undergraduate training in either TCM (acupuncture and Chinese herbal medicine) or acupuncture. The websites of individual universities and schools should be consulted for further information.

The Chinese Medicine Registration Act 2000 gives the CMRB powers to approve courses of study that provide qualifications for registration as Chinese medicine practitioners in Victoria. A student graduating from an approved course is eligible for registration as an acupuncturist and/or Chinese herbal medicine practitioner, and would not be required to sit an examination. All the Chinese medicine schools in Victoria now offer CMRB-approved Chinese medicine courses. The Board has not yet issued course approval guidelines related to the registration of dispensers. The trend in Chinese medicine education in Australia is currently toward bachelor-level training, with the main privately operated schools of natural medicine upgrading their diploma or advanced diploma level training to bachelor degrees over the past few years.

The National Academic Standards Committee (NASC), which includes over 40 members from educational institutions, profes-

sional associations representing Chinese medicine practitioners, and other stakeholders, published the *Australian Guidelines for Traditional Chinese Medicine Education* in 2001 [7]. This publication outlines criteria and minimum requirements for primary qualifying courses of study in Chinese medicine in Australia.

The NASC established the Australian Council for Chinese Medicine Education (ACCME) in 2003. The main purposes of the ACCME are to approve and review Chinese medicine education programs in Australia and provide standards for education providers to assist in the establishment and review of Chinese medicine education programs [7]. (See also "Chinese Medicine Education in Australia," p. 208, Education.)

Chinese Medicine Workforce

There are no up-to-date statistics on the Chinese medicine workforce in Australia. It was estimated that in 2002 there were approximately 2000 Chinese medicine practitioners who belonged to the two largest professional associations representing Chinese medicine practitioners [8]. In addition, an estimated 15 % of Australian general medical practitioners practice acupuncture [9].

In Australia, acupuncture performed by a registered (Western) medical practitioner is covered under the national government health scheme, Medicare. It is not, however, covered if performed by a traditionally trained acupuncturist (who is not a Western medical practitioner). Many private health insurance companies in Australia now cover acupuncture and Chinese herbal medicine consultations provided by approved providers.

Under the Goods and Services (GST) Act, the supply of certain complementary and alternative medicine (CAM) services may be GST-free. One of the stipulations for this to occur is that the supplier is a "recognized professional" in relation to the services provided. In order for CAM practitioners to retain or obtain GST-free status for certain services, they need to be "recognized professionals" [10].

With the exception of Victoria, which has statutory regulation, Chinese medicine practitioners need to be a member of a recognized professional association body that has, amongst other requirements, uniform national registration requirements (in order to fulfill the definition of "recognized professional") [10]. There is no single peak body representing Chinese medicine practitioners in Australia. The report *Towards a Safer Choice* identified 23 professional associations representing Chinese medicine practitioners in 1995 [1].

Research in Chinese Medicine in Australia

A significant problem facing CAM research in Australia is the general lack of research funding. For example, in 2001 the total funding by the National Health and Medical Research Centre (NHMRC), one of the major funding bodies for medical research in Australia, was A\$216 249 026, out of which A\$104 328 was allocated to CAM research projects [10]. Nevertheless, several Australian universities are actively conducting research into acupuncture and Chinese herbal medicine. Examples of research activities include:

Monash University
- Clinical research: randomized controlled trial (RCT) into the efficacy of Chinese herbal medicine in treatment of hypercholesterolemia and other cardiovascular risk factors.
- Laboratory research: study of prevention of atherosclerosis with Chinese herbal medicine in a mouse model; study investigating the effects of a Chinese herbal medicine on cardiomyocytes.

RMIT University
- Clinical research (acupuncture and herbs), focusing on allergy and chronic pain.
- Pharmacological research in Chinese herbal medicine, focusing on anti-allergy and anti-inflammatory effects of Chinese herbal medicine.
- Chinese herbal medicine farming, including

DNA fingerprinting and chemical analysis for authentication of herbal medicine.
- Knowledge management of Chinese medicine and socio-economic research on complementary medicine.

University of Western Sydney
- Development of a Chinese herbal medicine toxicology database.
- Clinical research includes evaluation of Chinese herbal medicine for treatment of endometriosis, functional dysmenorrhoea, menopausal vasomotor flushing, irritable bowel syndrome (IBS), chronic hepatitis C, evaluation of acupuncture for treatment of hypertension, and depression.
- Health economic research into complementary medicine.

University of Technology
- Clinical research includes: reliability study of tongue diagnosis; RCT on effect of acupuncture and Chinese herbs on sperm parameters; studies evaluating the effect of needle techniques and acupoint combinations on pressure pain threshold; RCT on the effect of acupuncture in patients with hepatitis C; the effectiveness of acupuncture as an adjunct treatment to existing alcohol and other drug treatment programs.
- Survey on workcover (Patients' State health insurance scheme) use by New South Wales acupuncturists.
- Database development for acupuncture and Chinese herbal medicine.

Victoria University
- Clinical research includes; treatment of gynecological patterns of disharmony with Chinese herbal medicine; the effectiveness of acupuncture in decreasing levels of anxiety in drug detoxification clients; the effect of *tai qi* on health, in particular bone density.
- Research into the teaching and learning of Chinese medicine in post-modern Western society.
- Research into the practice of Chinese medicine in the West.

Professional Developments, Legislation, and Regulation

The Development, Regulation, and Practice of Traditional East Asian Medicine in Australia

References

1. Bensoussan A, Myers SP. *Towards a Safer Choice*. Sydney: University of Western Sydney; 1996.
2. Chinese Medicine Registration Act 2000, Act No. 18/2000. Government Printer for the State of Victoria; 2000.
3. Committee on the Health Care Complaints Commission. *Report into Traditional Chinese Medicine*. Sydney: NSW Parliament; November 2005. Report No. 9/53.
4. Western Australia Department of Health. Regulation of practitioners of Chinese medicine in Western Australia. Discussion paper. Western Australia Department of Health; 2005.
5. Chinese Medicine Registration Board of Victoria. *Safe Access to Chinese Herbs*. 2004. Available at URL: www.cmrb.vic.gov.au.
6. Guidelines for levels and kinds of evidence to support claims for non-registrable medicines, including complementary medicines, and other listable medicines. Canberra: Therapeutic Goods Administration; 2001.
7. McDonald J. Introducing the Australian Council for Chinese Medicine Education. World Federation of Acupuncture. Conference Proceedings, Goldcoast, Queensland, Australia; 2005.
8. O'Brien K, Komesaroff P. Options for the establishment of a Victorian complementary and alternative medicine research centre. A discussion paper. Melbourne: Monash University and Baker Medical Research Institute; 2001.
9. Easthope G, Beilby J, Tranter B. Acupuncture in Australian general practice: practitioner characteristics. *MJA*. 1998;169:197–200.
10. O'Brien KA. Complementary and alternative medicine: the move into mainstream healthcare. *Clinical and Experimental Optometry*. 2004;87(2):110–20.

Contact Details

Kylie O'Brien, PhD
Victoria University, Melbourne, Australia

Further information on the regulation of Chinese medicine in Victoria and the CMRB may be found at www.cmrb.vic.gov.au.

Organizations and Associations in the USA

Deirdre Courtney, MTCM, CAc (China), Dublin, Ireland

Traditional East Asian medicine in the USA, like most other countries and jurisdictions, has not evolved in a coherent linear way. Rather, it has emerged in clusters around schools that were originally set up in the 1970s and 1980s to develop into the burgeoning practice it is today. There are currently at least 20 000 practitioners of traditional East Asian medicine in the USA. In this initial survey of the extent of the contemporary practice in the USA we outline the framework of practice, organization, and legislation that has emerged to date. Of its nature this is a work in progress and we anticipate with the help of readers and users of the Almanac that the information contained here will develop into a comprehensive overview of the practice in the USA. Below you will find listings of national bodies, state bodies, and the states that have licensing requirements.

National Associations/Organizations

- Accreditation Commission for Acupuncture and Oriental Medicine (ACAOM)
  www.acaom.org
- Acupuncture and Oriental Medicine Alliance (AOM Alliance)
  www.aomalliance.org
- Acupuncture and Oriental Medicine National Coalition (AOMNC)
  www.aomnc.com
- American Academy of Medical Acupuncture (AAMA)
  www.medicalacupuncture.org
- American Academy of Veterinary Acupuncture (AAVA)
  www.aava.org
- American Academy of Veterinary Medical Acupuncture (AAVMA)
  www.aavma.org

- American Association of Oriental Medicine (AAOM)
  www.aaom.org
- American Chinese Medicine Association (ACMA)
  www.americanchinesemedicine-association.org
- American Herbal Products Association (AHPA)
  www.ahpa.org
- American Herbalists Guild (AHG)
  www.americanherbalistsguild.com
- American Organization for Bodywork Therapies of Asia (AOBTA)
  www.aobta.org
- Council of Acupuncture and Oriental Medicine Associations (CAOMA)
  www.acucouncil.org
- Council of Colleges of Acupuncture and Oriental Medicine (CCAOM)
  www.ccaom.org
- Federation of Acupuncture and Oriental Medicine Regulatory Agencies (FAOMRA)
  www.faomra.com
- International Veterinary Acupuncture Society (IVAS)
  www.ivas.org
- National Acupuncture Detoxification Association (NADA)
  www.acudetox.com
- National Acupuncture Foundation (NAF)
  www.nationalacupuncturefoundation.org
- National Certification Commission for Acupuncture & Oriental Medicine (NCCAOM)
  www.nccaom.org
- National Oriental Medicine Accreditation Agency (NOMAA)
  www.nomaa.org
- National Qigong (Chi Kung) Association (NQA)
  www.nqa.org
- North American Society of Acupuncture and Alternative Medicine

- Qigong Association of America
  www.qi.org
- Society for Acupuncture Research (SAR)
  www.acupunctureresearch.org
- The Herb Society of America
  www.herbsociety.org
- United States Traditional Chinese Medicine
  Alumni Association

State Associations/Organizations

- Acupuncture and Oriental Medicine
  Association of Minnesota (AOMAM)
  www.aomam.org
- Acupuncture Association of Colorado (AAC)
  www.acucol.com
- Acupuncture Society of New York (ASNY)
  www.asny.org
- Acupuncture Society of Virginia (ASVA)
  www.acusova.com
- Acupuncture Society of Washington, DC
  (ASDC)
  www.dcacupuncture.org
- Alabama Association of Oriental Medicine
  www.acuphysician.com
- Arizona Society of Oriental Medicine and
  Acupuncture (AzSOMA)
  www.azsoma.org
- Association for Professional Acupuncture
  in Pennsylvania (APA)
  www.acupuncturepa.org
- California Alliance of Acupuncture Medicine
  (CAAM)
  www.caaminfo.com
- California State Oriental Medical
  Association (CSOMA)
  www.csomaonline.org
- Florida Association of Oriental Medicine
- Florida State Oriental Medical Association
  (FSOMA)
  www.fsoma.com
- Florida Toyohari Acupuncture Association
  http://toyohari.org/florida
- Georgia State Oriental Medicine Association
- Hawaii Acupuncture Association
- Idaho Acupuncture Association
  www.idahoacupuncture.org

- Illinois Association of Acupuncture
  and Oriental Medicine (ILaaom)
  www.ilaaom.org
- Indiana Association of Acupuncture
  and Oriental Medicine (IAAOM)
  www.iaaom.org
- Maine Association of Acupuncture
  and Oriental Medicine (MAAOM)
  www.maaom.org
- Maryland Acupuncture Society (MAS)
  www.maryland-acupuncture.org
- Michigan Association of Acupuncture and
  Oriental Medicine (MAAOM)
  www.michiganacupuncture.org
- New Hampshire Association for
  Acupuncture and Oriental Medicine
  (NHAAOM)
  http://nhaaom.org
- New Jersey Association of Acupuncture
  and Oriental Medicine
- North Carolina Association of Acupuncture
  and Oriental Medicine (NCAAOM)
  www.ncaaom.org
- Ohio Association of Acupuncture
  and Oriental Medicine (OAAOM)
  www.oaaom.org
- Oklahoma Acupuncture Association
- Oregon Acupuncture Association (OAA)
  www.oregonacupuncture.org
- Oriental Medicine Association
  of New Mexico (OMANM)
  www.omanm.org
- Rhode Island Society of Acupuncture
  and Oriental Medicine (RISAOM)
  www.risaom.org
- Texas Association of Acupuncture
  and Oriental Medicine (TAAOM)
  www.taaom.org
- United California Practitioners
  of Chinese Medicine (UCPCM)
  http://ucpcm.org
- Washington Acupuncture and Oriental
  Medicine Association (WAOMA)
  www.waoma.org
- Wisconsin Society of Certified
  Acupuncturists (WISCA)
  www.acupuncturewisconsin.org

Acupuncture and Oriental Medicine Regulatory Agencies

The following states have regulations specific to the practice of acupuncture or oriental medicine:

- Alaska
- Arizona
- Arkansas
- California
- Colorado
- Connecticut
- Florida
- Georgia
- Hawaii
- Idaho
- Illinois
- Indiana
- Iowa
- Kansas
- Louisiana
- Maine
- Maryland
- Massachusetts
- Minnesota
- Missouri
- Montana
- Nebraska
- Nevada
- New Hampshire
- New Jersey
- New Mexico
- New York
- North Carolina
- Ohio
- Oregon
- Pennsylvania
- Rhode Island
- South Carolina
- Tennessee
- Texas
- Utah
- Vermont
- Virginia
- Washington
- Washington, DC
- West Virginia
- Wisconsin

The following states do not have legislative codes at this time specific to acupuncture or oriental medicine:

- Alabama
- Delaware
- Kentucky
- Michigan
- Mississippi
- North Dakota
- Oklahoma
- South Dakota
- Wyoming

Acupuncture Laws, Codes, and Acts

In the following states, acupuncture or oriental medicine may not be practiced without a license:

- Alaska
- Arizona
- California
- Colorado
- Connecticut
- Florida
- Hawaii
- Idaho
- Illinois
- Indiana
- Iowa
- Louisiana
- Maine
- Massachusetts
- Minnesota
- New York
- Ohio
- Oregon
- Rhode Island
- Utah
- Vermont
- Washington
- West Virginia
- Wisconsin

Licensed Practitioners in the USA

The NCCAOM (www. nccaom.org) was established in 1982 and is incorporated as a nonprofit organization under Section 501(c)(6) of the Internal Revenue code. Over 17 000 Diplomates are currently certified through NCCAOM, which is a member of the National Organization for Competency Assurance and which is accredited by the National Commission for Certifying Agencies (NCCA). The American Academy of Medical Acupuncture has in the region of 2500 members and the American Academy of Veterinary Acupuncture reports a membership of 800.

Iran Center of Complementary and Alternative Medicine (ICCAM)

Farid Nikbin, MD, Teheran, Iran

The Iran Center of Complementary and Alternative Medicine (ICCAM) is the first CAM center in an Iranian hospital (Milad) and it employs a team of medical doctors who are trained in different branches of the complementary/alternative medical field. This article will introduce the center.

Main Team

1. Farid Nikbin, MD, is a homeopath, acupuncturist, and laser therapist, and is also trained in different energy therapy and healing systems such as reiki (mastery), pranic healing, spiritual human yoga, and Kirlian photography by means of GDV bioelectrography. He is Dean of Complementary and Alternative Medicine at Milad Hospital.
2. Mitra Hajizadeh, MD, is an internist, laser therapist, and pranic healer, and is also

trained in magnified healing, ayurveda, and hypnotism. She is Dean of Internal Medicine at Milad Hospital.
3. Kiarash Saatchi, MD, is a laser therapist, reiki master and teacher, and pranic healing teacher, and is also trained in magnified healing and ayurveda.

Our Past and Present Projects

1. Founding the first unique CAM center in an Iranian hospital (Milad Hospital) (see below for more details).
2. University projects:
   - FCAM (Fundamentals of Complementary and Alternative Medicine) courses: six-month and one-year unique courses on the main aspects, philosophy, and skills of more than 15 main branches of CAM as an introductory course for medical students, specialists, and other medically educated people who are interested in these kinds of approaches to medicine.
   - MT (Mental Techniques) courses: two month-courses on mental techniques and mind/body medicine. The main program is focused on different meditation and relaxation techniques, guided imagery, and NLP.
3. Books, articles, and lectures:
   - *Beyond the Calmness*: a book in the Persian language including 18 chapters on CAM's main branches and their applications in stress reduction and management (now a reference book for university courses). There are other books about to be published.
   - More than 30 articles about energy medicine, acupuncture, internal medicine, music therapy, vibrational medicine, homeopathy, and so on.

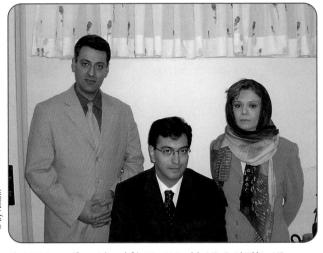

© by Nikbin

The ICCAM team (from right to left): Mitra Hajizadeh, MD; Farid Nikbin, MD; Kiarash Saatchi, MD.

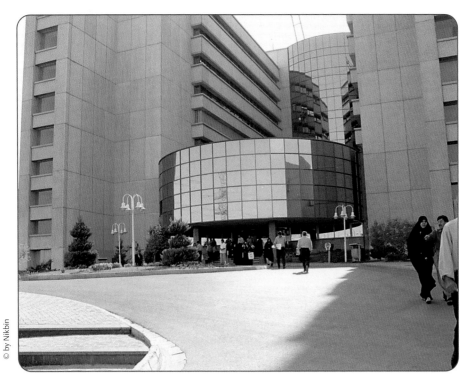

The Milad Hospital, Teheran

© by Nikbin

- More than 100 lectures and presentations on different parts of CAM in national and international congresses.
4. Other educational projects:
  - TV and radio programs: our team is also very active in the introduction of CAM and its applications as diagnostic and therapeutic ways to better health especially through an integrative medical approach (more than 100 TV and radio programs on five channels).
  - Stress management seminars and courses: in different companies, based on both psychotherapy and CAM methods.
  - Founding the central CAM internet site in Iran (www.cam.ir) as a unique center for the relationship between doctors, therapists, and patients. We have also begun electronic and distance education programs through this site.

Active Branches of CAM in ICCAM

Up to now there are only a few branches of CAM that are active in our department, but we hope to be able to activate other methods in future (see below). The currently active departments are:
- homeopathy
- acupuncture
- low-level laser therapy (LLLT) (and also some serial combinatory approaches of magnet, laser, and incoherent light like quantum therapy)
- energetic medicine (healing, GDV bioelectrography, auricular diagnostics, and other therapeutic approaches).

About the Milad Hospital

The Milad Hospital is the biggest hospital in both Iran and the Middle East with 1000 beds, 32 departments, and 24 surgery rooms, with more than 96 000 square meters of building space. It is used as a referral center for many other hospitals. More than 500 000 outpatients are treated each year in this hospital and we also treat nearly 55 000 inpatients each year.

Our Mission, Vision, and Future Plans

We hope to become a first-rank CAM center and a unique and pioneering department of integrative medicine (CAM and Western medicine) in Iran and the Middle East, based on WHO strategies for TM/CAM. Our vision is to provide the best methods for prevention, diagnosis, and treatment of disease. We hope to activate the following departments in the future:

- Traditional Iranian medicine (TIM) (and especially some of its approaches like traditional Iranian herbalism, cupping, and blood letting)
- Herbal medicine (Eastern and Western)
- Chiropractic therapy (and other type of manual therapies)
- Ayurveda (and especially some of its cleansing methods like panchakarma)
- Some forms of vibrational medicine (like MORA, RIFE, etc.).

Welcome to all Colleagues and Friends From Around the World

As an international institute (Health Pioneers Institute) and hospital department, we welcome all specialists in different branches of CAM who are interested in joining us, to work together and to create mutually beneficial relationships in different fields of CAM like education (short- and long-term courses), congresses and seminars, diagnostic and therapeutic approaches to special kinds of diseases.

Contact Details

Dr F. Nikbin may be contacted by email: drnikbin@yahoo.com

Perspectives on Traditional Acupuncture by Senior Blind Practitioners in Japan—Two Interviews

Stephen Birch, PhD, LAc, Amsterdam, the Netherlands

The following is an interview with the last President Akihiro Takai and current President Toshio Yanagishita of the Toyohari Igakukai, the East Asian Needle Therapy Medical Association. Toyohari is a form of *Keiraku Chiryo* or Japanese Meridian Therapy. Meridian Therapy has been practiced as a traditional system of acupuncture since the 1930s (predating Traditional Chinese Medicine acupuncture by about 15 years) [1]. Meridian Therapy is said to be the dominant form of traditional acupuncture in Japan. It was initiated in the 1920s–1930s by Sorei Yanagiya, Shinichiro Takeyama, Keiri Inoue, and Sodo Okabe. Toyohari arose out of this tradition in 1959, initially as a study group for blind Meridian Therapists, led by the founding President Kodo Fukushima, and evolving from that time to become one of the leading Meridian Therapy associations in Japan.

The interview was conducted in Tokyo one evening at the Toyohari Meridian Therapy Summer School in July 2005. It is interesting to hear about the history of blind people practicing acupuncture in Japan and to hear about the traditional acupuncture system of Meridian Therapy. About half the current Japanese Toyohari members are blind; most of the senior instructors are blind and have been practicing for many years. There are about 300 Toyohari members outside of Japan, and there are plans to start training blind acupuncturists in the USA. It is also interesting to hear the views of such traditional pragmatic practitioners on scientific research.

Interview with Akihiro Takai

To begin with, could you tell us a little about yourself and when you became President of the Toyohari Association?
My name is Akihiro Takai and I was born in 1928. I was a high school teacher after the Second World War. I had my first symptoms of Behçet disease in 1953 and, as a result of this disease, went fully blind in 1957. In 1959 I went to a school for the blind, studying for three years. This was a government-sponsored special institution for people who became blind later in life rather than being born blind. I got my acupuncture license in 1962. I joined the Toyohari Association in 1964 and have been a member since then, becoming President in 1994.

Could you say something about the history of blind people practicing acupuncture in Japan?
I heard that during the Tokugawa Era (1600–1853), during the third shogun, a high-ranking official went blind. Although it is not clear, this person may have been associated with the first blind acupuncturist in Japan. However, it is clear that during the fifth shogunate (late 1600s), the shogun had a kind of neurotic disease that nobody could treat. Waichi Sugiyama was the first established blind acupuncturist who was able to help him, and he was therefore recognized and elevated to a high position by the shogun. Because Sugiyama cured the shogun he was given support to establish a blind school to train acupuncturists, the Shinji Gakumonsho, "the study place to learn needling." Since it was a government-sanctioned school, it became the highest-level acupuncture school in Japan. It was there that future teachers were trained and sent around Japan.

Sugiyama Waichi also wrote a book, the *Sugiyama Ryu Sanbusho* (Sugiyama's Book in Three Parts), which he gave to the shogun. Because of Sugiyama's elevated status, it became a highly revered text. Students had to listen to the book read to them while they bowed down, and each passage was read to them only three times. (Ed.: Since those studying with Sugiyama were blind and there was as

Akihiro Takai

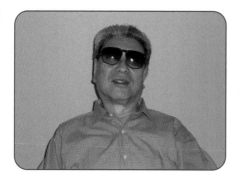

riod Western science became dominant in health care and was introduced into the training of acupuncturists. There were a lot of changes during that time, but I'm not familiar with all the details. However, I do know that there was an apprenticeship system for training non-blind, non-physician practitioners that was regulated by the police. This system was in place until the Second World War and was replaced in 1947 with the establishment of a national examination and national licensing by Douglas MacArthur and his occupying forces.

yet no Braille, the text could only be studied through being read aloud combined with rote learning.)

There have been blind practitioners since that time, but when did the numbers of blind practitioners in Japan suddenly increase? Was there a change associated with the Meiji reformation in the late 1800s?
Sugiyama Waichi was only able to teach 20 students in total. However, each of them taught others around Japan, so naturally the numbers of blind acupuncturists kept growing from that time. In the 1870s the Meiji government did not know what to do with the blind practitioners. Eventually, because of the established 200-year tradition of training blind practitioners, they decided to focus on building more schools to teach acupuncture and *anma* and to more blind people through regional blind institutions rather than solely through acupuncture schools.

During that time, wasn't acupuncture restricted because of the drive to establish Western medicine as the standard of health care? I have heard that the practice of acupuncture was restricted to blind people or medical doctors trained in the West. In the world of acupuncture, Japan is unique on account of its high percentage of blind practitioners. By the turn of the 20th century, acupuncture was practiced exclusively by blind practitioners or physician practitioners. Isn't it true that today a large percentage of acupuncturists in Japan is blind?
Before the Meiji government, traditional medicines were popular. But during the Meiji pe-

I imagine that the training programs for blind and sighted students are quite different. Could you comment a little on the differences? I ask this question because many Westerners may feel that it is strange to teach acupuncture to blind people. Also, there is a growing interest among some practitioners to start teaching acupuncture to blind people in the West.
Blind people are taught acupuncture in either a specialized acupuncture school or in one of the state-sponsored regional blind institutions. Many blind people are taught acupuncture in these nonspecialized blind institutions. So one difference is that in the blind institutions almost all the teachers are blind, yet in sighted acupuncture schools they are almost all sighted. But recently, with the increase in the number of sighted people studying acupuncture, some of the sighted acupuncture schools have hired some blind teachers, although they only teach practical skills. Since most of the training programs for teaching acupuncture to blind people are inside regular state-sponsored blind institutions, many Toyohari members have started studying acupuncture in these blind institutions. In fact, some members are instructors at these blind institutions.

Another difference in terms of the training is that many of the specialized acupuncture schools in Japan run day-time and some night-time programs. But the blind institutions are usually boarding schools. Students do not study only in day or evening programs, they study much more since they need more time to study.

I can imagine that one difference between the blind and sighted practitioners is that the sighted tend to be a bit more theoretical, whereas blind practitioners tend to be more practical and hands-on. Is that correct?
Blind people's sense of touch is definitely better, especially those who have been blind for a long time. Training through reading Braille helps a lot as well, particularly those who have only ever read using Braille. There is a big difference in pulse diagnosis skills between Toyohari practitioners and other acupuncturists, partly because of this phenomenon among the blind Toyohari members.

I also imagine that another big difference is that sighted people will be more interested in technological styles of treatment, more intellectually stimulating approaches, whereas blind practitioners are more likely to prefer working with their hands during treatment.
Yes, that's true. Acupuncture started by touching, so it is naturally important for acupuncture to touch the patient. At the beginning acupuncturists started placing the hands, then they started using bones and stones, and finally, with the development of metal needles, they started inserting needles.

Could you say something about Meridian Therapy and how it is different from other styles of acupuncture?
The origins of Meridian Therapy can be seen in ancient Chinese ideas, but in China they had to reject many traditional ideas after the Revolution and especially during the Cultural Revolution as part of the change necessary for modern adaptation—while in Japan different cultural forces were at work. Also, there are major weather differences between China and Japan that will also be reflected in the practice in the two countries. Further, Japan has been modernized very quickly and machines do a lot of the work. Thus people have become weaker, less physical, while in China, most people still do hard manual labor, and their bodies are more physically conditioned.

This factor is probably influential, as the Chinese prefer more physically stimulating needling methods and the Japanese more gentle and less physically stimulating needling methods.

What, in one sentence, would you say is the main focus of Meridian Therapy?
The *honchiho* (root treatment) used in the Toyohari Association is not used to cure the body, but to give the body a mild stimulus so that it heals itelf.

Interview with Toshio Yanagishita

Could you please first introduce yourself?
My name is Toshio Yanagishita. I was born in 1932 and am currently President of the Toyohari Association. I started studying acupuncture in 1946 at state-sponsored blind institutions, finishing my basic acupuncture education in 1954. I started studying *Keiraku Chiryo*, Meridian Therapy, in 1950 and became a member of the Toyohari Association about 10 years later.

Could you say something about the nature of Meridian Therapy?
Around 1930 a group of people in Japan were re-examining the classical Chinese texts and methods. From them they extracted ideas and methods that became the system of Meridian Therapy, which was clearly distinguishable from other styles of acupuncture of the day. Meridian Therapy is a system of acupuncture that tries to closely follow the classical ideas interpreted in the modern context.

How does this system differ from the system of acupuncture popular in China today, namely Traditional Chinese Medicine (TCM)?
After the Revolution in China they started using acupuncture strongly based on Western medical ideas. They also started interpreting the classics based on modern ideas as well. Therefore, in the current system of acupuncture in China, the concepts of *qi*, blood, etc. are being de-emphasized. Some people may feel I am overstating or exaggerating this dif-

*Toshio
Yanagishita*

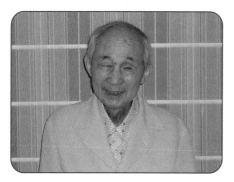

ful for a broader range of problems and diseases than is currently recognized. Even with
developments in modern medicine, there are
always patients and problems that cannot be
helped. We feel that this kind of therapy that
deals with the patient's *qi* can be helpful for
many of such patients. That is my vision.

This kind of Meridian Therapy is very
much favored by patients because it is very
comfortable, not difficult to apply to patients,
and can be very effective for a wide range of
problems. This we think will make it a very
useful therapy in the future.

ference, but this is what I feel after hearing
and reading about TCM.

*Could you say something about the difference
between Toyohari and other styles of Meridian
Therapy?*
A big difference between Toyohari and other
styles of Meridian Therapy is the use of the
inserted *chishin*, or "inserted and retained"
needle technique. In Toyohari we use non-
inserted needle techniques to regulate *qi*,
while other styles tend to use the inserted
and retained needle method to do this.

*What do you think about Toyohari in Japan
having about 300 members in branches outside
Japan? For example, it seems to have a larger
membership of non-Japanese members than
any other traditional acupuncture association
in Japan.*
Japanese people tend to like things imported
into Japan from the West. So, as more people
in the West study Toyohari, gradually more
people in Japan will turn toward it as a system
of therapy.

*Given these kinds of influences and devel-
opments going on here in Japan, what do you
see as the future of Toyohari acupuncture?
What are your hopes for the future?*
In the Toyohari Association, we find that this
style of Meridian Therapy treatment is able to
treat many diseases, even those that Western
medicine has difficulty treating. We hope that
this will eventually become better recognized.
Meridian Therapy, Toyohari, is a system of
treatment that deals with *qi* and can be help-

*Given these high ideals for Meridian Therapy
what do you think about the idea of doing research into Toyohari? In the modern period
research is seen as being important for showing
the value of a therapy. What do you think
about the role of research in a system such as
Toyohari?*
It is generally difficult for clinicians in Japan
to do research. Research that is not explicable
in Western medical terms is usually not acceptable. Therefore, what they could try doing
is setting up a system to collect their clinical
data systematically and then report
on this.

*If we could develop a model from which we
could start to examine Toyohari on its own
terms so that the traditional methods and ideas
were explored themselves and then do this
systematically in various locations outside and
within Japan, how would that sound as a
means to start addressing this issue?*
I think that it sounds like a good idea, but
I would have to ask the Board to lend its support. It would help to have a short summary
of what such a model would look like to present to them. And I want to be kept informed
about all the possibilities and projects that
come up.

Reference

1. Birch S, Felt RL. *Understanding Acupuncture.*
    Edinburgh: Churchill Livingstone; 1999:47–60.

Acupuncture in Japan—A Brief Look

Stephen Birch, PhD, LAc, Amsterdam, the Netherlands

The following is a very introductory summary of the acupuncture scene in Japan around the end of 2005. Thanks to Michitaka Tokunaga for helping to track down the information.

There are 89 acupuncture schools (university-based, vocational, and junior college) that train sighted students. There are 62 schools for teaching acupuncture to blind people (including regional centers that train blind people).

As of 2004, it was not clear how many of the more than 270 371 physicians in Japan practice acupuncture and moxibustion.

There are thought to be about 9077 hospitals and 97 051 general medical centers that provide acupuncture and moxibustion. (Doctors and dentists work only with outpatients, or mostly outpatients and no more than 19 inpatients.)

The practice of acupuncture and moxibustion in Japan is extremely diverse, with many different styles, theories, methods, and schools of thought.

If we compare the figures in 2004 to those in 1984, we can see a major change in some of the numbers. Since the Japanese population has fewer blind people than previously (owing to improved diet, lifestyle, healthcare, the departure of more elderly blind practioners,

etc.), the number of blind practitioners has decreased compared to the 1980s. We see the relative number of blind practioners dropping from around 35 % to around 19 %. At the same time, acupuncture has become increasingly popular, in part owing to its more modern appearance (because of an increase in scientific data and results). A result of the increasing popularity is that a larger percentage of sighted practitioners have entered the profession. We see the total number of acupuncturists rising from almost 52 794 to over 76 641 in a 20-year period. The number of sighted practitioners represents the largest portion of that increase, 33 562 to 62 168.

Blind people are strongly recommended to become acupuncturists and massage therapists. Sighted people choose these professions for quite different reasons.

One of the present trends is that traditional medicine as a whole is slowly declining in popularity in Japan (just as it is throughout the whole of Asia; see also "Education and Practice of Chinese Medicine in Taiwan," p. 151.). Thus we see a migration towards acupuncture not for its traditional theories and values but more likely because it has increasing scientific recognition.

Change in numbers of practitioners over a 20-year period in Japan[1]

Number of licensees[2]	Sighted practitioners 1984	Blind practitioners 1984 (% of total)	Sighted practitioners 2004	Blind practitioners 2004 (% of total)
Acupuncture	33 562	19 232 (36.4 %)	62 168	14 473 (18.9 %)
Moxibustion	33 339	18 092 (35.5 %)	59 899	15 201 (20.2 %)
Massage	–	–	72 349	25 799

[1] The 1984 data is quoted from: Sonoda K. *Health and Illness in Changing Japanese Society.* Tokyo: University of Tokyo Press; 1964, p. 23. See also: Birch S, Ida J. *Japanese Acupuncture: A Clinical Guide.* Brookline, MA: Paradigm Publications; 1998. The 2004 data was supplied by Michitaka Tokunaga, who contacted the licensing authorities in Japan in 2005.
[2] Many people have more than one license. A typical practitioner has all three.

The European Traditional Chinese Medicine Association (ETCMA)

Albert L. de Vos, Utrecht, the Netherlands and Michael McCarthy, MA (ThB), LAc, Dip CHM, Dublin, Ireland

History

The European Traditional Chinese Medicine Association (ETCMA) is an umbrella organization for professional associations that represent the different fields within Traditional Chinese Medicine (TCM). With the continuing integration of the European political and social landscape toward the end of the millennium, the need for a more pan-European approach to the organization of Traditional Chinese Medicine practice within Europe was becoming more evident. It was out of this milieu that the idea for the ETCMA was born and in 2001 it had its inaugural meeting.

Today the Association has members in nine different countries and it is still growing with applications continuing to come in from TCM organizations in the other countries. Each member association is made up of individual practitioners, and with a current practitioner membership of nearly 6000 it is fast becoming the major player on the European Chinese medicine professional practitioner scene.

The Association has had regular meetings and symposia since its inauguration and continues to promote its core aims of wider recognition and acceptance of TCM therapies by European governments and the public alike. The Association is also a forum for the exchange of views and experiences over matters of mutual interest, such as the statutory regulation of our therapies and the development of educational programs. Through its association with other groups in the health care field the ETCMA is actively engaged in influencing the shape of health care policy and regulation in Europe, especially insofar as it impacts on the TCM profession and on its clients/patients.

Aims and Objectives of the ETCMA

- To exchange information. The ETCMA collectively holds a wealth of experience, which can be shared for the benefit of every member. We regularly inform each other of the latest political developments affecting TCM therapies in our respective countries and give each other updates on educational developments etc.
- To develop and promote high standards of education. The ETCMA works toward developing accreditation systems for TCM education programs within Europe. We seek to establish minimum criteria for proficient professional practice, and also to define criteria for the practice of different TCM therapies. We would like to strengthen international academic exchanges and to assist in the development of academic collaboration with European colleges and universities.
- To lobby EU bodies and institutions. The ETCMA lobbies for the common interests of its members. We do this by seeking a voice on relevant EU committees and forums concerned with complementary therapies in order to influence health care policy and provision, with particular reference to TCM therapies.
- To promote research. The ETCMA wishes to see appropriate scientific research into the safety, validity, usefulness, and efficacy of TCM therapies: research that respects the integrity of TCM and helps gain its wider recognition and acceptance throughout Europe.
- To promote recognition of TCM. The ETCMA lobbies for TCM therapies provided by qualified practitioners to be included in the national health systems of European countries, and also for the coverage of TCM therapies by social and/or private insurance companies.

The Board and Executive of the ETCMA

President: Jasmine Uddin, UK
Chief Executive Officer: Albert L. de Vos,
The Netherlands
Treasurer: Johan Roose, Belgium

Board Members

Birte Nielsen, Denmark
Ing-Marie Lagerstrom, Sweden
Michael McCarthy, Ireland
Nils von Below, Germany
Petra Kostamo, Finland
Simon Becker, Switzerland

Member Organizations of the ETCMA

BELGIUM
**EUFOM Federation for Acupuncturists
(EUFOM Beroepsorganisatie Acupunctuur)**
Kerkhoflaan 19
3740 Eigenbilzen
Phone +32 89 511 037
Email info@eufom.com
www.eufom.com

DENMARK
**PA—Association of Acupuncture Practitioners
(Praktiserende Akupunktører)**
Bytoftevej 14
Slimminge
4100 Ringsted
Phone +45 5687 9011
Fax +45 5687 9001
Email bn@aku-net.dk
www.aku-net.dk

FINLAND
**FinnAcu—Finnish Traditional Chinese Medicine
Society of Acupuncture and Herbs
(Suomen perinteisen kiinalaisen lääketieteen
yhdistys ry)**
Rummunlyöjänkatu 2 A 5
02600 Espoo
Phone +358 41 528 2134
Fax +358 45 677 0096
www.finnacu.fi

GERMANY
**AGTCM—Association for Classical Acupuncture
and TCM (Arbeitsgemeinschaft für klassische
Akupunktur und Traditionelle Chinesische
Medizin e.V.)**
Wisbacher Straße 1
83435 Bad Reichenhall
Phone +49 8651 690 919
Fax +49 8651 710 694
Email sekretariat@agtcm.de
www.agtcm.de

THE NETHERLANDS
**NVA—Dutch Association for Acupuncture
(Nederlandse Vereniging voor Acupunctuur)**
Postbus 2198
3800 CD Amersfoort
Phone +31 33 461 6141
Fax +31 33 465 4062
Email nva@acupunctuur.nl
www.acupunctuur.nl

REPUBLIC OF IRELAND
**IRCHM—Irish Register of Chinese Herbal
Medicine**
5 Lower Mount Street
Dublin 2
Phone +353 1 611 4819
Email info@irchm.com
www.irchm.com

SWEDEN
**SAATCM—Swedish Acupuncture Association
for Traditional Chinese Medicine
(Svenska Akupunkturförbundet Traditionell
Kinesisk Medicin)**
Ystadsvägen 67
SE-121 51 Johanneshov
Phone +46 8 600 0230
Fax +46 8 600 0230
Email info@akupunkturforbundet.se
www.akupunkturforbundet.se

SWITZERLAND
SPO-TCM—Swiss Professional Organization for Traditional Chinese Medicine (SBO-TCM—Schweizerische Berufsorganisation für Traditionelle Chinesische Medizin; OPS-MTC—Organisation Professionnelle Suisse de Médecine Traditionnelle Chinoise)
Kähstrasse 8
9113 Degersheim
Phone   +41 71 372 0111
Fax   +41 71 372 0119
Email   sekretariat@sbo-tcm.ch
www.sbo-tcm.ch

UK
BAcC—British Acupuncture Council
63 Jeddo Road
London W12 9HQ
Phone   +44 20 8735 0400
Fax   +44 20 8735 0404
Email   info@acupuncture.org.uk
www.acupuncture.org.uk

How to Join the ETCMA

Applications for membership are welcomed from all not-for-profit practitioner associations that support the aims and objectives of the ETCMA. Further information is available at www.etcma.org.

Contact Details

European Traditional Chinese Medicine Association
Chief Executive Officer:
Albert L. de Vos
Hobbemastraat 18
3583 CX Utrecht
The Netherlands
Phone   +31 30 251 5340
Mobile   +31 65 356 3160
Email   contact@etcma.org

European Register of Organizations of Traditional Chinese Medicine (EuroTCM)

Subhuti Dharmananda, PhD, Portland, Oregon, USA

The European Register of Organizations of Traditional Chinese Medicine (EuroTCM) is an association of Chinese medicine organizations across Europe comprising schools, distributors, suppliers, manufacturers, and practitioners.

The organization's stated aims are: "through (the) joint effort of its members, to improve the standard of TCM in Europe namely by promoting common regulations, professional approach of practitioners, common codes of ethics and practice, standardisation of educational requirements and validation of the qualifying examinations, and transparency for the lay public." Below is a table of current member organizations. (See also the section Education, p. 193.)

Member organizations of EuroTCM

Country	Abbreviation	Full name	Type
Austria	MED CHIN	Medizinische Gesellschaft für Chinesische Gesundheitspflege in Österreich	College
	PROTCM	Österreichischer Berufsverband der TCM-Therapeuten	Professional org.
Belgium	BAF	Belgian Acupunctors Federation	Professional org.
	BATCM	Belgian Association for Traditional Chinese Medicine	Scientific org.
	FCAO	–	Snr. Students club
	OTCG	Opleidingsinstituut voor Traditionele Chinese Geneeswijzen	College
Bulgaria	BAAPT	Bulgarian Acupuncture Association of Physical Therapists	Professional org.
Czech Republic	CSBS	Ceskoslovenská Sinobiologická Spolecnost	College
	CSBSPTCM	Praktici TCM	Acupuncture org.
	NBJ	Foundation of the White Crane	Professional org.
	TCMB	TCM Bohemia— Klinika Tradicní Cínské Medicíny	Clinic
England	BC	Bodyharmonics Centre	College
	LCTA	London College of Traditional Acupuncture and Oriental Medicine	College
France	ELM	École Lü Men de Médicine Chinoise	College
Germany	ABZ Süd	Ausbildungszentrum Süd	College
Greece	AAGTCM	–	College
	EIOM	European Institute of Oriental Medicine & Natural Therapies	College
	ESPKI	Elleniko Sillogos Paradosiakis Kinezikis Iatrikis	Professional org.
	HAOTCM	Hellenic Academy of TCM	College
Hungary	H.SH.T	Hungarian Shaolin Temple	College
Ireland	ACMO	Acupuncture and Chinese Medicine Organisation	Professional org.

Country	Abbreviation	Full name	Type
Italy	SIA	Società Italiana di Agopuntura	College
Netherlands	DDF	Dutch Dao Foundation	Professional org.
	HTUTCM	Hwa To University of Traditional Chinese Medicine	College
	OC	International Oriental College	College
	ZHONG	Nederlandse Vereniging Traditionele Chinese Geneeskunde	Professional org.
Romania	RNQF	–	Professional org. and college
Russia	SJA	Su Jok Academy	College
Serbia/Montenegro	DOROTEJ	–	College
	RHCI	Railway Health Care Institute	Professional org.
	SJC	Balkan Su Jok College	College
Slovac Republic	SINBIOS	Slovenská SinoBiologická Spolecnost	College
Slovenia	SAATCM	Slovenian Association of Acupuncture and TCM	Professional org.
Sweden	NJA	Nei Jing College	College

The International Council of Medical Acupuncture and Related Techniques (ICMART)

Bryan Frank, MD, DABMA, Edmond, Oklahoma, USA

The International Council of Medical Acupuncture and Related Techniques (ICMART) is an international organization comprising more than 80 medical acupuncture societies worldwide. It includes over 30 000 conventionally trained medical doctors practicing acupuncture and related techniques.

ICMART sponsors/organizes a world congress most years with local host associations in different countries worldwide. It has been doing this since 1983. The organization has active involvement in developments with local and international groups and promotes sponsorship of prizes for conference lectures and posters etc. for members, from commercial organizations supplying the profession.

ICMART also has a website, which contains information on the member associations and links to their own websites, plus congress information and abstracts. As with other professional traditional East Asian Medicine bodies, contact is maintained with WHO and contributions are made to the International Guideline on Trial Methodology and standardizing acupuncture nomenclature. The organization also publishes a newsletter for its members.

ICMART promotes the idea:

- that an orthodox medical diagnosis is made prior to treatment with acupuncture and/or related techniques;
- that the general orientation of its members is a scientific approach through evidence-based medicine even though much data is still in its infancy;
- that traditional approaches are very much respected and included in its scope;
- and that evidence-based approaches can equally be applied to Traditional Chinese Medicine and acupuncture, although there is still much work to be done in this field.

Further information regarding the activities of ICMART is available on its website: www.icmart.org.

ICMART Members List (February 2006)

ARMENIA

Armenian Association of Traditional and Alternative Medicine
President: Dr M.N. Avagyan
49/4 Komitas Avenue
Yerevan 375051
Phone +374 (8) 1 237 134 or 239 044
Fax 374 (8) 1 230 191
Email vgma@web.am

AUSTRALIA

Australian Medical Acupuncture College (AMAC)
ICMART delegate: Dr Chin Chan
(Federal Vice President)
PO Box 7930
60 Ashmore Road
Bundall
Queensland 4217
Phone +61 7 5592 6699
Fax +61 7 5592 6770
Email bbundall@bigpond.net.au
chan4217@ozemail.com.au
cchan@bigpond.net.au

Dr Daniel Traum
(Immediate Past Federal President)
1429 Malvern Road
Malvern 3144
Phone +61 3 9824 6388
Fax +61 3 9824 6377
Email danjo@netspace.net.au
www.acupunctureaustralia.org

AUSTRIA
Austrian Association of Acupuncture
President: Prof. Helmut Nissel
Schlosshoferstrasse 49
1210 Vienna
Fax   +43 1 278 7272 7
Email   helmut.nissel@akupunktur.at
www.akupunktur.at

ICMART delegate: Dr Helmut Liertzer
Bahnstrasse 4
2340 Mödling
Phone   +43 223 6865 251
Fax   +43 223 6865 2514
Email   ordination@liertzer.at
www.akupunktur.at

Austrian Medical Society for Neuraltherapy
President: Dr Wolfgang Ortner
Tannenweg 5
2451 Hof am Leithaberge
Phone/Fax   +43 2168 63999
Email   wolfgang.ortner@acw.at

ICMART delegate: Dr Linda Kluger
Blaselgasse 3
1180 Vienna
Phone/Fax home   +43 1 4705 369
Phone office   +43 1 4791 471
Fax office   +43 1 4786 252
Email   linda.kluger@utanet.at

Office address   Simone Paumann
Bahnhofbichl 13
6391 Fieberbrunn
Phone   +43 5354 52120
Fax   +43 5354 5300 731
Email   oenr@tirol.com
www.neuraltherapie.at

AZERBAYCAN (AZERBAIJAN)
Azerbaycan National Acupuncture Association
President: Dr Ehtibar Kazimov
Moskova Cad. No. 82/1
Baku
Phone home   +994 (8) 1266 5151
Phone office   +994 (8) 1266 9877
Fax   +994 (8) 1247 9878
Email   inam_med@mail.az

BELARUS
Belarus Acupuncture Association
President: Dr Alexander Sivakov
Masherova Street 47/1–170
220035 Minsk
Phone home   +375 (8) 172 23 50 58
Fax   +375 (8) 172 45 52 35

BELGIUM
Belgian Association of Medical Acupuncturists
President and ICMART delegate:
Dr Gilbert Lambrechts
Everselstraat 11
3580 Beringen
Phone   +32 11 424 480
Email   bvga@skynet.be
www.acupuncture.be

BRAZIL
Brazilian Medical Association of Acupuncture
Rua Carlos Steinen no. 578
Paraiso
04004-012 Sao Paulo-SP

President: Dr Ruy Tanigawa
Rua Estella 515
Bloco H
Cj. 191
04011-002 Villa Mariana-SP
Phone   +55 11 5572 1666
Email   ruy_tanigawa@hotmail.com.br
          Secretaria.amba@terra.com.br
www.amba.org.br

ICMART delegate:
Prof. Jorge Cavalcanti Boucinhas
Av. Rui Barbosa 90
Tirol CP 1239
59015-290 Natal-RN
Phone   +55 84 2015 372
Fax   +55 84 2112 646
Email   boucinhas@natal.digi.com.br

Medical Society of Acupuncture of Sao Paulo
President: Dr Hong Jin Pai
Alameda Jaú 687
01420-001 Sao Paulo-SP
Phone   +55 11 3284 2513 or 3284 9393
Phone/Fax   + 55 11 3284 5947 or 3284 6307
Email   hongpai@uol.com.br

BULGARIA
Bulgarian Association of TCM
President: Dr Emil Iliev
PO Box 33
1463 Sofia
Phone home   +359 2 514 797
Phone office   +359 2 9526 191
Fax   +359 2 9520 241
Email   emil.iliev@gmx.net

CANADA
Canadian Medical Acupuncture Society
President: Dr Steven Aung
9904-106 Street
Edmonton
Alberta T5K 1C4
Phone home   +1 (1) 780 434 8102
Phone office   +1 (1) 780 426 2764
Fax   +1 (1) 780 426 5650
Email   draung@aung.com

CROATIA
Croatian Medical Acupuncture Association
President: Dr Jasna Lukic-Nagy
Krajiska 16/IV
41000 Zagreb
Phone home   +385 1 3707 159
Phone/Fax   +385 1 4830 317
Email   jasna.lukic-nagy@zg.hinet.hr

CYPRUS
Pancyprian Medical Society of Acupuncture
President: Dr St. G. Martoudis
57 Aeschylos Street
Nicosia
Phone   +357 2 764 202
Fax   +357 2 767 829

CZECH REPUBLIC
Czech Medical Acupuncture Society (CZMA)
President: Dr Ladislav Fildán, MD
Tyrsova 56
61200 Brno
Phone   +420 541217726
Email   fildan.ladislav@quick.cz

DENMARK
Danish Medical Association of Acupuncture
President: Dr Ruth Kirkeby
Nellikevej 1
6400 Sønderborg
Phone   +45 74 433 718
Fax   +45 73 623 050
Email   kirkeby@dadlnet.dk
www.acumed.dk

ESTONIA
Estonian Association of Acupuncture and Traditional Chinese Medicine
President: Dr E. Hanniotti
ICMART delegate: Dr Anatoly S. Levitan
Tammsaare 87-75
13416 Tallinn
Phone   +372 6 520 889
Fax   +372 6 011 193

Estonian Acupuncture Association
President: Dr Malle Lilleberg
Hobusepea 2–206
10133 Tallinn
Phone   +372 5090706
Email   d.trisong@neti.ee
Personal email   info@akupunktuur.ee
                 lilleberg@akupunktuur.ee
www.akupunktuur.ee

FINLAND
Finnish Medical Acupuncture Society
President: Dr Seppo Y. T. Junnila
Punakorvaantie 10
24800 Halikko
Phone   +358 2772 3650
Fax   +358 2772 3230
Mobile   +358 50 590 2600
Email   seppo.junnila@halikko.salonseutu.fi

FRANCE
French Medical Acupuncturist Federation for Continuous Medical Training (FAFORMEC)
President: Dr Christian Mouglalis
1 Place Delorme
44000 Nantes
Phone   +33 240 482 631
Email   c.mouglalis@free.fr
www.acupuncture-medic.com

ICMART delegate: Dr Heidi Thorer
Chemin du Bois Durand
85300 Soullans
Phone +33 251 682 131
Email Heidi.thorer@wanadoo.fr

GERMANY
German Medical Association of Acupuncture (DÄGfA)
President: Dr Walburg Maric-Oehler
Louisenstr. 15–17
61348 Bad Homburg
Phone +49 61 7221 038
Fax +49 61 7269 0441
Email maric-oehler.daegfa@t-online.de
www.daegfa.de

German Society of Acupuncture and Neural Therapy (DGfAN)
President: Dr Rainer Wander
Friedenstrasse 47
07985 Elsterberg-OT Coschütz
Phone office +49 36621 20314
Phone home +49 36621 29025
Fax office +49 36621 28104
Fax home +49 36621 29026

ICMART delegate: Dr Horst Becke
Walter-Rathenau-Str. 106
14974 Ludwigsfelde/Berlin
Phone/Fax home +49 3378 871 694

Office of DGfAN
Mühlweg 11
07368 Ebersdorf/Thüringen
Phone/Fax +49 3378 871 614
Email dgfan@t-online.de
       Drwander@t-online.de
www.dgfan.de

German Research Institute of Chinese Medicine
President: Dr Claus Schnorrenberger
Karl-Jaspers-Allee 8
4020 Basel
Switzerland
Phone home +41 61 312 5585
Phone office +41 61 295 8887
Fax +41 61 312 5587

International Association and Network for Yamamoto New Scalp Acupuncture
President: Dr Susanna Schreiber
Montanusstr. 1
51429 Bergisch Gladbach
Phone +49 2204 530 81
Fax +49 2204 530 84
Email info@ian-med.de

GREECE
Medical Acupuncture Society of Northern Greece
President: Ass. Prof. Dimitrios Vasilakos
M. Alexandrou 102
55236 Panorama
Thessaloniki
Phone/Fax +30 2310 342 627
Email vasilakos@acupuncture.gr

ICMART delegate: Dr Charisios Karanikiotes
Egnatia Str. 54
54624 Thessaloniki
Phone +30 2310 253 193
Fax +30 2310 253 191
Mobile +30 6944 757 495
Email webmaster@icmart.org
       karanik@acupuncture.gr
http://users.med.auth.gr/~karanik

Hellenic Medical Acupuncture Society
ICMART delegate: Dr Miltiades Karavis
54 Vas. Sofias Avenue
11528 Athens
Phone +30 210 7220 542
Fax +30 210 7293 345
Email karavis@ath.forthnet.gr
www.mediacus.gr

Panhellenic Medical Acupuncture Society
President: Dr Christos G. Markopoulos
34 Solonos Street
10673 Athens
Phone +30 210 3637 064

HUNGARY
Hungarian Medical Acupuncture Association
President: Dr Gabriella Hegyi
Petôfi u. 79
1196 Budapest
Phone/Fax +36 (06) 1 281 3035
Email drhegyi@hu.inter.net

IRELAND

Irish Medical Acupuncture Society

ICMART delegate: Dr Diarmaid O'Connel

Belvedere Surgery

Douglas Road

Cork

Phone   +353 21 4294 777

Fax   +353 21 4294 056

ISRAEL

The Israel Association of Medical Acupuncture

President: Dr Libon

Fax   +972 09 7722255

Email   libon521@netvision.net.il

The Medical Society of Acupuncture of the Israeli Medical Association (MSAIMA)

President: Dr E. Dvorkin

32 Mahrazet Street

PO Box 3167

Bat-Yam 59 131

Phone home   +972 50 84213

Fax   +972 50 65616

ITALY

Research Institute in Clinical Homeopathy, Acupuncture, and Psychotherapy (CSOCAP)

President: Dr Osvaldo Sponzilli

Via Sabotino 2

00195 Rome

Phone office   +39 06 3751 6391

Fax   +39 06 3724 797

Email   csocap@tiscalinet.it

Drosvaldosponzilli@virgilio.it

Italian Association of Manual Medicine and Neuroreflexotherapy (AIMAR)

President: Dr Tiberiu Brenner

Via Emilia Est 18/1

41100 Modena

Phone/Fax home   +39 059 386 071

Phone office   +39 059 222 445

Mobile   +39 0335 6184 707

Italian Medical Association of Acupuncture (AMIA)

President and ICMART delegate: Prof. F. Negro

Piazza Navona 49

00186 Rome

Email   amia@byworks.com

Fondazione Mateo Ricci

ICMART delegate: Prof. Lucio Sotte

Corso Garibaldi 160

62012 Civitanova Marche (MC)

Phone   +39 0733 770 654

Fax   +39 0733 168 91

Email   rivitmtc@tin.it

Associazione Terapie Naturale (A. Te. Na)

President and ICMART delegate: Dr Mauro Cucci

Piazza Wagner 8

20145 Milan

Phone/Fax   +39 02 468 798

Email   mfrcu@tin.it

JAPAN

International Section of Japanese Society of Ryodoraku Medicine

ICMART delegate: Dr T. Yamamoto

1-10-15 Chuodori

Nichinan

Miyazaki 887

Phone home   +81 985 583 141

Phone office   +81 987 234 815

Fax   +81 987 235 923

Email   YNSA@mnet.ne.jp

col-3633@mnet.ne.jp

Japanese Society of Veterinary Oriental Medicine

ICMART delegate: Dr Noriko Shimizu

377-15 Nakamachi

Kodaira City

Tokyo 1870042

Phone   +81 42 343 9219

Fax   +81 42 342 5340

Email   fwny9250@mb.infoweb.ne.jp

LATVIA

Latvian Medical Society. Association of Acupuncture and Related Techniques

President: Prof. Nickolay A. Nickolaev

Office   Dzirciema Str. 16

Riga LV-1007

Phone   +371 (8) 7 366 345

Fax   +371 (8) 7 205106

Home   Dubultu Ave. 102
Jurmala LV-2008
Phone/Fax   +371 (8) 7 767 198
Mobile   +371 (8) 95 34567
Email   tcmlv@e-apollo.lv

LITHUANIA

**Lituanian Medical Doctors Association
of Acupuncture and Traditional Medicine**
President: Dr Essertas Aris
Postfach 233 007
Akademieklinik
Kaunas
Email   eskes@kaunas.omniphone.net

LUXEMBOURG

**Luxembourg Medical Association
of Acupuncture**
President: Dr Guy Vinandy
4–6 Avenue de la Gare
1610 Luxembourg
Phone   +352 402 226
Fax   +352 495 630
Email   guydoc@pt.lu
www.acupuncture.lu

THE NETHERLANDS

**Dutch Medical Acupuncture Association
(NAAV)**
Presidents: Dr H. H. Van der Meiden,
Dr A. Doorgeest
ICMART delegates: Dr Robert van Bussel,
Dr D. Kopsky
NAAV Office
PO Box 1203 12103
3501 AC Utrecht
Phone   +31 30 2474630 or 2524006
Fax   +31 30 2474439 or 2524009
Email   info@naav.nl
www.naav.nl

NEW ZEALAND

Medical Acupuncture Society of New Zealand
ICMART delegate: Dr Wellington Tan
Meadowbank Medical Centre
2 Blackett Crescent
Meadowbank
East Auckland
Phone   +64 09 528 4242

NORWAY

**Norwegian Society of Medical Acupuncture,
Physician's Section**
Chairman of the Educational Board and ICMART
delegate: Dr Holgeir Skjeie
Hellemyr Legekontor
PO Box 7067
4674 Kristiansand
Phone   +47 3801 9880
Fax   +47 3801 9881
Email   holgeir@medisinsk-akupunktur.no

POLAND

Polish Acupuncture Association
President: Dr Piotr Wozniak
Instytut Centrum Zdrowie Matki Polki
ul. Rzgowska Street 281/289
93-338 Lodz
Email   president@akupunktura.org
         wozniakp@mazurek.man.lodz.pl
www.akupunktura.org

ICMART delegate: Dr Olgierd Kossowski
Winnicka Street 10
02-093 Warsaw
Phone/Fax   +48 22 659 8323 or 659 8266

PORTUGAL

Medical Acupuncture Society of Portugal
President: Dr Jorge Goncalves
Rua Goncalo Cristovao
84–5° E
4000 Porto
Phone   +351 931 9445 371
Email   jorgedr@netcabo.pt

ROMANIA

Romanian Acupuncture Society
Str. Ionel Perlea 10
Bucharest 70754
Phone   +40 314 1062
Fax   +40 312 1357
Email   amr@itcnet.ro

President: Prof. Dumitru Constantin
Central Military Hospital
Str. Calea
Plevnei 188
Bucharest 1
Phone +40 1 3122 534
Mobile +40 94 380 232
Email prof.dc@k.ro
        dumitruconstantindulcan@yahoo.com

**Transylvanian Association
of Integrated Quantum Medicine**
President: Dr Joseph Mezei
Ilarie Chendi Street 24
545400 Sighisoara
Phone +40 265 772 304
Email qmed@gbnet.ro

RUSSIA

**Russian Association of Acupuncture
and Traditional Medicine**
President: Dr Alexander Kachan
2 Kostushko Street
196247 Saint Petersburg
Phone office +7 812 555 9933
Phone home +7 812 552 5329
Fax +7 812 273 0039 or 251 7228

Russian Association of Integrative Medicine
President: Prof. Gavaa Luvsan
Executive Director: Prof. Oleg Zagorulko
2 Abrikosovsky per.
119992 Moscow
Phone +7 095 248 1052
Email ozag@mail.ru
        ozag@med.ru

SERBIA

**The Section for Acupuncture and Traditional
Medicine of the Medical Doctors Association
of Serbia**
President: Assoc. Prof. Ljubica Konstantinovic
Klinika za rhabilitaciju
Sokobanjska 13
11000 Beograd
Phone +381 11 660 755/ext. 199
Mobile +381 0633 23996
Email const@ptt.yu
        mandicd@eunet.yu

SLOVAK REPUBLIC

**Slovak Medical Society of Acupuncture
in the Slovak Medical Association**
President: Dr Jozef Smirala
Fibichova 9
82105 Bratislava
Phone +421 7 4329 2396
Fax +421 7 4333 8287

ICMART delegate: Dr Ondrej Bangha
Krajinska 101
82556 Bratislava

**National Institute of TB
and Respiratory Diseases**
Krajinska 91
82556 Bratislava
Phone +421 2 4025 1658
Email bangha@appollo.sk

SLOVENIA

**Slovenian Association of Acupuncture
and Traditional Chinese Medicine**
Vice President and ICMART delegate:
Dr Primoz Rozman
Polanskova 3
1231 Ljubljiana
Phone office +386 1 5438 100
Phone private +386 1 5613 788
Mobile +386 41 669 156

SPAIN

**Scientific Association
of Medical Acupuncturists of Sevilla**
President: Dr Rafael Cobos Romana
Avenida de la Borbolla 47
41013 Seville
Phone +34 95 423 1990
Fax +34 95 423 6050
Email rcobos@acmas.com
www.acmas.com

Grupo Master Universitario de Acupunctura
President: Dr Juan Carlos Crespo de la Rosa
Calle Virgen de Consolacion 14
3°D
41011 Seville
Phone +34 95 4276 570
Mobile +34 9395 35785
Fax +34 95 4278 711
Email jccrespo@cica.es
        medbiol@arrakis.es

Acupuncturist Section,
Official College of Physicians, Barcelona
President: Dr Isabel Giralt
Diagonial 400
4° 2a
08037 Barcelona
Phone +34 934 582 975
Email isagiralt@menta.net

SWEDEN
Swedish Medical Acupuncture Society
President: Dr Christer Carlsson
Florencekliniken
Masvagen 14
22733 Lund
Phone home +46 46 211 0818
Phone office +46 46 389 040
Fax home +46 46 157 512
Fax office +46 46 389 093
Email akusyd@swipnet.se

TURKEY
The Turkish Academic Acupuncture Society
President: Dr Mehmet Fuat Abut
Gazeteciler Mh
Saglamfikir s No. 23
80300 Esentepe
Istanbul
Phone home +90 212 212 3092
Phone office +90 212 212 3152
Fax +90 212 266 7039
Email bilgi@akademikakupunktur.org

Turkish Acupuncture Association
President: Dr Abdulkadir Erengul
Phone +90 216 355 2432

Secretary: Dr Baki Dokme
Rumeli Cad. Efe Sk. 18/2
Osmanbey
Istanbul
Phone/Fax +90 212 233 0800
Mobile +90 532 266 5109
Email bakidokme@hotmail.com
www.istakupder.8m.com

UK
British Medical Acupuncture Society
BMAS House
3 Winnington Court
Northwich
Cheshire CW8 1AQ
Phone +44 1606 786 782
Fax +44 1606 786 783
Email admin@medical-acupuncture.org.uk

President: Dr Jonathan Rae
Royal London Homoeopathic Hospital
Greenwell Street
London W1W 5BP
Phone +44 20 7387 9642
Fax +44 20 7387 9643

ICMART delegate: Dr Jacqueline Filshie
18 Dryburgh Road
Putney
London SW15 1BL
Phone home +44 208 788 3512
Email jacqueline.filshie@btinternet.com

British Dental Acupuncture Society
ICMART delegate: Dr Palle Rosted
200 Abbey Lane
Sheffield S8 0BU
Phone +44 114 236 0077
Fax +44 114 262 0491
Email prosted@aol.com

UKRAINE

**Ukranian Association of Acupuncture
and Reflexotherapy**

President: Dr Eugenia Macheret

ICMART delegate: Dr Taras Usichenko

Anaesthesiology and Intensive Care Department

University of Greifswald

Friedrich-Loeffler-Str. 23b

17487 Greifswald

Germany

Email   usichenko@gmx.de
        macheret@ukr.net

USA

**American Division of the International College
of Acupuncture and Electro-Therapeutics
(American College of Acupuncture
and Electro-Therapeutics)**

President: Prof. Yoshiaki Omura, MD, ScD

800 Riverside Drive (8-1)

New York, NY 10032

Phone   +1 212 781 6262

Fax   +1 212 923 2279

**American Academy of Medical Acupuncture
(AAMA)**

4929 Wilshire Boulevard

Suite 428

Los Angeles, CA 90010

Phone   +1 323 954 5514

Fax   +1 323 954 0959

Email   jdowden@prodigy.net

www.medicalacupuncture.org

ICMART delegate: Dr Bryan L. Frank, MD, DABMA

PO Box 30415

Edmond, OK 73003-0007

Mobile   +1 405 623 7667

Fax   +1 405 341 5342

Email   bfrankmd@aol.com

Dr Marshal Sager

191 Presidential Blvd

Suite C-130

Bala Cynwyd, PA 19004

Phone   +1 610 668 2400

Email   drmhs@verizon.net

Regulation and Developments in the Republic of Ireland

Celine Leonard, PhD, MBAc, Dublin, Ireland

Nature of Regulatory Environment

The regulation of Chinese medicine in Ireland is in the nature of voluntary self-regulation. Ireland is unique in that relatively few professions are regulated by law. Historically, herbalists and acupuncturists in Ireland, as in the UK, have practiced under a system of law known as common law. Essentially, this means that unless there is a statute prohibiting an activity then it is permissible to engage in that activity. This has created a body of professionally trained non-conventional practitioners of medicine in a way that the Napoleonic Code prevalent in most of the rest of Europe has not permitted. Under Common Law, any member of the public has the right to choose to attend a practitioner and the practitioner has the right to practice and prescribe herbal medicines. The adverse effect of Common Law practice has been that there is no official state recognition of herbalism or acupuncture as professions and therefore no distinction between professionally trained and untrained practitioners.

However, the vast majority of Chinese medicine practitioners in Ireland are members of self-regulating bodies, where there are approximately 600 professionally qualified Chinese medicine practitioners in Ireland. There are six schools offering either acupuncture training and/or Chinese herbal training on a three- and four-year weekend release basis.

Professional Registers of Chinese Medicine and Acupuncture

The main independent professional bodies are as follows:

- Irish Register of Chinese Herbal Medicine (IRCHM).
- Association of Chinese Herbalists in Ireland (ACHI).
- The Traditional Chinese Medicine Council of Ireland (TCMCI), which has recently been formed from the amalgamation of the following three organizations:
  - Acupuncture and Chinese Medicine Organisation
  - Acupuncture Foundation of Ireland Professional Association
  - Association of Irish Acupuncturists.

There is one practitioner body that is directly associated with a private college. This is called the Professional Register of Traditional Chinese Medicine.

Recent Developments

Recently we have seen the establishment of a government-sponsored forum in relation to complementary and alternative medicine (CAM), which led to the forming of a National Working Group to look into the regulation of CAM. Whilst regulation in relation to acupuncture practice is not at a critical juncture at this point, the battle for recognition of herbal medicine as a profession began properly in 1999 with the decision of the Irish Medicines Board to make hypericum and ginko biloba prescription-only medicinals in view of increasing reports of interaction with conventional medicines. Members of the public instantly lost access to over-the-counter (OTC) supplies of hypericum and ginkgo. Furthermore, given the absence of any state recognition, herbalists also lost them from their materia medica. Ironically, since these substances had no medicines license, they were effectively made unavailable, even to those few doctors who might have had adequate herbal medicine training to prescribe them in the first place. Herbalists and their supporters were galvanized into action because they saw this as evidence of a new European-wide regulatory process, which was ignorant of herbalism as a profession and judged the action of herbal substances purely in terms of pharmaceutical products rather than complex substances used either in isolation or in combination as dictated by traditional practice.

The Irish Herbal Practitioners Association was formed at that time to act as a representative umbrella body for herbal organizations and to lobby in Ireland and through the European Herbal Practitioners Association (EHPA) in the EU in the interests of its members. Its ultimate aim was to have the practice of herbal medicine recognized and regulated as a unique modality in its own right in Ireland. Statutory Regulation (SR) was seen as the only way to protect herbalism as a profession and to protect herbalists' access to their materia medica. This struggle has been ongoing for over 15 years against a background where the harmonization of European medicines legislation threatens the very existence of the common law nature of herbal practice. With the passing of 65/65 EEC, herbalists were suddenly made subject to Medicines Legislation. It seems that the practice and principles of traditional herbal medicine were either misunderstood or ignored. Given the lack of regulatory bodies in Ireland this left herbalists subject to legislation but with none of the privileges that regulation might have offered. Furthermore, this happened against a background where the cooperation of national medicines regulatory bodies meant that the misuse or non-traditional use of a herbal substance resulting in adverse effects notifications meant that these substances were suddenly made unavailable in many European countries.

For much of that time and against increasing difficulty, herbalists in Ireland have been building relations with relevant Irish regulatory bodies, such as the Irish Medicines Board and especially the Department of Health and Children, which is ultimately responsible for medicines legislation. As early as 2000 we had the stated support of the then Minister of Health and Children. In November 2001, it

was stated as part of the New National Health Strategy that complementary health practices should be regulated. The Minister's support was invaluable to us in that regulatory bodies were forced to accept our lobbying for our profession and to include us in medicines provisions. In October 2002 we succeeded in having a derogation for herbal medicines written into pharmaceutical regulations. Although this failed to give the official recognition to herbalism and herbal practice that we had been seeking, it did create the necessary legal means for us to continue to practice on an individual basis with patients. Furthermore, it allowed for the creation of a specialized list, whereby hypericum and ginko were once again made available to herbalists.

The Irish Government took the position that it would be first to implement the incoming Traditional Herbal Medicinal Products Directive (THMPD). Herbalists were included in the Committee that drew up an interim Licensing Scheme. This Committee made a strong case for the Regulation of Herbal Practitioners in its final report. However, because of the speed with which the THMPD went through the European Parliament, the interim licensing scheme has been rendered redundant and herbalists in Ireland face the same threat to their practice as any herbalist with non-medical training in the rest of Europe.

Meanwhile, the support of the Minister of Health and Children brought about the creation of a National Working Group on the Regulation of Complementary Practitioners (NWG). Its express remit was to consider appropriate regulatory frameworks that would guarantee public safety in seeking treatment from complementary practitioners. This group began its work in May 2003. Three herbalists sat on the NWG, all making a strong case for the necessity of SR to protect the public and to guarantee good practice in herbal medicine. Our final report was given to the new Minister of Health in December of last year.

When the NWG first began its work, it was stated explicitly that the Department of Health and Children would only deal with unified practitioner bodies. As with other complementary/alternative professions, the fields of acupuncture and herbal medicine have been rife with competing groups and competing commercial interests. There have been no common standards and no proper accreditation procedures to guarantee adequate standards of training. The status of the NWG has given impetus to the forces of cooperation, which has led to the creation of the National Herbal Council (NHC) in autumn 2005 from five herbal practitioner organizations and the creation of the Traditional Chinese Medicine Council of Ireland (TCMCI) from three existing acupuncture and Chinese medicine organizations. The National Herbal Council launched the first National Register of Herbal Practitioners on 1st February, 2006.

The NWG launched its report in May 2006, so we look to the future, hopefully better organized and in a better position to influence our development as a profession.

Contact Details

Celine Leonard, PhD
Irish Register of Chinese Herbal Medicine
Dublin, Ireland
www.irchm.com

Acupuncture in Germany in 2006

Gabriel Stux, MD, Düsseldorf, Germany

In Germany, with the emergence of the problem of low quality acupuncture treatment exposed by clinical studies, acupuncture providers have been working together with other competent partners on acupuncture quality initiatives in order to ensure acupuncture therapy is of the best quality and value. This initiative goes by the slogan "Acupuncture according to all the rules of the art". Seven guidelines or standards for acupuncture quality were compiled in the form of a consent paper on the quality of acupuncture treatments.

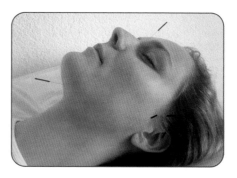

Fig. *1* Ex-1 yin tay *for headache.*

As a result, a uniform acupuncture Quality Mark has arisen, which consists of the application of these guidelines for acupuncture practice as well as the basic practitioner training and annual post-graduate training. Physicians (practitioners) can access the national Quality Mark via the website (German language) www.akupunktur-qualitaet.info. Here they can access appropriate documents as well as Quality Marks to be applied in practice.

How is acupuncture used in practice? Frequently, it is used in a Western influenced reductionistic form, that is, symptomatically: in the form of simple needling of specific acupuncture points, e. g. LI-4, *hegu*, instead of prescribing Diclophenac. Otherwise, acupuncture is used according to the rules of the art based on Chinese differential diagnosis and Chinese medical principles and theory and now perhaps on the seven guidelines or standards for acupuncture quality.

Recently, a German acupuncture study (GERAC) with 3400 patients tested acupuncture for arthrosis of the knee, chronic low back pain, migraine, and tension headache (for the national compulsory health insurance scheme). The studies showed sensational results for acupuncture in comparison with standard Western therapies. These were the largest controlled clinical trials of acupuncture ever conducted.

For back pain, even after six months, acupuncture was almost twice as effective in its long-term result as standard Western therapies. In the case of arthrosis of the knee joint it was three times more effective. In the case of migraines, a six week acupuncture therapy, made up of eleven individual treatments, was more effective than a continuous six-month's medical prophylactic therapy.

Professor Hans-Christoph Diener, MD, the German "headache Guru" summarized: "Acupuncture represents an effective and low-risk addition of the therapeutic repertoire for chronic headache, which justifies application of acupuncture in the context of pain-therapy treatment."

With both forms of headache (migraine and tension) there was also no clear evidence of verum acupuncture being better than sham acupuncture.

In sub-group analysis, however, verum acupuncture achieved a greater reduction in the number of days of headache compared to sham acupuncture in both studies. The sub-group analyses show that both acupuncture forms (verum and sham) contain a non-specific acupuncture component, whilst only verum acupuncture contains specific components.

The Acupuncture Randomized Trials (ART) with 900 patients showed a very significant difference in the three examined diagnoses in the acupuncture group versus waiting list control. There was a considerable difference between the acupuncture and "minimal acupuncture" groups in the treatment of arthrosis of the knee joint. This also becomes noteworthy in the case of back pain in the ART study, if one compares the responder rates of 50 % pain reduction. This responder rate, however, was not defined as a primary outcome, though it is a frequent outcome criterion in other studies.

Evaluation of the study results by the medical establishment was guided by the specific interests of the different groups. Now, acupuncture was established as a routine treatment for public health insured patients for only two diagnoses, low back pain and osteoarthritis of the knee.

In 1993, Kersken and Molsberger determined that the quality of the application of acupuncture technique in controlled clinical trials is usually inferior even if the study design is judged to be good. It is interesting that this may also have occurred in these large clinical studies. Within these studies, monitoring was primarily focused on data acquisition, not on the quality of the application of acupuncture technique. It appears that Western forms of the application of acupuncture technique have primarily been practiced, as often occurs in the context of a physicians busy clinical practice. Frequently Chinese diagnoses are used in very few cases. While TCM acupuncture was discussed in the GERAC study, in reality this also was used in only a few cases, as suggested by Molsberger, because "the bird wings had to be supported". The majority of physicians practicing acupuncture in the GERAC study had received training of only 140 hours. Fundamentally this means that in such cases a basic Chinese diagnosis is not possible.

In addition, the reduction in the number of treatments from 10 to 12, even in the case of chronic illnesses, would not lead to optimal long-term treatment successes. The effects of Western acupuncture are clearly greater for simple illnesses, such as arthrosis of the knee joint related conditions, than with migraine, which requires the rigorous application of Chinese acupuncture. If we look at the currently available treatment results from clinical studies, expert opinions seem to be unanimous in the view that Chinese acupuncture based on a Chinese diagnosis shows clearly better success rates, even in the case of chronic illnesses.

Those who see acupuncture and Chinese medicine as part of a holistic energetic medicine across a wide spectrum of indications, and who want to practice acupuncture at a high level, will train further in acupuncture and Chinese medicine beyond the physicians' diploma.

Our website www.akupunkturaktuell.de (German language) brings up-to-date acupuncture news and information every two weeks and has been available for over six years. We have also been conducting a forum inviting contributions on the interpretation and discussion of the results of the clinical study results. (See also "Acupuncture Quo Vadis?," p. 219; "Comments on the German Acupuncture Studies," p. 37, Research; and "Acupuncture in Western Europe," p. 137, Professional Developments, Legislation, and Regulation.)

Contact Details

Gabriel Stux, MD
German Acupuncture Society Düsseldorf
(Deutsche Akupunktur Gesellschaft, Düsseldorf, DAGD)
Düsseldorf, Germany
www.akupunktur-aktuell.de
akupunktur@arcor.de

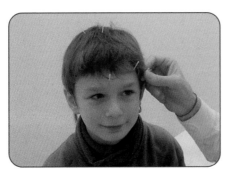

Fig. 2 10-year-old boy with headache treatment.

Education

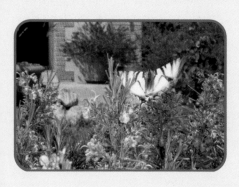

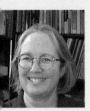

Felicity Moir

Introduction

Welcome to the educational section of the Thieme Almanac.

In this section we are attempting to list all the colleges, schools, and courses of Chinese medicine worldwide, and more detail in respect of a selection of these. Within Chinese medicine we include the systems that have developed in other countries in East Asia—Japan, Korea, Vietnam, etc. As acupuncture and Chinese medicine seem to be taught in most countries of the world, the outlook is global, with education throughout the world from China and Japan to Australia, Europe, and the USA, to name just a few. We hope to include the complete range of what is known as Chinese medicine—acupuncture, herbal medicine, tui na, qi gong, dietary therapy—and also cover medical acupuncture, anatomical acupuncture, and biomedical acupuncture.

The ideas and focus in this issue have come about primarily as a result of the interests of the people involved in the origins of this Almanac and of those who have responded to requests. The focus has in some instances been dictated by this editors' knowledge and experience, by what has been translated, and by responses to requests for information. The Almanac can therefore be seen as work-in-progress. Our hope is that the areas covered here will stimulate debate and provide an avenue for you, the readers, to let us know what is happening in your countries, regions, schools, and colleges. Over time we should build up a larger and more comprehensive picture of the diversity of practice around education. We therefore welcome you to send us articles and comments, update our knowledge, and clarify our understanding. We apologize in advance if any information is incorrect or out of date. The World Wide Web, one of our sources of the basic information about schools and courses, is a wonderful tool, but human input or lack of updated material limits its use.

In this section we have included basic information about educational practices in a number of countries, with comments on accreditation processes in operation, entry requirements, years of training, and lists of schools and courses. We also investigate specific areas around the issue of education that seem to be interesting and different. The aim is not to be comprehensive but to provide a flavor of practice in education and issues confronting educators. In each Almanac we will also give a brief synopsis of the history of Chinese medicine education in one particular country. This year we have looked at the USA.

We offer you the possibility to announce your continuing education events in our online calendar on the Almanac website: www.thieme.com/almanac.

Bearing in mind that the overall aim of what we are trying to do is to teach acupuncture and Chinese medicine in a better way and to maintain and develop standards of education, we hope that the Almanac will become a forum for the dissemination of information and will stimulate ideas that can be shared by all.

Felicity Moir, MSc, BAc, DipCHM, MBAcC
School of Integrated Health, University of Westminster, London, UK

A Brief History of Acupuncture and Chinese Medicine Education in the USA

Thanks to Changzhen Gong for his article in *The European Journal of Integrated Eastern and Western Medicine* (February 2005) and to the Report of the Working Group Meeting on Quality of Academic Education in Traditional Medicine, convened by the World Health Organization Regional Office for the Western Pacific, Melbourne, Australia, 22nd to 24th November, 2003.

1970s Key original teachers and founders of courses:
Dan Bensky, Ted Kaptchuk, and John O'Connor studied in Macao.
Miles Roberts, Dan Kenner, Peter Thompson, and others graduated from the three-year program at the Meiji Oriental Institute, Japan, and then passed the Japanese national licensure examination.
Robert Duggan, Dianne Connelly, and 36 others studied with Professor J.R. Worsley in the UK.
Bill Prensky, Steven Rosenblatt, and David Bresler founded the Institute of Taoist Studies in Los Angeles.

1972 President Nixon visited China. His personal physician, Dr Kenneth Riland, observed the practice of acupuncture and reported positively, and a *New York Times* columnist, James Reston, reported benefits of an acupuncture treatment he had received while in China.

1973 Nevada was the first state to adopt a system for licensure for non-physician acupuncturists.
The *American Journal of Acupuncture* and *American Journal of Chinese Medicine* were started.

1974 Oregon conducted the first formal examination of acupuncture candidates.

1975 The New England School of Acupuncture (NESA), the oldest school of acupuncture and Oriental medicine in the USA, was founded by the late master acupuncturist James Tin Yau So, with the help of several of his students.
Tai Sophia course was started.
New York adopted a standard for licensure.

1981 The American Association of Oriental Medicine (AAOM) (formerly the American Association of Acupuncture and Oriental Medicine [AAAOM]) was founded for promoting public education about acupuncture and advocacy for the profession.

1982 The Council of Colleges of Acupuncture and Oriental Medicine (CCAOM) was formed for the purpose of advancing the status of acupuncture and Oriental medicine in the USA.
The Accreditation Commission for Acupuncture and Oriental Medicine (ACAOM) (formerly the National Accreditation Commission for Schools and Colleges of Acupuncture and Oriental Medicine [NACSCAOM]) was established by the Council of Colleges of Acupuncture and Oriental Medicine (CCAOM).

1984 The National Certification Commission for Acupuncture and Oriental Medicine (NCCAOM) (formerly the National Commission for the Certification of Acupuncturists [NCCA]) was chartered for examining and licensing acupuncture practitioners.

1985 The NCCAOM administered the first national exam.
Tai Sophia (formerly the Traditional Acupuncture Institute [TAI]) was the first school accredited by the NACSCAOM.

1987 The American Academy of Medical Acupuncture (AAMA) was established for training conventional medical doctors to practice acupuncture.

1990 By the fall of 1990, ACAOM had achieved its original aims: recognition by the US Department of Education for accreditation of acupuncture programs at the professional master's degree level, and recognition by the prestigious Council on Post-Secondary Accreditation (COPA).

1993 Establishment of the UCLA Center for East–West Medicine, the first major US medical school with such a center.

1994 The Food and Drug Administration (FDA) passed the Dietary Supplement and Health Education Act (DSHEA) to regulate herbs as dietary supplements.

1998 Conference on Acupuncture, convened by the National Institutes of Health, concluded: " … there is sufficient evidence of acupuncture's value to expand its use into conventional medicine and to encourage further studies of its physiology and clinical value."

2003 Doctoral programs in acupuncture and Oriental medicine (AOM) were developed by ACAOM.
The Oregon College of Oriental Medicine began the first doctoral program in acupuncture and Oriental medicine in the USA.

2005 In June, ACAOM's Doctoral Task Force completed its work in developing a list of professional competencies, including the knowledge, skills, and attitudes (KSAs), expected of graduates of an entry-level, first-professional doctoral program in AOM.

2006 Currently, ACAOM has over 50 schools and colleges with accredited or candidacy status with NCCAOM.

See www.acaom.org for a list of accredited schools and colleges and links to their websites.

Contemporary Education in Chinese Medicine within a Strategy of Standardization

Professor Wang Yulai and Zhao Yonglie, PhD, Beijing, China
(English translation by R. M. Bloom, Los Angeles, California, USA)

Abstract

Standardization is the foundation of industrial modernization, for specialization and for the attendant development of norms and guarantees of quality, both in production and in delivery of services. It is also the means by which an orderly movement of scientific and technological progress to the marketplace is ensured. Standardization permeates every facet of life in present-day society. The system of standardization is one of vast and worldwide scope. The standardization of Traditional Chinese Medicine (TCM) is part and parcel of the modernization and internationalization of Chinese medicine. Indeed, standardization is the crucial basis for the continued growth and development of Chinese medicine. Standardization of education in Chinese medicine consists of the regulation of the marketplace of Chinese medical education, in order to guarantee a sound and orderly growth of Chinese medical education internationally, and to provide the impetus to delivering Chinese medicine to the wider world. The standards in contemporary education in Chinese medicine, which we shall consider below, touch on the following: conditions of the schools, qualifications of the instructors, development of goals, design of the curriculum, content of instruction, course syllabuses, development of instructional materials, implementation of instructional requirements, etc.

Keywords

Strategy of standardization, strategic standardization, standards, standardization, Chinese medicine, Traditional Chinese Medicine (TCM), education in Chinese medicine, Chinese medical education.

Introduction

In recent years, Chinese medicine has come to be accepted by people throughout the world, and its international status has achieved significant elevation. Chinese medical education is a bridge to people's understanding and grasp of Chinese medicine, and to their familiarity and interaction with it. International education in Chinese medicine is currently making great strides past Chinese borders, and it is proceeding along the path already laid by the internationalization of Chinese advanced higher education. How will the strategy of standardization be employed to develop norms for a standardized education in Chinese medicine, to regulate the market in Chinese medical education, to guarantee the sound and orderly international development of Chinese medical education, and thus to spur on the movement of Chinese medicine toward the world at large?

Advantages of Standardization for the Development of Chinese Medicine

Standardization in Chinese medicine is a timely requirement, on both a national and international scale.

In recent years, the growth of TCM has received both the concerted interest of people worldwide and the serious attention of world health organizations. Owing to its increasingly rapid growth and popularity, there has been lively activity in academic research in Chinese medicine. In many nations, the regulatory apparatus has begun to take an interest in Chinese medicine, and in more than a few countries Chinese medicine has already achieved legal status. Under these happy circumstances, our work toward modernization and standardization of Chinese medicine is motivated by a deep commitment to the historical mission of facilitating the entrance of Chinese medicine into the worldwide scene, and to bringing Chinese medicine into the mainstream of systematic medical science. There are, however, problems inherent in the process of promoting Chinese medicine worldwide.

Chinese medicine operates in the context of an extremely long and rich historical and cultural background, and it is coextensive with various unique aspects of Chinese traditional culture. The content of Chinese medicine is vast, and, with respect to its particular linguistic modalities, it possesses an especially pronounced inflection deriving from traditional Chinese culture; moreover, its theoretical system is *sui generis*. The propagation of this theoretical system within the international arena is received, and then practiced, in different nations, among different peoples in different cultural settings, within the scope of different religious traditions, and by those of different educational backgrounds.

Despite the rapid increase in the growth and popularity of Chinese medicine in many nations, full legal status has nevertheless not yet been achieved in the majority of nations, where both official legal and regulatory apparatus and strong and effective administrative control of the practice of Chinese medicine, are lacking. As a result, inadequate controls regarding the training and practice of practitioners of Chinese medicine are undermining its reputation, as well as the health and economic interests of patients.

Because of this, the matter of the standardization of Chinese medicine by the Chinese medical authorities and organizations of different nations, using a common terminology and language, emerges as an especially prominent and important problem. Furthermore, standardization can help to harmonize the scope and boundaries of Chinese medicine with that of other health and medical professions, not only by linking Chinese medicine with a wider sphere, but also by incorporating advanced technology and methods of administration into Chinese medicine, thus promoting the advancement of Chinese medicine.

The World Federation of Acupuncture-Moxibustion Societies (WFAS) and the World Federation of Chinese Medicine Societies (WFCMS) have been charged with the formulation and promotion of the legal status for international standards in Chinese medicine. In the formulation of standards for the internationalization of Chinese medicine, China occupies a position of indisputable advantage, and the country carries a responsibility that cannot be ignored. In constructing the standardization of Chi- nese medicine, we draw upon our plentiful experience, and a vast accumulation of empirical data, in every respect. We can rely upon the success of having already developed standards in China, and of transforming these standards, one step at a time, into international standards, while at the same time having a direct hand in formulating and promoting international standards for Chinese medicine.

The Crucial Role of Standardization in Chinese Medical Education

International education in Chinese medicine has become one aspect of the globalization of higher education. Respective levels of Chinese medical education in different countries (and in different regions within countries), however, differ greatly. This has had a deleterious influence on the dissemination of Chinese medicine and has affected its international reputation. How to employ the strategy of standardization, how to set up international standards for Chinese medical education, how to eliminate below-par or unsound entities from the international market in Chinese medical education, how to guarantee the sound and orderly growth of Chinese medical education within the international stage, and how to promote the further advance of Chinese medicine internationally, are important issues that have to be resolved. The following aspects will be discussed: conditions of the schools; qualifications of teachers; development of goals and objectives; design of the curriculum; organization of the course syllabus; development of textbooks; and the implementation of teaching requirements and goals.

Current Developments in Standardization of Chinese Medical Education

Educational Facilities and Educators in China

According to the National Chinese Medicine Administrative Board's 2003 statistics, there are 23 institutes of higher education in Chinese medicine in China that occupy a total physical area of 14 070 282 m², with a total collection of 10 065 000 books, a total of 540 074 electronic books, 15 816 educational computers, and material capital assets of 4 224 540 000 Yuan (approx. 530 million USD). A relatively stable, well-structured contingent of educators specializing in Chinese medicine, of excellent political and professional quality, has already been built up. Within the 23 institutes of Chinese medical education, there are a total of 20 210 educational professionals employed, of which 1152 are senior faculty, 4435 associate senior faculty, 5813 intermediate rank faculty, and 3873 junior faculty. There are a total of 9230 full-time regular faculty, of which 588 hold doctoral degrees, 2285 master's degrees, and 6088 undergraduate degrees. There are 3417 graduate advisors, of which 338 are doctoral candidate advisors, 2812 master's candidate advisors, and 267 advisors to both doctoral and master's candidates.

The Structure of Educational Levels and Educational Goals

Policies for fostering the growth of institutes of education in Chinese medicine must be oriented toward modernization and toward the world at large. These policies must foster the development of high-quality practitioners of Chinese medicine, who are able to adapt to the needs of the new century and must elevate quality in traditional Chinese medical education to a more prominent and important position. Modern higher education in Chinese medicine has an already established system of individual educational degree systems: the

three-year junior college system; the bachelor's and comprehensive bachelor's and master's seven-year system; the second bachelor's degree; the non-medical specialty master's–doctoral five-year system; and the master's, doctoral, and post-doctoral degrees; as well as other levels in the educational system.

Chief among the educational goals of higher education in Chinese medicine is to foster the development of ideals, ethics and culture, and the development of individuals who can carry on the task of building socialism. Students will have cultivated a systematic grasp, both scientific and cultural, of foundational knowledge in Chinese medicine (basic concepts, basic principles, basic methods, basic technique, and basic theoretical knowledge.) Additionally, there will be a good grounding in basic practical knowledge (effective training in basic experimental method and technique, and related practical ability in Chinese medicine, as well as training in the fundamental elements of scientific research and its practical application).

Fields of Study and the Curriculum

Modern education in Chinese medicine is fairly broad in the choice of specializations, majors, and their respective curricula. The undergraduate curriculum in Chinese medicine includes course offerings in TCM, Acupuncture, Acupressure, Orthopedics, Mongolian Traditional Medicine, Tibetan Traditional Medicine, Foundational TCM, the Literature of TCM, Surgery, Organ System Diagnostics, Rehabilitative Medicine, and other subjects. In pharmacy, the undergraduate curriculum offers courses in Chinese Herbal Medicine, Medicinal Preparation, Medicinal Authentication and Identification, Theory of Chinese Herbal Medicine, the Natural Ecology of Chinese Herbal Medicine, and other subjects. Additionally, there are related course offerings in Public Health Administration, Pharmaceutical Manufacture and Administration, Commercial and Industrial Management, Biomedical Engineering, Technical Translation, Library and Information Science, Nursing,

Law, Computer Science, and other technological specialties.

The graduate level major consists of the following series of course offerings. There are seven core courses: Basic Theory of Chinese Medicine, Foundations of Clinical Chinese Medicine, Historical Sources of Chinese Medicine, Pharmacology and Prescribing, Clinical Chinese Herbal Medicine, Diagnostics, and Integrated Chinese and Western Medicine. There are eight courses in clinical medicine: Internal Medicine, Surgery, Gynecology, Pediatrics, Orthopedics and Bone-Setting, Acupuncture and Acupressure, Integrated Chinese and Western Clinical Practice, and Integrated Chinese and Western Orthopedics in Clinical Practice. There are also five courses in herbal medicine: Clinical Chinese Herbal Medicine, Chinese Herbal Pharmacochemistry, Chinese Herbal Pharmacology, Preparation and Production of Chinese Herbal Medicine, and Biochemistry in Chinese Herbal Medicine. Additional curricula include Management, as it relates to enterprises in acupuncture and acupressure, likewise Administration in Social Medicine, Public Health and Nursing, and other areas. Other general required courses include for example: Education in Political Thought and Culture (Marxism and the Present-day Technological Revolution, Theory of Scientific Socialism, Natural Dialectics). The basic core courses include for example: Foreign Languages, Biostatistics, Concepts and Methods of Scientific Research, and Practical Computing.

Development of Texts, Their Content and Methodology

The composition of texts used for higher education in Chinese medicine has gradually conformed to a standard. Seven editions of a national standard series of texts have been published, one after another. The series currently covers 46 topics in Chinese medicine. There is now a program underway to implement the development of standard texts apropos the main body of the curriculum, in which the required basic curriculum is pared down and elective courses are added. Recently, a new series of texts for undergraduate instruc-

tion in Chinese Herbal Medicine, Preparation of Herbal Medicine, Acupuncture, Orthopedics, etc., has been compiled under the auspices of the Chinese Medical Science and Technology Publishing House, The Scientific Press Publishing House, and the Normal School Publishing House.

Future Prospects

The project of developing standards for education in Chinese medicine comprises a process of successive and increasing refinement, ranging from the simple to the complex. We have to employ appropriate and effective strategies to establish a high water mark for standards in education in Chinese medicine, in order to promote the transmission of Chinese medicine to the world at large, and better to foster and provide free play to the process of internationalization of education in Chinese medicine.

Overseas Students of Chinese Medicine in China

According to statistical surveys, the number of foreign students in China pursuing studies in Chinese medicine is second only to those who come to study Chinese. According to the Chinese National Graduate Student Foundation Administrative Committee survey data of overseas students in China in the year 2003 (released in February 2004), it was found that those pursuing studies in medical science numbered 7184, accounting for 9.23 % of all overseas students; of these, 4183 were pursuing studies in Chinese medicine, those studying the natural sciences dominating overall.

Overseas students with their different cultural and educational backgrounds, language abilities, religious beliefs, and so forth, comprise a diverse and complex whole. While pursuing their studies in Chinese medicine, students inevitably encounter difficulties in getting rid of certain preconceptions. This makes for difficulties in their appreciation of the theoretical aspects of Chinese medicine.

Consequently, in clinical practice, students are often able to adopt only a mechanical approach, and with this it is hard to achieve a good clinical outcome. In addition, overseas students from different countries have their own mother tongue. Despite the fact that the majority of these students are able to attain a certain proficiency in English, there is nevertheless considerable difference among them with respect to the degree of comprehension and expression that they exhibit. Moreover, Chinese medicine is a science with a strongly traditional Chinese flavor. Owing to its long historical and cultural background, and its exceedingly rich content and terminology, the phraseology and idioms of Chinese medicine possess an especially pronounced inflection and color unique to traditional Chinese culture. The rendering of the associated vocabulary and terms of art into English cannot be treated as an exercise in purely literary translation. There also exists a certain number of students among those studying Chinese medicine who do so out of an intense and blind desire to obtain possession, during the limited time devoted to study, of certain so-called "esoteric knowledge," "ready recipes," "special techniques," and the like. These students view Chinese medicine as mere technique, ancillary to the greater whole of clinical medical practice, and they neglect the study and research into the theoretical foundations of this technique. In fact, Chinese medicine is, properly speaking, a branch of the natural, empirical sciences, and cannot be understood through the mere grasp of certain "ready recipes." Without a true understanding of its theoretical system, Chinese medicine cannot be applied correctly and effectively. How overseas students from differing sociological, linguistic, and religious backgrounds can be helped to understand Chinese medicine correctly and study it in an appropriate manner is, therefore, an especially difficult problem currently facing the system of education in Chinese medicine.

Education Goals and Specialization in New Student Enrollment

With regard to their various objectives in study, their different cultural and educational backgrounds, their level of proficiency in Chinese, as well as other factors, entering students are directed into one of three groups of course offerings. These are the undergraduate core course sequence, the undergraduate preparatory sequence, and the supplementary and refresher course sequence. The undergraduate core course offerings include the following: Chinese Medicine, Acupuncture, Chinese Herbal Medicine, Chinese Herbal Pharmaceutical Production and Engineering, Medical Enterprise Management and Administration, Pharmaceutical Enterprise Business Management, Nursing, Clinical Medicine, and Acupressure, all of which are taught entirely in Chinese. The preparatory course sequence offerings consist mainly of courses in medical Chinese and basic theoretical concepts in Chinese medicine, which are taught in Chinese. The supplementary and refresher course offerings comprise Chinese Medicine, Acupuncture, Herbal Medicine, Orthopedics and Bone-Setting, Acupressure, *Qi Gong*, Chinese Medical Dietetics, Aesthetics and Weight-Reduction, Basic Theory of Chinese Medicine, Clinical Medicine, and Clinical Acupuncture. Courses are taught in Chinese, English, Korean, and other languages as required.

Contact Details

Professor Wang Yulai
Director of First Clinical Hospital
Beijing University of Chinese Medicine
Beijing, China

Zhao Yonglie, PhD
Clinical Department
Beijing University of Chinese Medicine
Beijing, China

Contemporary Education in Chinese Medicine within a Strategy of Standardization: A Response

Volker Scheid, PhD, FRCHM, MBAcC, London, UK

In "Contemporary Education in Chinese Medicine within a Strategy of Standardization" (see p. 198), Wang Yulai and Zhao Yonglie outline the strategies that currently guide the development of Chinese medicine in the People's Republic of China (PRC). If those who at present control this development have their way, the very same strategies will soon shape the future of Chinese medicine throughout the world. The purpose of this brief riposte is to ask whether or not this is desirable and, if so, for whom.

Wang and Zhao themselves do not consider such questions. For them, modernization and standardization are progressive and therefore, by definition, intrinsically good. Intellectually, this position has its roots in the ideologies of modernization that have dominated Chinese politics, culture, and medicine throughout the twentieth century. It assumes that history necessarily progresses from primitive society to the modern nation state, and from traditional to modern forms of social life. It views the increasing regulation, bureaucratization, and standardization of life made possible by the powers of a strong nation state, and its ability to establish institutions of surveillance and control, as both progressive and desirable. It maintains that science is the only appropriate model for understanding the world, and the only legitimate tool for solving its problems [1, 2].

The influence of these ideologies is visible in all areas of contemporary Chinese medicine. It is seen in the transmission of knowledge through standardized textbooks and nationwide exams in modern educational institutions; in the hospitalization of Chinese medicine that has increased the distance between doctor and patient; and in the creation of standardized categories for diagnosis and treatment that shift authority from individual physicians to regulatory bodies. In an age of increasing globalization, a further aspect of standardization is the transformation of Chinese medicine from a practice embedded in specific local cultures into a marketable commodity that can be easily moved to different locations across the world [3, 4].

Like all ideological commitments, Wang and Zhao's assumption that standardization constitutes an intrinsically desirable attribute reveals itself to be extremely one-sided, once it is opened up to closer scrutiny. For any process of transformation implies that gains made in one area must be paid for by losses in another. Max Weber, the famous German sociologist, pointed out long ago that modernity is not necessarily liberating. It enslaves us in an "iron cage" of rationalization and bureaucratization, by reducing autonomy, by shifting control of decisions away from individuals toward institutions, and by reducing experiences of authenticity that humans find essential for a fulfilling life. If the growth of alternative medicine in the West during the 1970s and 1980s was inspired by attempts to reclaim such autonomy, then embracing standardization as advocated by Wang, Zhao, and the PRC implies cutting Chinese medicine in the West loose from these roots.

Standardization, of course, has never been either an intrinsic or essential aspect of the Chinese medical tradition. Its core text, the *Huang Di Nei Jing* (The Yellow Emperor's Classic of Medicine) is a prototype of non-standardized knowledge, if ever there was one. A collection of texts by different authors who agree with each other only on the most basic of terms, its very diversity inspired later generations of physicians and provided them with a canvas onto which they could project their own ideas [5]. Viewed from this perspective, the growth of medical knowledge within the Chinese medical tradition was helped rather than hindered by the polysemous nature of its foundational texts and the unregulated spaces in which physicians could debate them.

Not surprisingly, the ideal of the scholar physician in imperial China was the very antithesis of the regulated and controlled technician imagined by Wang and Zhao. "Each doctor," as the medical historian Nathan Sivin explains, "was expected to arrive at his own synthesis through the interaction of deep book-learning and practice. The goal was to be fully responsible for his very limited power over life and death, not to become a technician manipulating bodies" [6, 7]. If that is true, then we must ask ourselves to what extent the standardization of Chinese medicine that is currently taking place in the name of developing tradition is actually achieving its opposite.

My own position is that, like *yin* and *yang*, standardization and individual self-development do not need to be regarded as polar opposites, but rather as mutually supportive processes. This, too, is something we can learn from history. Only at one other time during the entire history of Chinese medicine, in the Song dynasty, did the state become involved in facilitating and regulating its practice [8, 9, 10]. This initiated a period of unprecedented growth and development that defined the core paradigms and styles of practice of élite medicine for centuries to come. State intervention made this growth possible by creating an infrastructure for learning, collating, and disseminating medical knowledge. It was left to individual physicians, however, to use these resources to develop their medical tradition along multiple and diverse currents.

Regulation and standardization by their very nature inhibit diversity, and thus the growth of medical knowledge. In a limited way they can help to disseminate knowledge and create a space in which vibrant communities of medical practitioners can discuss and debate their different visions of what it means to be a good physician. That is what we can learn from the Song transformation of Chinese medicine. It is also the balanced perspective on modernization that we should embrace today.

References

1. Hui W. The fate of "Mr Science" in China: the concept of science and its application in modern Chinese thought. In: Barlow TE, ed. *Formations of Colonial Modernity in East Asia*. Durham: Duke University Press; 1997 [1995].
2. Kwok DWY. *Scientism in Chinese Thought 1900–1950*. New Haven and London: Yale University Press; 1965.
3. Andrews BJ. *The Making of Modern Chinese Medicine, 1895–1937* [PhD dissertation]. Cambridge; 1996.
4. Scheid V. *Chinese Medicine in Contemporary China: Plurality and Synthesis*. Durham: Duke University Press; 2002.
5. Unschuld PU. *Huang Di Nei Jing Su Wen* [The Yellow Emperor's Classic of Medicine]: *Nature, Knowledge, Imagery in an Ancient Chinese Medical Text, With an Appendix. The Doctrine of the Five Periods and Six qi in the Huang Di Nei Jing Su Wen*. Berkeley: University of California Press; 2003.
6. Sivin N. *Traditional Medicine in Contemporary China*. Ann Arbor: The University of Michigan Center for Chinese Studies; 1987.
7. Ibid.: 25–26.
8. Goldschmidt, A. *The Transformation of Chinese Medicine During the Northern Song Dynasty (AD 960–1127)*. [PhD dissertation]. University of Pennsylvania; 1999.
9. Goldschmidt, A. Changing standards: tracing changes in acumoxa therapy during the transition from the Tang to the Song dynasties. *East Asian Science, Technology, and Medicine*. 2001; 18:75–111.
10. Hinrichs, TJ. *The Medical Transforming of Governance and Southern Customs in Song Dynasty China (960–1279 CE)*. [PhD dissertation]. Harvard University; 2003.

Contact Details

Volker Scheid, PhD, FRCHM, MBAcC
Senior Research Fellow
School of Integrated Health
University of Westminster, London, UK
www.wmin.ac.uk

Teaching Traditional Chinese Medicine in China: Colleges and Universities

Currently in China there are professional Traditional Chinese Medicine (TCM) universities, colleges, and secondary schools, a master–apprentice education system, and clinical training conducted in hospitals. In addition, there is vocational schooling at various levels, including continuing education, postgraduate training, correspondence courses, and independent study.

At the end of 2003, there were 32 colleges and universities and 45 secondary schools teaching TCM in China. There were also TCM specialized departments in 184 health schools, 58 medical colleges and universities. These include 13 doctoral specializations and 23 additional graduate specializations.

Colleges and Universities of TCM in China

Anhui College of TCM
103 Meishan Road
Hefei
Anhui Province 230038
Phone   +86 551 516 9009/5
Fax   +86 551 281 9950
www.ahtcm.edu.cn

Beijing University of Chinese Medicine
President: Zheng Shouzeng
11 Bei San Huan
Dong Lu
Chao Yang District
Beijing 100029
Phone   +86 10 6421 3841
Fax   +86 10 6421 3817
www.bjucmp.edu.cn

Changchun College of TCM
President: Wang Zhihong
Boshuo Road 1035
Jingyuetan
Changchun
Jilin Province 130117
Phone   +86 431 617 2513
Fax   +86 431 617 2345
www.ccutcm.com.cn

Chengdu University of TCM
President: Zhu Bao De
37 Shierqiao Road
Chengdu
Sichuan 610075
Phone   +86 28 776 8611
Fax   +86 28 776 3471
www.cdutcm.edu.cn/html/etcm.html

Fujian University of TCM
President: Du Jian
282 Wusi Road
Fuzhou
Fujian Province 350003
Phone   +86 591 357 0322
Fax   +86 591 357 0746
www.fjtcm.edu.cn

Gansu College of TCM
President: Liu Yanzhen
35 Dingxi Road
Lanzhou
Gansu Province 730000
Phone   +86 931 861 9329
Fax   +86 931 862 7950
www.gszy.edu.cn

Guangxi College of TCM
President: Wang Naiping
179 Mingxiu Road
Nanning
Gangxi Autonomous Region 530001
Phone   +86 771 313 5848
Fax   +86 771 313 0664
www.gxtcmu.edu.cn

Guangzhou University of TCM
President: Feng Xinsong
12 Airport Road
Guangzhou
Guangdong Province 510405
Phone   +86 20 3659 5233
Fax   +86 20 3659 4735
www.gzhtcm.edu.cn

Guiyang College of TCM
President: Liang Guangyi
1 Eastern Road
Guiyang
Guizhou Province 550002
Phone   +86 851 565 2099
Fax   +86 851 565 2638
www.gyctcm.edu.cn

Heilongjiang University of TCM
President: Kuang Haixue
24 Heping Road
Dongli District
Harbin
Heilongjiang Province 150040
Phone   +86 451 8211 2786
Fax   +86 451 8211 2786
Email   hljutcm@yahoo.com.cn
www.hljucm.net

Henan College of TCM
President: Pengbo
1 Jinshui Road
Zhengzhou
Henan Province 450008
Phone   +86 371 594 5879
Fax   +86 371 594 4307
www.hactcm.edu.cn

Hubei College of TCM
President: Wanghua
1 Tanhualin
Wuchang
Wuhan
Hubei Province 430061
Phone   +86 27 8891 0230
Fax   +86 27 6888 9170
www.hbtcm.edu.cn

Hunan College of TCM
President: You Zhaoling
1 Shaoshan Road
Changsha
Hunan Province 410007
Phone   +86 731 560 0508
Fax   +86 731 550 4879
www.hnctcm.edu.cn

Jiangxi College of TCM
President: Liu Hongning
1 Yunwan Road
Wanli District
Nanchang
Jiangxi Province 330004
Phone   +86 791 711 8822/55
Fax   +86 791 711 8800
www.jxtcmi.com

Liaoning College of TCM
President: Ma Ji
79 Chongshan Road
Huanggu District
Shenyang
Liaoning Province 110032
Phone   +86 24 8684 1637
Fax   +86 24 8684 1382
www.lnutcm.edu.cn

Nanjing University of TCM
President: Xiang Ping
282 Hanzhong Road
Gulou District
Nanjing
Jiangsu Province 210029
Phone   +86 25 8679 8167
Fax   +86 25 8679 8168
www.njutcm.edu.cn

Shandong University of TCM
President: Wang Xinlu
53 Jingshi Road
Jinan
Shandong Province 250014
Phone   +86 531 261 3011
Fax   +86 531 296 3364
www.sdutcm.edu.cn

Shanghai University of TCM

President: Yan Shiyun

1200 Cailun Road

Zhangjiang

Hi-Tech Park

Pudong New District

Shanghai 201203

Phone   +86 21 5132 2274

Fax   +86 21 5132 2276

Email   english@shtcm.com

www.shtcm.com

Shanxi College of TCM

President: Tao Gongding

169 Jinci Road

Taiyuan

Shanxi Province 030024

Phone   +86 351 604 2281

Fax   +86 351 604 2276

www.sxtcm.com

Tianjin College of TCM

President: Zhang Boli

88 Yuquan Road

Nankai District

Tianjin 300193

Phone   +86 22 2305 1023

Fax   +86 22 2305 1066

www.tjutcm.edu.cn

Yunnan College of TCM

President: Li Qingsheng

88 Shuangqiao Road

Kunming

Yunnan Province 650011

Phone   +86 871 715 0982

Fax   +86 871 715 0982

www.yntm.edu.cn

Zhejiang College of TCM

President: Xiao Luwei

548 Bin Wen Road

Bing Jiang District

Hangzhou

Zhejiang Province: 310053

Phone   +86 571 8661 3501

Fax   + 86 571 8661 3500

www.zjtcm.net

Chinese Medicine Education in Australia

State Legislation

In most states and territories in Australia there is no statutory legislation controlling the practice of Chinese medicine, and therefore no statutory requirements from the Department of Health concerning the training. There are universities providing training in acupuncture and Chinese herbal medicine, which therefore come under the Office of Higher Education legislation. Some of these courses have affiliate links with private schools with the university that provide the health sciences and research training, and the private schools provide the training in Chinese medicine, including clinical training. There are also private schools and colleges covering training in acupuncture and Chinese herbal medicine. There are courses in acupuncture for doctors, physiotherapists, and nurses, some of which are recognized by their professional bodies as postgraduate training.

The state of Victoria has developed regulations governing the practice and training of Chinese medicine.

Accrediting Organizations

Other than in the Registration Board of Victoria, although there is currently no statutory regulation governing Chinese medicine, most of the full-time teaching institutions have been proactive in developing voluntary accreditation. The Australian Acupuncture and Chinese Medicine Association (AACMA), the largest professional association in Australia, recognizes graduates of established four- to five-year Australian bachelor degree programs in acupuncture, and/or Chinese herbal medicine, as well as some sub-degree programs that are currently applying for bachelor level accreditation or for articulation with a recognized

bachelor degree program. The association does not recognize primary qualifying programs offered by correspondence/distance mode.

(See also p.157, Professional Developments, Legislation, and Regulation.)

Length of Courses

Most courses are four- to five-year undergraduate programs, including acupuncture and/or herbal medicine; some include *qi gong, tui na*, and Chinese language. All courses include training in health sciences, professional practice and ethics, and research. Contact hours are approximately 2500.

AACMA-Recognized Course List

Entry requirements are normally a tertiary entrance qualification; subjects include biology, chemistry, and English.

Australian College of Natural Medicine
362 Water Street
Fortitude Valley
Queensland 4006
Phone   +61 7 3257 1883
Email   info@acnm.edu.au
www.acnm.edu.au
Bachelor of Health Science (Acupuncture)
Acupuncture

Melbourne College of Natural Medicine
Level 1
368 Elizabeth Street
Melbourne
Victoria 3000
Phone   +61 3 9662 9911
Email   info@mcnm.edu.au
Bachelor of Health Science (Acupuncture)
Acupuncture

RMIT University
Royal Melbourne Institute of Technology
Chinese Medicine Unit
Plenty Road
Melbourne
Victoria 3083
Phone +61 3 9925 7745
Email charlie.xue@rmit.edu.au
www.rmit.edu.au
Bachelor of Applied Science (Chinese Medicine)/
Bachelor of Applied Science (Human Biology)—
double degree award
Acupuncture and Chinese Herbal Medicine
Advanced Diploma of Traditional Chinese Medicine
(provisional recognition)
Acupuncture and Chinese Herbal Medicine

Sydney Institute of Traditional Chinese
Medicine
92–94 Norton Street
Leichardt
New South Wales 2040
Phone +61 2 9550 9906
Email administration@sitcm.edu.au
Diploma of TCM Remedial Massage (Anmo-tui na)
TCM Remedial Massage
Bachelor of Health Science in Traditional Chinese
Medicine Acupuncture and Chinese Herbal
Medicine

University of Technology Sydney
PO Box 123
Broadway
Sydney
New South Wales 2007
Phone +61 2 9514 2500
Email bob.hayes@uts.edu.au
www.uts.edu.au
Bachelor of Health Science in TCM
Diploma of TCM Remedial Massage (Anmo-tui na)
TCM Remedial Massage

University of Western Sydney
PO Box 555
Campbelltown
New South Wales 2560
Phone +61 2 9685 9087
Email study@uws.edu.au
www.uws.edu.au

Bachelor of Applied Science (Traditional Chinese
Medicine)
Acupuncture and Chinese Herbal Medicine
Bachelor of Health Science (Chinese Medicine)—
Acupuncture (major Acupuncture)

Victoria University of Technology
PO Box 14428
MCMC
Melbourne
Victoria 3000
Phone +61 3 9688 4110
Email ccs@vu.edu.au
www.vu.edu.au
Bachelor of Health Science (Chinese Medicine)—
Chinese Herbal Medicine (major Chinese Herbal
Medicine)

The above courses cover the states of Victoria, New South Wales, and Queensland.

Medical Acupuncture

All recognized general practitioners practicing medical acupuncture must be accredited by the Joint Consultative Committee for Medical Acupuncture (JCCMA) and participate in on-going Continuing Professional Development (CPD) requirements to maintain their eligibility with Medicare Australia.

Contact Details

AACMA-recognized course list: for an update on this list, refer to www.acupuncture.org.au.

For further details of courses recognized by other professional organizations, refer to Australian Natural Therapists Association: www.anta.com.au.

For details of courses in Chinese medicine approved by the Registration Board of Victoria, contact: www.cmrb.vic.gov.au/registration/approvedcourses.

For medical acupuncture courses accredited by the JCCMA, refer to: www.racgp.org.au.

Chinese Medicine Education in New Zealand

State Legislation

Education providers must be accredited by the qualifications authority before they can offer programs of education and training. Programs are assessed against unit standards. Accredited providers assessing against unit standards must engage with the moderation system that applies to those unit standards.

Entrance Qualifications

A tertiary entrance qualification is normally required; useful subjects include biology, chemistry, and English. Chinese language courses are also useful.

Length of Courses

A minimum of four years of full-time study in Traditional Chinese Medicine, including Western anatomy, physiology, and pathology, as well as acupuncture. All colleges teach acupuncture, some teach herbal medicine and some *tui na* and *qi gong*.

- Four years of study (3600 total hours of study, which may include up to 720 hours of supervised clinical training) of acupuncture and Traditional Chinese Medicine; or
- Postgraduate training (1200 total hours of study, which may include up to 360 hours of supervised clinical training) of which Traditional Chinese Medicine diagnosis and acupuncture theory are the focus.

Professional Body

The New Zealand Register of Acupuncturists is the main professional body.

Members of the Register have been trained at recognized places and/or have shown equivalent standards of proficiency through their clinical practice and by examination.

New Zealand School of Acupuncture and Traditional Chinese Medicine
PO Box 11076
Wellington 6015
Wellington Campus
Level 1057
Willis Street
CBD
Wellington 6001
Phone   +64 4 473 9005
Fax   +64 4 473 9040

Auckland Campus
1/272 Jervois Parade
Herne Bay
Auckland 1002
Phone   +64 9 361 1161
Fax   +64 9 361 2481
Email   admin@acupuncture.co.nz
www.acupuncture.co.nz
Acupuncture, herbs, qi gong, tui na

Christchurch College of Holistic Healing
PO Box 18788
New Brighton
Christchurch 8030
Campus   183 Shaw Street
New Brighton
Christchurch 8007
Phone   +64 3 388 2333
Fax   +64 3 388 2287
Email   info@holistichealing.co.nz
www.holistichealing.co.nz
Acupuncture

Auckland College of Natural Medicine
PO Box 49011
Mt Roskill
South Auckland 1030
Campus   Level 1
321C Great South Road
Greenlane
Auckland 1005
Phone   +64 9 580 2376
Fax   +64 9 580 2379
Email   acnm@xtra.co.nz
www.acnm.co.nz
Acupuncture, herbs, tui na

New Zealand College of Oriental Medicine Ltd
PO Box 19423
Hamilton 2015
Campus   227 Baverstock Road
Nawton
Hamilton
Phone   +64 7 849 2008
Fax   +64 7 849 0003
Email   dean@nzom.ac.nz
www.nzom.ac.nz
Acupuncture, herbs

Contact Details

Details of the National Diploma of Acupuncture can be found on the website at www.nzqa.govt.nz/framework.

New Zealand Register of Acupuncturists:
www.acupuncture.org.nz

Chinese Medicine Education in Norway

The accrediting body for higher education in Norway is the Norwegian Agency for Quality Assurance in Education (NOKUT).

In 2003, the Department of Health in Norway provided a status report on the situation relating to acupuncture education in Norway. Its conclusion concerning education in traditional classical acupuncture was that the minimum standard that should be provided was a four-year full-time bachelor degree course in acupuncture.

There are many organizations in Norway that provide courses in acupuncture, which are of varying length (and quality). The Norwegian Acupuncture Association (NAFO) recognizes two of these organizations. Both are independent and private, and do not receive any funds or other support from the education authorities.

Since 1999, the Norwegian College of Acupuncture has offered a five-year part-time course for people who have completed their high school education, and/or have other general skills, such as four years in general work practice. This is the same entry requirement as for any higher education in colleges or universities in Norway. The five-year course includes anatomy, physiology, functional anatomy, assessment methods, and pathology. These elements have comprised the main content of the first two years of study.

Three- and five-year part-time courses for health personnel, such as doctors, physiotherapists, nurses, dentists, and chiropractors, are also offered.

Students from these two courses are "merged" after the second year of the five-year course, and subsequently they more or less follow the same course.

The Norwegian College of Acupuncture is applying for a BSc validation.

The Nordic Acupuncture College offers both a three- and a five-year part-time course for health personnel such as doctors, physiotherapists, nurses, homeopaths, and dentists.

Norwegian College of Acupuncture

St. Olavsgt. 12
0165 Oslo
Phone +47 2 2988 140
Fax +47 2 2361 853
www.akhs.no

Nordic Acupuncture College (Nordisk Akupunkturhøgskole)

Kongsvelen 30
0193 Oslo
Phone +47 2 6754 0607
Fax + 47 2 6756 5676
www.nahs.no

Contact Details

Norwegian Agency for Quality Assurance in Education:
www.nokut.no/sw335.asp

Norwegian Acupuncture Association:
www.akupunktur.no

Chinese Medicine Education in the UK

At the moment there is no statutory legislation controlling the practice of Chinese medicine in the UK, and therefore no statutory requirements from the Department of Health concerning the training.

There are:

- universities providing training in acupuncture and Chinese herbal medicine that come under higher education legislation from the Department of Education;
- private schools and colleges covering training in acupuncture and Chinese herbal medicine, some of which are validated by universities, and therefore coming under Higher Education legislation;
- private schools and colleges that are not affiliated with universities;
- courses in acupuncture for doctors, physiotherapists, and nurses, some of which are recognized by their professional bodies as postgraduate training.

While there is currently no statutory regulation governing Chinese medicine, most of the full-time teaching institutions have been proactive in developing voluntary accreditation, and this allows graduates to join a professional body.

The two accrediting bodies described below are the main, but not the only, bodies with robust procedures of accreditation. Educational programs are evaluated, based on institutional processes, educational policy and procedures, content, length of program, and outcomes. Indicators are used to determine if educational programs meet the criteria.

The British Acupuncture Accreditation Board (BAAB)

The BAAB was founded in 1990, and graduates of accredited courses are eligible to join the British Acupuncture Council (BAcC).

The course should be a minimum of three years full-time, or the part-time equivalent of 3600 hours, of which at least 1200 must be structured time with a member of staff, and comprising no fewer than 400 hours of clinical instruction, of which 200 hours must be in taking direct responsibility for all aspects of patient care.

All programs include traditional Chinese medicine physiology, pathology and diseases, point location and acupuncture techniques, biological and clinical sciences, communication skills, practitioner–patient relationship, ethics, and practice management and research.

The European Herbal Practitioners Association (EHPA)

The EHPA was founded in 1994. Graduates of accredited courses of Chinese medicine join the Register of Traditional Chinese Medicine.

The course should comprise a minimum of 2560 hours, of which one-third must be structured time with a member of staff, and with no fewer than 400 hours of clinical instruction, of which 200 hours must be in direct responsibility for all aspects of patient care. All programs include Traditional Chinese Medicine physiology, pathology and diseases, herbs and formulae, quality assurance and control, biological and clinical sciences, communication skills, practitioner–patient relationship, ethics, and practice management and research.

With the exception of Middlesex University, all the courses listed below teach Chinese medicine acupuncture on their full-time undergraduate programs. Their Chinese herbal medicine courses are taught as separate programs, either at undergraduate or postgraduate level. Middlesex University runs a four-year program, which includes training in acupuncture and Chinese herbal medicine. Some of the courses include *tui na* courses, either concurrently or as further training.

For an update, refer to the BAcC website (www.acupuncture.org.uk).

Entry requirements are normally secondary school qualifications, such as five GCSEs, including English, maths, and preferably biology or combined science, plus A levels.

College of Integrated Chinese Medicine
(Affiliated to the University of Kingston)
19 Castle Street
Reading RG1 7SB
Phone +44 118 950 8880
Fax +44 118 950 8890
www.cicm.org.uk

College of Traditional Acupuncture (UK)
(Affiliated to Oxford Brookes University)
Haseley Manor
Hatton
Warwick
Warwickshire CV35 7LU
Phone +44 1926 484 158
Fax +44 1926 484 444
www.acupuncture-coll.ac.uk

International College of Oriental Medicine UK
(Affiliated to the University of Brighton)
Green Hedges House
Green Hedges Avenue
East Grinstead
West Sussex RH19 1DZ
Phone +44 1342 313 106/7
Fax +44 1342 318 302
www.orientalmed.ac.uk

London College of Traditional Acupuncture and Oriental Medicine
(Affiliated to the University of Portsmouth)
60 Ballards Lane
Finchley
London N3 2BU
Phone +44 20 8371 0820
Fax +44 20 8371 0830
www.lcta.com

Northern College of Acupuncture
(Affiliated to the University of Wales)
61 Micklegate
York YO1 6LJ
Phone +44 1904 343 303
Fax +44 1904 330 370
www.chinese-medicine.co.uk

School of Five Element Acupuncture
13 Mandela Street
London NW1 0DU
Phone   +44 20 7383 5553
Fax   +44 20 7383 5503
www.sofea.co.uk
(SOFEA are not enrolling any new undergraduate students)

University of Salford
School of Community Health Sciences and Social Care
5th Floor, Allerton Building
Frederick Road Campus
Salford
Greater Manchester M6 6PU
Phone   +44 161 295 2372
www.chssc.salford.ac.uk

University of Westminster
Department of Complementary Therapies
School of Integrated Health
115 New Cavendish Street
London W1W 6UW
Phone   +44 20 7911 5082
www.westminster.ac.uk

Courses at Stage Two Accreditation
Middlesex University
School of Health and Social Sciences
Enfield Campus
Queensway
Enfield
Middlesex EN3 4SA
Phone   +44 208 411 5000
Phone (admissions)   +44 208 411 5161
www.mdx.ac.uk

University of Lincoln
School of Health and Social Care
Brayford Pool
Lincoln LN6 7TS
Phone +44 1522 837 419
Fax +44 1522 886 791
www.lincoln.ac.uk

British Medical Acupuncture Society (BMAS)

The BMAS offers training to healthcare professionals who are registered by statute in the UK. This includes doctors, dentists, nurses, midwives, health visitors, physiotherapists, osteopaths, chiropractors, and podiatrists.

The organization provides a foundation course that covers the basic concepts of acupuncture. This is run over a period of four to five days. There are then further training days: a post-foundation training day and an intermediate training program that covers the entire field of medical acupuncture through six days of weekend courses, attended over a period of three years.

Acupuncture Association of Chartered Physiotherapists (AACP)

Basic membership of the AACP is granted only on evidence that a physiotherapist has completed at least 40 hours of training on courses approved by the AACP.

Accredited membership of the AACP is granted only on evidence that a physiotherapist has completed at least 80 hours of training on courses approved by the AACP.

Advanced members of the AACP are only awarded their status after a minimum of 200 hours training, on extended courses approved by the Education Committee of the AACP, or in holding an MSc in Acupuncture.

The British Academy of Western Medical Acupuncture

The Academy runs practical comprehensive courses for those with suitable medical qualifications. The courses are in the style of postgraduate studies, and the academic year is from September to April over 15 days.

Contact Details

Acupuncture Association of Chartered Physiotherapists:
www.aacp.uk.com

British Academy of Western Medical Acupuncture:
www.acupuncture-medical.co.uk

British Acupuncture Accreditation Board:
www.acupuncture.org.uk/content/baab/baab.html

British Acupuncture Council:
www.acupuncture.org.uk

British Medical Acupuncture Society:
www.medical-acupuncture.co.uk

European Herbal Practitioners Association:
www.users.globalnet.co.uk/~ehpa

Register of Chinese Herbal Medicine:
www.rchm.co.uk

Chinese Medicine Education in the USA

Forty-one states and the District of Columbia either license, certify, or register practitioners, thus statutorily recognizing the practice of acupuncture, and therefore have legislation over the standards of training. Michigan and Kansas allow non-physician acupuncturists to practice under the supervision of a licensed medical doctor. In the remaining seven states, either acupuncture is unregulated, no determination has been made, or it is determined to be the practice of medicine.

The National Commission for the Certification of Acupuncture and Oriental Medicine (NCCAOM)

An attempt is being made to set minimal competency standards throughout the USA through certification by the NCCAOM. Several thousand practitioners have already become certified, and some states have adopted the NCCAOM examination as part of their licensing criteria. California and a few other states have set higher standards and do not recognize the NCCAOM-certified "diplomates" membership status. California conducts its own state licensing examination.

The Accreditation Commission for Acupuncture and Oriental Medicine (ACAOM)

The Council of Colleges of Acupuncture and Oriental Medicine (CCAOM) established the ACAOM in June 1982. It is a private, non-profit organization recognized by the US Department of Education as a specialized and professional accrediting agency. The US Department of Education periodically reviews the ACAOM to ensure its compliance. Each state may also choose to set additional eligibility criteria (usually additional academic or clinic hours). Texas and California, for example, are two states with additional requirements. A small number of states have additional jurisprudence or practical examination requirements, such as passing the Clean Needle Technique (CNT) examination.

As an independent body, the ACAOM accredits first professional master's degree and professional master's level certificate and diploma programs in acupuncture, and first professional master's degree and professional master's level certificate and diploma programs in Oriental medicine, with a concentration in both acupuncture and herbal therapies. The commission fosters excellence in acupuncture and Oriental medicine education by establishing policies and standards that govern the accreditation process for acupuncture and Oriental medicine programs. The accrediting process requires programs to examine their goals, activities, and outcomes; to consider the criticism and suggestions of a visiting team; to determine internal procedures for action on recommendations from the Commission; and to maintain continuous self-study and improvement mechanisms.

The ACAOM does not require an acupuncture/Oriental medicine program to acquire degree-granting authorization from its State Board of Higher Education in order to be eligible for accreditation. The practical result of this policy is that some ACAOM-certified programs confer degrees, while others confer diplomas or certificates. Currently, the ACAOM has over 50 schools and colleges with accredited or candidacy status with the Commission.

Entry requirements for courses include a prerequisite of two years' college education.

The ACAOM's acupuncture program requirements include a minimum three-year (27-month) program of 1905 hours and 105 semester credits.

The ACAOM's Oriental medicine program requirements include a minimum four-year (36-month) program of 2625 hours and 146 semester credits.

The ACAOM's Doctoral program requirements include 4000 hours and 1200 hours beyond that of the master's degree, and 650 clinical hours.

Only institutions already offering accredited master's level programs are allowed to develop doctoral degrees.

The California State Legislature and the California Acupuncture Board

To obtain a license to practice acupuncture in California, you must qualify for and then take a written examination administered by the Acupuncture Board. This can be done by:

- completing the necessary curriculum requirements and graduating from a school approved by the Acupuncture Board;
- completing a tutorial program approved by the Acupuncture Board (similar to an apprenticeship);
- completing a foreign education training program, equivalent to the curriculum required at a school approved by the Acupuncture Board.

In California, acupuncturists are considered a primary health care profession. Thus, they need to meet a common standard of competence expected of all primary health care professions, such as the ability to recognize serious diseases that may require immediate referral to a specialist.

The CCAOM has established that minimum standards of training for full acupuncture and oriental medicine training programs should be 3200 hours, following 500 hours of college level training in basic science.

There are currently 30 schools/training programs approved by the board (16 in California and 14 in other states).

Medical Acupuncture

Medical doctors (MDs), certified in "medical acupuncture" by the American Academy of Medical Acupuncture (AAMA), are required to take 200 hours of didactic training in acupuncture and 100 hours of clinical training. Several medical schools now include acupuncture courses.

NCCAOM-Accredited Courses

Academy of Chinese Culture and Health Sciences
1601 Clay Street
Oakland, CA 94612
Phone   +1 510 763 7787
Fax   +1 510 834 8646
Email   info@acchs.edu
www.acchs.edu
Master of Science in Traditional Chinese Medicine
  program

Academy for Five Element Acupuncture
1170A E. Hallandale
Beach Blvd
Hallandale Beach, FL 33009
Phone   +1 954 456 6336
Fax   +1 954 456 3944
Email   info@acupuncturist.edu
www.acupuncturist.edu
Master of Acupuncture program

Academy of Oriental Medicine at Austin
2700 West Anderson Lane
Suite 204
Austin, TX 78757
Phone   +1 512 454 1188
Fax   +1 512 454 7001
Email   info@aoma.edu
www.aoma.edu
Master of Acupuncture and Oriental Medicine
  program

Acupuncture and Integrative Medicine College, Berkeley
2550 Shattuck Avenue
Berkeley, CA 94704
Phone   +1 510 666 8248
Fax   +1 510 666 0111
Email   info@aimc.edu
www.aimc.edu
Master of Science in Oriental Medicine program

Acupuncture and Massage College
(Formerly Southeast Institute of Oriental Medicine)
10506 North Kendall Drive
Miami, FL 33176
Phone   +1 305 595 9500
Fax   +1 305 595 2622
Email   admissions@amcollege.edu
www.amcollege.edu
Master of Science in Oriental Medicine program

American Academy of Acupuncture and Oriental Medicine
1925 West County Road B2
Roseville, MN 55113
Phone   +1 651 631 0204
Fax   +1 651 631 0361
Email   tcmhealth@aol.com
www.aaaom.org
Master of Science in Acupuncture and Oriental Medicine program

American College of Acupuncture and Oriental Medicine
9100 Park West Drive
Houston, TX 77063
Phone   +1 713 780 9777
Fax   +1 713 781 5781
Email   info@acaom.edu
www.acaom.edu
Master of Acupuncture and Oriental Medicine program

American College of Traditional Chinese Medicine
455 Arkansas Street
San Francisco, CA 94107
Phone   +1 415 282 7600
Fax   +1 415 282 0856
Email   info@actcm.edu
www.actcm.org
Master of Science in Traditional Chinese Medicine program

Arizona School of Acupuncture and Oriental Medicine
4646 East Fort Lowell Road
Suite 104
Tucson, AZ 85712
Phone   +1 520 795 0787
Fax   +1 520 795 1481
Email   asaom@dakotacom.net
www.asaom.edu
Master of Acupuncture program
Master of Acupuncture and Oriental Medicine program

Atlantic Institute of Oriental Medicine
100 E. Broward Blvd
Fort Lauderdale, FL 33301
Phone   +1 954 763 9840
Fax   +1 954 763 9844
Email   atom@atom.edu
www.atom.edu
Master of Science in Oriental Medicine program

Bastyr University
14500 Juanita Drive N.E.
Kenmore, WA 98028-4966
Phone   +1 425 823 1300
Fax   +1 425 823 6222
Email   admiss@bastyr.edu
www.bastyr.edu
Master of Science in Acupuncture program
Master of Science in Acupuncture and Oriental Medicine program

Colorado School of Traditional Chinese Medicine
1441 York Street
Suite 202
Denver, CO 80206-2127
Phone +1 303 329 6355
Fax +1 303 388 8165
Email cstcm-admin@traditionalhealing.net
www.traditionalhealing.net
Master of Science in Traditional Chinese Medicine program

Dongguk Royal University
440 Shatto Place
Los Angeles, CA 90020
Phone +1 213 487 0110
Fax +1 213 487 0527
Email info@dru.edu
www.dru.edu
Master of Science in Oriental Medicine program

Dragon Rises College of Oriental Medicine
901 N.W. 8th Avenue
Suite B-5
Gainesville, FL 32601
Phone +1 352 371 2833
Fax +1 352 371 2867
Email info@dragonrises.net
www.dragonrises.net
Master of Acupuncture and Oriental Medicine program

East West College of Natural Medicine
3808 N. Tamiami Trail
Sarasota, FL 34234
Phone +1 941 355 9080
Fax +1 941 355 3243
Email registrar@ewcollege.org
www.ewcollege.org
Master of Science in Oriental Medicine program

Eastern School of Acupuncture and Traditional Medicine
427 Bloomfield Avenue
Suite 301
Montclair, NJ 07042
Phone +1 973 746 8717
Fax +1 973 746 8714
Email easternschoolacup@earthlink.net
www.easternschool.com
Diploma in Acupuncture program

Emperor's College of Traditional Oriental Medicine
1807B Wilshire Boulevard
Santa Monica, CA 90403
Phone +1 310 453 8300
Fax +1 310 829 3838
Email dsl@emperors.edu
www.emperors.edu
Master of Traditional Oriental Medicine program

Five Branches Institute: College and Clinic of Traditional Chinese Medicine
200 Seventh Avenue
Santa Cruz, CA 95062
Phone +1 831 476 9424
Fax +1 831 476 8928
Email tcm@fivebranches.edu
www.fivebranches.edu
Master of Traditional Chinese Medicine program

Florida College of Integrative Medicine
7100 Lake Ellenor Drive
Orlando, FL 32809
Phone +1 407 888 8689
Fax +1 407 888 8211
Email info@fcim.edu
www.fcim.edu
Master of Traditional Oriental Medicine program

Institute of Clinical Acupuncture and Oriental Medicine
Chinatown Cultural Plaza
100 North Beretania Street
Suite 203B
Honolulu, Hawaii 96817
Phone   +1 808 521 2288
Fax   +1 808 521 2271
Email   info@orientalmedicine.edu
www.orientalmedicine.edu
Master of Traditional Oriental Medicine program

Jung Tao School Of Classical Chinese Medicine
207 Dale Adams Road
Sugar Grove, NC 28679
Phone   +1 828 297 4181
Fax   +1 828 297 4171
Email   info@jungtao.edu
www.jungtao.edu
Diploma in Acupuncture program

Midwest College of Oriental Medicine—Chicago, IL
4334 North Hazel
Suite 206
Chicago, IL 60613
Phone   +1 773 975 1295
Fax   +1 773 975 6511
Certificate of Completion in Acupuncture program
Master of Science in Oriental Medicine program

Midwest College of Oriental Medicine—Racine, WI
6232 Bankers Road
Suites 5 & 6
Racine, WI 53403
Phone   +1 262 554 2010
Fax   +1 262 554 7475
Email   info@acupuncture.edu
www.acupuncture.edu
Certificate of Completion in Acupuncture program
Master of Science in Oriental Medicine program

Minnesota College of Acupuncture and Oriental Medicine
Northwestern Health Sciences University
2501 W. 84th Street
Bloomington, MN 55431
Phone   +1 952 885 5435
Fax   +1 952 887 1398
Email   mmckenzie@nwhealth.edu
www.nwhealth.edu
Master of Acupuncture program
Master of Oriental Medicine program

National College of Naturopathic Medicine
049 S.W. Porter Street
Portland, OR 97201
Phone   +1 503 552 1555
Fax   +1 503 279 9300
Email   admissions@ncnm.edu
www.ncnm.edu
Master of Science in Oriental Medicine program

New England School of Acupuncture
40 Belmont Street
Watertown, MA 02472
Phone   + 1617 926 1788
Fax   +1 617 924 4167
Email   info@nesa.edu
www.nesa.edu
Master of Acupuncture program
Master of Acupuncture and Oriental Medicine program

New York College of Health Professions
(Formerly New Center for Holistic Health Education, and Research)
6801 Jericho Turnpike
Syosset, NY 11791-4413
Phone   +1 516 364 0808
Fax   +1 516 364 0989
Email   info@nycollege.edu
www.nycollege.edu
Master of Science in Acupuncture program
Master of Science in Oriental Medicine program

New York College of Traditional Chinese Medicine

(Formerly New York Institute of Chinese Medicine)
155 First Street
Mineola, NY 11501
Phone   +1 516 739 1545
Fax   +1 516 873 9622
Email   nyicm@aol.com
www.nyctcm.edu
Master of Science in Acupuncture program
Master of Science in Oriental Medicine program

Oregon College of Oriental Medicine

10525 S.E. Cherry Blossom Drive
Portland, OR 97216-2859
Phone   +1 503 253 3443 ext. 111
Fax   +1 503 253 2701
Email   admissions@ocom.edu
www.ocom.edu
Master of Acupuncture and Oriental Medicine
*   program*

Pacific College of Oriental Medicine—Chigaco, IL

3646 North Broadway, 2nd Floor,
Chicago, IL 60613
Phone   +1 773 477 4822
Fax   +1 773 477 4109
Email   admissions-sd@pacificcollege.edu
www.pacificcollege.edu
Master of Traditional Oriental Medicine program

Pacific College of Oriental Medicine—New York, NY

915 Broadway
2nd Floor
New York, NY 10010
Phone   +1 212 982 3456
Fax   +1 212 982 6514
Email   admissions-ny@pacificcollege.edu
www.pacificcollege.edu
Master of Science in Acupuncture program
Master of Science in Traditional Oriental Medicine
*   program*

Pacific College of Oriental Medicine—San Diego, CA

7445 Mission Valley Road
Suite 105
San Diego, CA 92108
Phone   +1 619 574 6909
Fax   +1 619 574 6641
Email   admissions-sd@pacificcollege.edu
www.pacificcollege.edu
Master of Science in Traditional Oriental Medicine
*   program*

Phoenix Institute of Herbal Medicine and Acupuncture (PIHMA)

301 E. Bethany Home Road
Suite A-100
Phoenix, AZ 85012
Phone   +1 602 274 1885
Fax   +1 602 274 1895
Email   contactus@pihma.edu
www.pihma.edu
Master of Science in Acupuncture program
Master of Science in Oriental Medicine program

Samra University of Oriental Medicine

3000 South Robertson Blvd
4th Floor
Los Angeles, CA 90034
Phone   +1 310 202 6444
Fax   +1 310 202 6007
Email   info@samra.edu
www.samra.edu
Master of Science in Oriental Medicine program

Santa Barbara College of Oriental Medicine

1919 State Street
Suite 207
Santa Barbara, CA 93101
Phone   +1 805 898 1180
Fax   +1 805 682 1864
Email   email@sbcom.edu
www.sbcom.edu
Master of Acupuncture and Oriental Medicine
*   program*

Seattle Institute of Oriental Medicine
916 N.E. 65th Street
Seattle, WA 98115
Phone   +1 206 517 4541
Fax   +1 206 526 1932
Email   info@siom.edu
www.siom.edu
Master of Acupuncture and Oriental Medicine program

Sophia Institute
(Formerly Traditional Acupuncture Institute)
7750 Montpelier Road
Laurel, MD 20723
Phone   +1 410 888 9048
Fax   +1 410 888 9004
Email   admissions@tai.edu
www.tai.edu
Master of Acupuncture program

South Baylo University
1126 N. Brookhurst Street
Anaheim, CA 92801
Phone   +1 714 533 1495
Fax   +1 714 533 6040
Email   admin@southbaylo.edu
www.southbaylo.edu
Master of Science in Acupuncture and Oriental Medicine program

Southern California University Of Health Sciences
16200 E. Amber Valley Drive
PO Box 1166
Whittier, CA 90604
Phone   +1 562 947 8755
Fax   +1 562 902 3332
Email   admissions@scuhs.edu
www.scuhs.edu
Master of Acupuncture and Oriental Medicine program

Southwest Acupuncture College— Albuquerque, NM
7801 Academy Road N.E.
Albuquerque, NM 87109
Phone   +1505 888 8898
Fax   +1 505 888 1380
Email   abq@acupuncturecollege.edu
www.acupuncturecollege.edu
Master of Science in Oriental Medicine program

Southwest Acupuncture College— Boulder, CO
6620 Gunpark Drive
Boulder, CO 80301
Phone   +1 303 581 9955
Fax   +1 303 581 9944
Email   boulder@acupuncturecollege.edu
www.acupuncturecollege.edu
Master of Science in Oriental Medicine program

Southwest Acupuncture College— Santa Fe, NM
1622 Galisteo Street
Santa Fe, NM 87505
Phone   +1 505 438 8884
Fax   +1 505 438 8883
Email   sfe@acupuncturecollege.edu
www.acupuncturecollege.edu
Master of Science in Oriental Medicine program

Swedish Institute College of Health Sciences
226 West 26th Street
PO Box 11130
New York, NY 10001
Phone   +1 212 924 5900
Fax   +1 212 924 7600
Email   acupuncture@swedishinstitute.edu
www.swedishinstitute.edu
Master of Science in Acupuncture program

Texas College of Traditional Chinese Medicine
(Formerly Texas Institute of Traditional Chinese Medicine)
4005 Manchaca Road
Suite 200
Austin, TX 78704

Phone +1 512 444 8082
Fax +1 512 444 6345
Email texastcm@texastcm.edu
www.texastcm.edu
Master of Acupuncture and Oriental Medicine
*   program*

Tri-State College of Acupuncture
80 8th Avenue
Suite 400
New York, NY 10011
Phone +1 212 242 2255
Fax +1 212 242 2920
Email TSITCA@aol.com
www.tsca.edu
Master of Science in Acupuncture program
Master of Science in Oriental Medicine program

Traditional Chinese Medical College of Hawaii
65–1206 Mamalohoa Highway,
Building 3
Suite 9
Kamuela, HI 96743
Phone +1 808 885 9226
Fax +1 808 885 9227
Email tcmch@tcmch.edu
www.tcmch.edu
Master of Science in Oriental Medicine program

World Medicine Institute
(Formerly Tai Hsuan Foundation)
College of Acupuncture and Herbal Medicine
PO Box 11130
Honolulu, HI 96828
Phone +1 808 949 1050
Fax +1 808 955 0118
Email worldmedicine@cs.com
www.acupuncture-hi.com
Master of Acupuncture and Oriental Medicine
*   program*

University of East West Medicine
970 W. El Camino Real
Sunnyvale, CA 94087
Phone +1 408 733 1878
Fax +1 408 992 0448
Email info@uewm.edu
www.uewm.edu
Master of Science in Traditional Chinese Medicine
*   program*

Yo San University of Traditional Chinese Medicine
13315 West Washington Blvd,
Los Angeles, CA 90066
Phone +1 310 577 3000
Fax +1 310 577 3033
Email info@yosan.edu
www.yosan.edu
Master of Acupuncture and Traditional Chinese
*   Medicine program*

Contact Details

For information on individual state legislation regarding Chinese medicine, go to: www.nccaom.org/StateData.htm or www.naturalhealers.com.

American Board of Medical Acupuncture (ABMA)
For ABMA-approved training programs, go to: www.dabma.org/programs.asp.

Accreditation Commission for Acupuncture and Oriental Medicine (ACAOM)
www.acaom.org

California State Board
For up-to-date information, go to: www.acupuncture.ca.gov/education/schools.htm.

Chinese Medicine Education in Canada

Other than in British Columbia, there is no statutory legislation at the present time controlling education in Chinese medicine in Canada. Each state has its own voluntary professional bodies and entry requirements.

Alberta

For acupuncture, the graduate must have completed a program of studies that has been approved by the Health Disciplines Board, or have satisfactorily completed an examination approved by the board in order to be regulated. There is no regulation relating to herbal medicine.

**Alberta College of Acupuncture
and Traditional Chinese Medicine**
125-4935 40th Avenue N.W.
Calgary
Alberta T3A 2N1
Phone   +1 403 286 8788
Fax   +1 403 247 4648
Email   info@acatcm.com
www.acatcm.com

Grant MacEwan College
PO Box 1796
Edmonton
Alberta T5J 2P2
Phone   +1 780 497 5040
Fax   +1 780 497 5001
Email   www.macewan.ca

British Columbia

British Columbia was the first state in North America to officially designate Traditional Chinese Medicine (TCM) practice. The College of Traditional Chinese Medicine Practitioners and Acupuncturists of British Columbia (CTCMA)

is an official professional licensing authority, established in 1996 by the Government of British Columbia, Canada to regulate the practice of TCM and acupuncture in the province. The college is a self-regulatory body that operates under the auspices of the provincial government and through the Health Professions Act: Traditional Chinese Medicine Practitioners and Acupuncturists Regulation and Bylaws. The college grants a title once an applicant with the appropriate educational training has passed the associated licensing examinations and safety courses.

TCM and acupuncture educational programs are evaluated based on institutional processes, content and length of program, and outcomes. Indicators are used to determine whether educational programs meet the criteria.

Five areas of an educational program are reviewed: institutional processes, curriculum, students and graduates, resources, program content.

Entry requirements are two years' university education or equivalent.

Acupuncture Program
The minimum requirement is 1900 hours in three academic years, including 450 hours minimum of clinical instruction.

All programs include TCM, point location and acupuncture techniques, biological and clinical sciences, communication skills, ethics, medical legal issues, and practice management.

Herbology Program
The minimum requirement is 1900 hours in three academic years, including 450 hours minimum of clinical instruction.

All programs include: TCM, herbology, biological and clinical sciences, communication skills, ethics, medical legal issues, and practice management.

224   THIEME Almanac 2007

The TCM Practitioner Program

This requires 2600 hours minimum in four academic years, including 650 hours minimum of clinical instruction.

The program is a combination of the acupuncture program, the herbology program listed above, and courses in *tui na*, *shi liao*, and Chinese rehabilitation exercises such as *tai ji quan* and *qi gong*.

The TCM Doctorate Program

This requires 3250 hours minimum in five academic years, including 1050 hours minimum of clinical instruction.

In addition to the TCM practitioner program listed above, the program consists of a minimum of 450 hours in modern clinical research in TCM, TCM classics, Western diagnostic information, other TCM treatment modalities—gerontology, psychology, advanced studies in acupuncture, herbal pharmacology—and a minimum of 150 hours of clinical instruction.

Academy of Classical Oriental Sciences
303 Vernon Street
Nelson
British Columbia V1L 4E3
Phone +1 250 352 5887
Toll Free 1 888 333 8868
Fax +1 250 352 3458
Email acos@acos.org
www.acos.org

Canadian College of Acupuncture and Oriental Medicine
551 Chatham Street
Victoria
British Columbia V8T 1E1
Phone +1 888 436 5111
Fax +1 250 360 2871
Email ccaom@islandnet.com
www.ccaom.com

Canadian College of Traditional Chinese Medicine
202–560 West Broadway
Vancouver
British Columbia V5Z 1E9
Phone +1 604 879 2365
Fax +1 604 875 0095

International College of Traditional Chinese Medicine (ICTCM)
769 Pandora Avenue
Victoria
British Columbia V8W 1N9
Phone +1 250 388 4266
Fax +1 250 380 6738
Email info@tcminternational.com
www.tcminternational.com

International College of Traditional Chinese Medicine of Vancouver
201–1508 West Broadway
Vancouver
British Columbia V6J 1W8
Phone +1 604 731 2926
Email info@tcmcollege.com

International Tai Shan College of Traditional Chinese Medicine
206–370 East Broadway
Vancouver
British Columbia V5T 4G5
Phone/Fax +1 604 872 6833
Email studytcm@taishancollege.com

Mission-Beijing College of Chinese Medicine and Pharmacology
200–2010 E. 48th Avenue
Vancouver
British Columbia V5S 1G7
Phone +1 604 301 0628
Fax +1 604 301 0681
Classes conducted in English and Mandarin

Oshio College of Acupuncture and Herbology
110–114 1595 Mckenzie Avenue
Victoria
British Columbia V8L 1A4
Phone +1 250 472 6601
Fax +1 250 472 6601
Email oshio@home.com

Shang Hai TCM College of BC Canada
212–4885 Kingsway
Burnaby
British Columbia V5H 4T2
Phone   +1 604 430 5838
Fax   +1 604 430 5878
Email   info@acupuncture-college.com
www.acupuncture-college.com

**Western Canadian Institute
of TCM Practitioners**
520–4400 Hazelbridge Way
Richmond
British Columbia V6X 3R8
Phone   +1 604 270 1818
Fax   +1 604 270 3998
www.tcm.bc

Ontario

There is currently no regulation of education
in Ontario, but the educational standard for
acupuncture/TCM is presently under review
by the provincial government. For further information, contact the Canadian Society of
Chinese Medicine and Acupuncture. Entry requirements to courses seem to be two years
of post-secondary education or training, or
working experience in related fields.

**Academy of Clinical Chinese Medicine
of Toronto (ACCMT)**
18 Wynford Drive
Suite 606
Don Mills
Ontario M3C 3S2
Phone   +1 416 385 2848
Fax   +1 416 510 2557
Email   accmt@hotmail.com

**Acupuncture and Traditional Chinese
Medicine Institute**
276 Willard Avenue
Toronto
Ontario M6S 3R2
Phone/Fax   +1 416 767 6266
Email   chengkoh@interlog.com

**Beijing Union University College of Chinese
Medicine and Pharmacology**
Branch of Canada
3443 Finch Avenue E.
Suite 302
Scarborough
Ontario M9C 2Y3
Phone   +1 416 493 8447
Fax   +1 416 493 9450

Canadian College of Holistic Health
10670 Yonge Street
Richmond Hill
Ontario L4C 3C9
Phone   +1 905 884 9141
Fax   +1 905 884 5889
www.cchh.org

Canadian College of Oriental Medicine
120 Eglinton Avenue E.
Suite 200
Toronto
Ontario M4P 1E2
Phone   +1 416 410 4986
Fax   +1 416 410 4986
Email   admissions@ccom.ca

Centennial College
651 Warden Avenue
Scarborough
Ontario M1L 3Z5
Phone   +1 416 289 5307
www.centennialcollege.ca

Huangdi College of Traditional Chinese Medicine
1560 Bloor Street W.
Unit 1
Toronto
Ontario M6P 1A4
Phone: +1 416 539 9998

**Institute of Acupuncture and Traditional
Chinese Medicine**
779 Chelsea Court
Unit no CL2
Brockville
Ontario K6V 6J8
Phone   +1 613 498 3906
Fax   +1 613 498 1886
Email   iatcm@ripnet.com
www.recorder.ca/acupuncture

Institute of Chinese Medicine and Acupuncture, Canada
154 Wellington Street
London
Ontario N6B 2K8
Phone   +1 519 642 1970
Fax   +1 519 642 2932
Email   icma@skynet.ca

Institute of Traditional Chinese Medicine
368 Dupont Street
Toronto
Ontario M5R 1V9
Phone   +1 416 925 6752
Fax   +1 416 925 8920

International University of Alternative Medicines
107 Leitch Drive
Grimsby
Ontario L3M 2T9
Phone   +1 877 3544 666
Fax   +1 905 563 8930
Email   zusanli 2000@yahoo.com
          or deqi 2000@yahoo.ca

Michener Institute for Applied Health Sciences
222 St Patrick Street
Toronto
Ontario M5T 1V4
Phone   +1 416 596 3117
Fax   +1 416 596 3180
Email   info@michener.ca
www.michener.ca

Ontario Academy of Traditional Chinese Medicine
94 Cumberland Street
Suite 416
Toronto
Ontario M5R 1A3
Phone   +1 416 968 9988

Ontario College of Acupuncture and Chinese Medicine
658 Danforth Avenue
Suite 413
Toronto
Ontario M4J 1L1
Phone   +1 416 560 2340

Ontario College of Traditional Chinese Medicine
145 Sheppard Avenue E.
Suite102
100 & 201 North York
Toronto
Ontario M2N 3A7
Phone   +1 416 222 3667
Fax   +1 416 646 3667
Email   info@octcm.com
www.octcm.com

Toronto Institute of Chinese Medicine and Acupuncture
212 Bathurst Street
Toronto
Ontario M5T 2R9
Phone   +1 416 603 0236
Fax   +1 416 603 7080

Toronto School of Traditional Chinese Medicine
2010 Eglinton Avenue W.
Suite 302
Toronto
Ontario M6E 2K3
Phone   +1 416 782 9682
Fax   +1 416 782 9681
Email   info@tstcm.com
www.tstcm.com

Quebec

The Acupuncture Program at Rosemont College is the only accredited program offered in Quebec. Those who successfully complete the examination l'Ordre des Acupuncteurs du Québec become registered acupuncturists and are granted a work permit in Quebec.

The program is three years and is made up of 1980 hours of classroom training. It contains courses in acupuncture, Western sciences, communication, and counseling techniques. It is aiming to upgrade to university level.

Collège de Rosemont
Departement d'acupuncture
6400 16ème Avenue
Montreal
Quebec H1X 2S9
Phone   +1 514 376 1620, poste 353
www.crosemont.qc.ca

Further information

**Canadian Society of Chinese Medicine
and Acupuncture (CSCMA)**
434 Dundas Street W.
Unit 303
Toronto
Ontario MRT 1G7
Phone   +1 416 597 6769
Fax   +1 416 597 0028
www.tcmcanada.org

**College of Traditional Chinese Medicine
Practitioners and Acupuncturists
of British Columbia (CTCMA)**
www.ctcma.bc.ca/index.asp

Professional Standards

Part of the development of state/governmental regulatory processes for Chinese medicine professionals is setting professional standards* of education. Standards are an attempt to define what it is that professionals can be expected to do, that is, they articulate the attributes and capabilities that describe good practice and are written to measure performance outcomes. They are not a detailed syllabus or curriculum. They are a source of information to:

- help individuals to improve performance;
- help people make informed decisions about the structure and content of education and training and related qualifications; and
- help workers and employers improve their services.

The following are extracts of professional standards from three countries that have them in writing. They are all written in different ways, and as such illuminate the various ways groups of professionals and educators have tried to capture the essence of what a professional of Chinese medicine does. Some have been written in relation to acupuncture and some for herbal medicine, but they could be superimposed with slight changes.

USA

In the USA, core competencies have been developed for the First Professional Master's level and also for the First Professional Doctorate. The Accreditation Commission for Acupuncture and Oriental medicine (ACAOM) has developed them, in conjunction with representatives from professional bodies, the Council of Colleges in the United States, and also the World Federation of Chinese Medicine Societies (WFCMS).

The First Professional Master's professional competencies can be viewed in the Accreditation Handbook Part 1: Structure, Scope, Process and Standards Essential Requirement 8.

The following are their headings for professional competencies (acupuncture program 1–7 and oriental medicine 1–10). Mostly they are written as statements of content, except for number 7, where they are given an outcome measure.

1. Collecting data and using the following examinations of the patient, in order to be able to make a diagnosis.
2. Formulating a diagnosis by classifying the data collected and organizing it according to traditional oriental medical theories of physiology and pathology. This skill implies comprehensive understanding of the following fundamental theories and concepts.
3. Determining treatment strategy based on the diagnosis formulated.
4. Performing treatment by applying appropriate techniques, including needles, *moxa*, manipulation, counseling, and the utilization of skills appropriate for preparation of tools and instruments.
5. Assessing the effectiveness of the treatment strategy and its execution.
6. Complying with practices as established by the profession and society at large, through:
   - application of a code of ethics;
   - practice of responsible record-keeping and patient confidentiality;
   - maintenance of professional development through continuing education;
   - maintenance of personal development by continued cultivation of compassion.
7. In order to be able to:
   - recognize situations where the patient

---

* Other expressions: national occupational standards, professional practice standards, subject benchmark statements, professional competencies requires emergency or additional care or care by practitioners of other health care (or medical) modalities, and to refer such patients to whatever resources are appropriate to their care and well-being;

- appropriately utilize relevant biomedical clinical science concepts and understandings to enhance the quality of oriental medical care provided;
- protect the health and safety of the patient and the health care provider related to infectious diseases, sterilization procedures, needle handling and disposal, and other issues relevant to blood borne and surface pathogens;
- communicate effectively with the biomedical community;

the student must have an adequate understanding of:

- relevant biomedical and clinical concepts and terms;
- relevant human anatomy and physiological processes;
- relevant concepts related to pathology and the biomedical disease model;
- the nature of the biomedical clinical process, including history taking, diagnosis, treatment, and follow-up;
- the clinical relevance of laboratory and diagnostic tests and procedures, as well as biomedical physical examination findings;
- relevant pharmacological concepts and terms, including knowledge of relevant potential medication, herb and nutritional supplement interactions, contraindications and side effects.

8. Making a diagnosis/energetic evaluation by:
   - identifying position, nature, and cause of the dysfunction, disorder, disharmony, vitality, and constitution. This evaluation is based on the 13 concepts below, plus knowledge of distinctive patterns of herbal combinations and recognition of medical emergencies.
9. Planning and executing an herbal treatment, using the following knowledge.
10. Understanding professional issues related to oriental herbs.

The First Professional Doctorate

The First Professional Doctorate has developed competency statements under the following key areas (domains). They assume the inclusion of the professional competencies as above, but are written as outcome measures:

1. Patient care
2. Professional development and currency
3. Professionalism
4. Systems-based practice

Under each of these headings are core competency statements, with subheadings of knowledge, skills, and attitudes. For example, under the domain of patient care there is the core competency of "ability to apply critical thinking." Within this competency comes:

- **Knowledge:** to understand and recognize appropriate methods of analyzing information that form the basis for clinical action.
- **Skills:** to engage in skillful, responsible thinking that facilitates good judgement because it (a) relies on criteria, (b) is self-correcting, and (c) is sensitive to context.
- **Attitudes:** to have an interest in using all available techniques and tools to derive the maximum information about the patient's care.

Contact Details

Accreditation Commission for Acupuncture and Oriental Medicine:
www.acaom.org

UK

In the UK, professional standards have recently come into the spotlight. With statutory regulation now on the government agenda for acupuncture and herbal medicine, and courses of Chinese medicine now established in state-sponsored universities, the development of standards has become timely. Further, as the Acupuncture Regulatory Working Group struggled with the different professional contexts within which acupuncture is practiced in the UK by different groups of healthcare professionals (lay practitioners, physiotherapists, doctors, nurses), a framework was seen as necessary to establish some form of equivalence. The government appointed Skills for Health (SfH), its approved standards-setting body for health-sector professions, to bring together the various stakeholders for consultation. Two groups were set up, one for herbal medicine and one for acupuncture.

From the outset, the British Acupuncture Council (BAcC) saw the process set by SfH as "top down" and rushed. Also, there was little deviation allowed from the generic structure that SfH used for all healthcare professional groups. This in no way illuminated what the profession saw as the artistry of professional practice, the often unpredictable complexity inherent in professional practice, and was more suited to Western medical practice and healthcare settings. As a result the BAcC set about writing its own "Standards of Practice for Acupuncture."

Below are a precis and extracts from two documents as a means of comparison. The first is the National Professional Standards for Herbal Medicine, which follow the structure set by SfH. The second are those written by the BAcC.

National Professional Standards for Herbal Medicine

Complementary medicine—herbal medicine
There are six units, with elements of competence within each. With each unit there is a:
- summary;
- set of statements of the knowledge and understanding expected;
- set of statements of the applied technical knowledge and understanding;
- set of statements of the professional and practice knowledge.

With each element of competence, there are performance criteria and scope statements.

Unit 1. Assess the needs of the client
HM1.1 Evaluate and process requests for herbal medicine
HM1.2 Prepare to assess the client
HM1.3 Assess the client

Unit 2. Provide a treatment and management plan to meet the needs of the client
HM2.1 Negotiate and formulate the treatment and management plan with the client
HM2.2 Evaluate the effectiveness of the herbal medicine treatment
HM2.3 Complete post consultation activities

Unit 3. Dispense herbal medicines and products
HM3.1 Receive and validate herbal prescription
HM3.2 Assemble and label required herbal medicine(s) or product(s)
HM3.3 Issue prescribed herbal medicine(s) or product(s)

Unit 4. Plan and maintain the growing of herbs
HM4.1 Plan and prepare the growing area
HM4.2 Establish herbs in the growing area
HM4.3 Maintain the development of herbs

Unit 5. Plan and maintain the harvesting of herbs
HM5.1 Plan the harvesting of herbs
HM5.2 Maintain the harvesting of herbs
HM5.3 Prepare harvested herbs

Unit 6. Prepare herbal medicines in batches
HM6.1 Prepare environment, equipment, and ingredients for the assembly or manufacturing process
HM6.2 Prepare, process, assemble, and pack the manufactured product
HM6.3 Complete the assembly or manufacturing process

Performance Criteria
Below is an example of performance criteria for Unit 1, Element HM1.3 (assess the client):
You will need to:
1. Respect the client's privacy and dignity throughout the consultation and ensure they are as comfortable as possible.
2. Conduct the consultation in a manner that encourages the effective participation of the client and meets their particular requirements.
3. Support the client to identify significant aspects of their lives and use this to inform the consultation.

4. Determine any contraindications or restrictions to physical examination and investigation and take appropriate action.
5. Use examination and investigation methods that are safe, appropriate to the client's presenting condition, and comply with professional and legal requirements.
6. Use systematic questioning and appropriate physical examination to establish a diagnosis.
7. Seek advice and support from an appropriate source when the needs of the client and the complexity of the case are beyond your own remit or capability.
8. Inform the client when additional information is required and obtain their consent to obtain the information.
9. Evaluate the information obtained for and during the consultation, and determine appropriate action.
10. Ensure records are signed, dated, and include all relevant details and any supporting information.

Contact Details

Skills for Health:
www.skillsforhealth.org.uk/view_framework

**BAcC Standards of Practice
for Acupuncture**
The standards are written under six key headings:

1. Practice Context
2. Diagnosis and Treatment
3. Communications and Interaction
4. Safety
5. Professional Development
6. Business Management

Within each of these there is an overall statement and a set of standards. Each standard is expanded further under three headings: *principles* (that articulate aspects of the main standard), *descriptors* (fuller descriptions to which practitioners can be expected to aspire), and *practitioner cues* (questions that serve as a stimulus for review and reflection, which the practitioner could ask themselves and others). For example:

Practice Context—Acupuncture practitioners recognize that they work within a specific context, or set of contexts, and that this necessarily plays a part in shaping their practice and influencing their relationships with patients, carers, colleagues, and other healthcare practitioners.

Standard 2—Acupuncture practitioners recognize and understand that they always operate within a set of contexts influenced by political, societal, and cultural considerations that will impact on their practice.

Table 1 Practice Context Standard 2

Principles	Descriptors	Practitioner cues
Acupuncture practitioners recognize that different belief systems in a multicultural society may influence therapeutic expectations and outcomes	We need to understand that words and ideas in traditional Chinese culture may have different meanings and values to those of the cultural background of the practitioner and patient or the cultural milieu in which the practitioner works, so that we can develop a language that is meaningful to the patient by creating a shared frame of reference for clinical discussion.	▪ What is your own definition of spirit, and what influences helped you shape it? ▪ Would it matter if a patient has a different understanding of the terms "spirit," "energy," or "wind," for example, to your own? ▪ Do you routinely communicate with patients what you mean by unity of mind, body, spirit, or balancing their *qi*? ▪ Do you generally use Chinese terminology with your patients to explain your diagnosis or describe what you are doing, or do you "translate"? What informs your choice?

Table 2 Diagnosis and Treatment Standard 1

Principles	Descriptors	Practitioner cues
Practitioners use the four examinations (*si zhen*) to discern the signs and symptoms of the patient.	As practitioners of Chinese medicine, we collect information on all aspects of patients—body, mind, and spirit—using the four examinations: looking, asking, listening/smelling, and palpation, and the specific techniques inherent in them. We collect information that is only relevant to inform our diagnosis and treatment strategy, and explain to patients why we might need to ask more intimate or indirect questions, or conduct specific examinations. We conduct the consultation with empathy and compassion.	▪ What methods of examination do you use routinely? Are there any you rely on more than others? Are there any you do not feel comfortable in doing? ▪ Are there any patients you do not feel comfortable with using a specific examination method? ▪ How do you check the sensitivity and accuracy of your examining methods? ▪ How much do you see informed consent entering into this phase of the therapeutic encounter?

Diagnosis and Treatment—Acupuncture practitioners, following the BAcC Education Guidelines (April 2000), make a diagnosis, formulate a treatment plan, and treat patients using needles and other techniques that have an impact on the flow of *qi* in the channels. Through the manipulation of *qi* within the body, acupuncture treatment is aimed at awakening the body's ability to protect and heal itself.

Standard 1—Acupuncture practitioners gather information from patients using the four examinations (*si zhen*).

Contact Details

British Acupuncture Council:
www.acupuncture.org.uk

State of Victoria, Australia

The description of the course of study is extremely detailed. The knowledge, skills, and attributes expected of graduates of approved courses of study in Chinese medicine are set out under knowledge, skills, attributes, and attitudes.

For example, graduates are expected to have the following attributes and attitudes necessary for professional practice:

▪ Respectful awareness and appreciation of human life, and the effect that illness and suffering can have on physical, social, and spiritual well-being.
▪ Open-minded sense of inquiry in the pursuit of excellence, relating to both professional and personal development.
▪ Commitment to ethical professional practice and a willingness to address ethical issues appropriately and sensitively.
▪ Awareness of the professional responsibility of a Chinese medicine practitioner, both to the client and the wider community.

The specific program content is defined under the following nine headings:
1. Chinese Medicine Theoretical Paradigm
2. Modalities of Chinese Medicine—Acupuncture
3. Chinese Herbal Medicine
4. *Tui na* (Chinese Therapeutic Massage)
5. Chinese Medicine Classic Literature
6. Basic and Biomedical Sciences
7. Clinical Chinese Medicine
8. Clinical Training—General Description
9. Professional Development—Other Areas of Study

Under each of these headings are a number of subsections, with a synopsis and learning outcomes under each. A number of examples are given below as a way of illustrating the document.
1. Chinese Medicine Theoretical Paradigm

(a) Terminology for Chinese Medicine
Upon completion of this area of study, students should be able to:
- Briefly outline the history, development, and structure of the Chinese language.
- Demonstrate the writing of simple Chinese characters used in the practice of Chinese medicine.

(b) (...)

(c) Principles of Chinese Medicine
Upon completion of this area of study, students should be able to:
- Explain *yin yang* theory and *wu xing* theory in general, and in relation to Chinese medicine.

(d) Diagnosis in Chinese Medicine
Upon completion of this area of study, students should be able to:
- Comprehend the guiding principles of Chinese medicine diagnosis.
- Understand the application of the four data-collection methods, including inspection, auscultation and olfaction, interrogation, and palpation.

2. Modalities of Chinese Medicine—Acupuncture
(a) Channel and Acupuncture Point Theory
This area of study should cover *jing luo* and point theory. This should include the composition and functions of the *jing luo* system and acupuncture points in sufficient detail to enable the naming/numbering of the points, the location of individual points, explanation of the classification, and an understanding of their therapeutic functions and clinical indications. 400 acupuncture points should be studied.
Upon completion of this area of study students should be able to:

- Outline the composition and function of the *jing luo* system, the distribution and connection of each of the various components of the system.

5. Chinese Medicine Classic Literature
(a) *Huang Di Nei Jing* (The Yellow Emperor's Classic of Medicine)
Upon completion of this area of study, students should be able to:
- Explain the current academic views of formation of the *Huang Di Nei Jing* corpus, and the methods used in studying the texts.

7. Clinical Chinese Medicine
(b) Gynaecology and Obstetrics
Upon successful completion of the area of study, students should be able to:
- Identify and explain any cautions and contraindications that need to be considered in the treatment of the main gynecological and obstetric disorders, including the complications which could arise from the particular disease; possible adverse reactions to the herbal formula; possible interactions between the formula and other medications commonly used for the particular disease; cautions and possible adverse reactions to be considered in performing the treatment using acupuncture, moxibustion, and/or *tui na*.

Contact Details

Chinese Medicine Registration Board of Victoria:
www.cmrb.vic.gov.au/registration/cmcoursestudy.html

The Bologna Process

The following is a brief summary of the key aspects of the Bologna Process, which is a European-wide attempt to rationalize higher education. As such, it is important to be aware of this initiative, as it will affect Chinese medicine courses within higher education institutions throughout Europe.

The Bologna Process is an intergovernmental initiative that aims to create a European Higher Education Area (EHEA) by 2010, and to promote the European system of higher education worldwide. It now has 45 signatory countries and is conducted outside the formal decision-making framework of the European Union (EU). Decision-making within the Bologna Process rests on the consent of all the participating countries.

It was launched in 1999, when ministers from 29 European countries met in Bologna and signed a declaration establishing what was necessary to create an EHEA by the end of the decade. The broad objectives of the Bologna Process became the following:

- to remove the obstacles to student mobility across Europe;
- to enhance the attractiveness of European higher education worldwide;
- to establish a common structure of higher education systems across Europe;
- to have the common structure based on two main parts: undergraduate and graduate.

In its aim to improve the quality of higher education and, in turn, human resources across Europe, the Bologna Process will play a key role in contributing to the EU's Lisbon Strategy goals, which aim to deliver stronger, lasting growth and to create more and better jobs.

Since 1999, ministers have met three times to assess progress towards the creation of the EHEA: in Prague in 2001, in Berlin in 2003, and in Bergen in 2005. The UK will host the next ministerial summit in London in 2007.

Following the success of the Bologna Process in higher education across Europe, the EU's Bruges–Copenhagen Process was launched to foster similar cooperation in vocational education and training.

The Europe Unit has produced its own guide to the Bologna Process.

The Ten Bologna Process Action Lines

Established in the Bologna Declaration of 1999

1. Adoption of a system of easily readable and comparable degrees.
2. Adoption of a system essentially based on two cycles.
3. Establishment of a system of credits.
4. Promotion of mobility.
5. Promotion of European cooperation in quality assurance.
6. Promotion of the European dimension in higher education.

Added After the Prague Ministerial Summit of 2001

7. Focus on lifelong learning.
8. Inclusion of higher education institutions and students.
9. Promotion of the attractiveness of the EHEA.

Added After the Berlin Ministerial Summit of 2003

10. Doctoral studies and the synergy between the EHEA and the European Research Area.

For the latest information please see:
www.bologna–bergen2005.no/

Recognition of Qualifications

The recognition of qualifications between European countries is vital to enable Europe's citizens to study and work in countries other than their own. A major obstacle to mobility has been the possibility that an individual's qualifications will not be recognized abroad.

The EU institutions have begun to address this problem by helping to remove these obstacles to mobility. The aim is to allow students and workers to use their qualifications and competencies as a "common currency," which can be "earned" in one setting and "spent" in another. It is fundamental to EU law that citizens should have the freedom to establish themselves and work anywhere in the EU. The new EU directive, simplifying the procedure for the mutual recognition of professional qualifications, will allow professionals such as doctors, dentists, and architects to provide services anywhere in the EU.

The Council of Europe's Convention on the Recognition of Qualifications concerning Higher Education in the European Region, usually referred to as the Lisbon Convention, came into being on 1st February 1999. It seeks to ensure that holders of a qualification from one European country have that qualification recognized in another European country, and refers to the Diploma Supplement.

The European Commission has set up a number of initiatives to facilitate recognition of qualifications: the Diploma Supplement, the European Credit Transfer and Accumulation System (ECTS), the Tuning Project, and Europass.

Contact Details

The Europe Unit and the Bologna Process:
www.europeunit.ac.uk/bologna_process/index.cfm

Also refer to:
The Bologna Process—Towards the European Higher Education Area:
www.bologna-bergen2005.no/EN/BASIC/Pros-descr.HTM

European Quality Assurance Standards:
www.bologna-bergen2005.no/

More information on the recognition of qualifications can be found on the websites of the European Commission and Council of Europe, as below:
European Commission— Recognition of qualifications:
www.europa.eu.int/comm/education/policies/rec_qual/rec_qual_en.html

Council of Europe— Recognition of qualifications:
www.coe.int/T/DG4/HigherEducation/Recognition/default_en.asp

Recognition of professional qualifications— EU legislation:
www.europa.eu.int/comm/internal_market/qualifications/future_en.htm

Lisbon Recognition Convention:
www.conventions.coe.int/Treaty/Commun/QueVoulezVous.asp?NT=165&CM=1&DF=8/16/04&CL=ENG

WHO Recommendations on Training in Acupuncture

According to the World Health Organization (WHO), independently trained acupuncturists should have a minimum of 2500 hours of training in addition to basic biosciences extending over two years. The WHO recommends that physicians complete 1500 hours of training to practice as a part of Oriental Medicine, but can become qualified to practice acupuncture as an adjunct to their other modalities with just 200 hours of training. WHO also recommends that chiropractors and other health care professionals complete a full 2500 hours of training or limit their practice to acupressure.

See WHO Guidelines for Basic Training and Safety in Acupuncture: www.acucouncil.org/reports/training_programmes.htm
Source: www.acucouncil.org/reports/who_contents.htm

Basic training in acupuncture

Category of personnel	Level of training	Acupuncture (ACU) Core syllabus			Modern Western Medicine (MED)	Official exami- nation	Certificate
		Theory	Clinical	Supervised practice	Theory & clinical		
Acupuncture practitioners (non-medical)	Full course of training	1000 hours	500 hours	500 hours	500 hours	ACU & MED	ACU
Qualified physicians	Full course of training	500 hours	500 hours	500 hours		ACU	
Qualified physicians	Limited training in ACU as a technique for clinical work	Not less than 200 hours				ACU	
Other health personnel	Limited training in ACU for use in primary health care	Varies according to application envisaged				ACU	

World Health Organization Guidelines for Quality Assurance of Traditional Medicine Education in the Western Pacific Region

For most interesting information on traditional medicine education in the Western Pacific Region (most of which is on Chinese Medicine and related subjects) go to: www.wpro.who.int/health_topics/traditional_medicine/publications.htm and open up the report of the Working Group Meeting on Quality Academic Education in Traditional Medicine.

Convened by: World Health Organization (WHO) Regional Office for the Western Pacific, Melbourne, Australia, 22nd to 24th November 2003.

Areas covered: traditional medicine education in Australia, China, Hong Kong, Japan, Korea, Vietnam, USA.

Also in the document are WHO Guidelines for Quality Assurance of Traditional Medicine Education in the Western Pacific Region and Teaching and Learning Strategies of Traditional Medicine Education.

Calendar

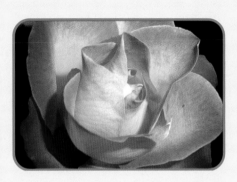

Introduction

Why a Congress Calendar?

We would be remiss in our aim to increase cooperation if we neglected to include information on that most basic and effective means of human communication: a physical meeting place for the exchange of ideas.

We have therefore included an overview of meetings taking place in the field of traditional East Asian medicine (TEAM) worldwide, from October 2006 through December 2007, as communicated to us by various professional societies or organizations, or found through our own research.

Your Cooperation Is Appreciated

A heartfelt thank you to all who responded to our requests for information. Without your cooperation we would not have been able to produce a congress calendar.

Despite our best intentions, our current calendar is far from complete. If your society or organization is not listed, please contact us so that we can include your upcoming meeting in the next edition of the Almanac.

We will continue to ask for information with regard to your current events. You can also contact us with your latest meeting news by mailing us at almanac@thieme.com, or by completing our response form found in the congress section of the Almanac website: www.thieme.com/almanac.

How to Use the Congress Calendar

The print version of the congress calendar is organized chronologically. Each entry contains the name of the event, topic, organizer, umbrella organization, date, location, language(s), website, and email address. To provide you with a handy pocket calendar, we have included a date book, where each page reflects one week. Major meetings are highlighted here, and two are introduced with a separate text.

The congress calendar can also be consulted online at www.thieme.com/almanac/calendar, where other means of cross-referencing are available. The online version will be augmented and updated monthly.

Furthermore, this section contains miscellaneous bits and pieces of information that always come in handy, and some of it is simply entertaining.

Accuracy and Improvements

Although to the best of our knowledge all the information provided is correct at the time of publication, the publisher asks that you please refer to the specific society or organization's URL address as the final source of information.

Our objective is to provide you with a useful resource, so please contact us with your ideas on how we can optimize the congress calendar.

List of Events

2006

Date **28 September–3 October**
Location **Freudenstadt, Germany**
Event 111. ZÄN-Kongress
Topic Komplementärmedizin zwischen Individualität und Wirtschaftlichkeit, Labor- und Komplementärmedizin
Organizer Zentralverband der Ärzte für Naturheilverfahren und Regulationsmedizin
Umbrella Organization Zentralverband der Ärzte für Naturheilverfahren und Regulationsmedizin
Language(s) German
Website www.zaen.org
Email info@zaen.org

Date **28 September–1 October**
Location **Sofia, Bulgaria**
Event 6th European Congress of Traditional Chinese Medicine
Topic Chinese Medicine from the Past to the Future
Organizer Bulgarian Acupuncture Association of Physical Therapists (BAAPT)
Umbrella Organization European Register of Organizations of Traditional Chinese Medicine EURO-TCM and Bulgarian Acupuncture Association of Physical Therapists (BAAPT)
Language(s) English
Website www.eccm-sofia.org/
Contact Person Emanuela Hristova
Email registration@ecm-sofia.org

Date **4–8 October**
Location **Lyon, France**
Event 5th International Symposium of Auriculotherapy and Auriculomedicine
Organizer Dr C. Vulliez – Dr R. Nogier – Dr Y. Rouxeville
Umbrella Organization GLEM – EIPN – AASF
Language(s) English
Website www.symposiumlyon2006.com
Email contact@symposiumlyon2006.com

Date **5–8 October**
Location **East Rutherford, NJ, USA**
Event Traditional Chinese Medicine World Foundation–Annual Conference
Topic Building Bridges of Integration for Traditional Chinese Medicine – Transformation: Spirit in Healing
Organizer Traditional Chinese Medicine World Foundation
Umbrella Organization Traditional Chinese Medicine World Foundation
Language(s) English
Website www.tcmconference.org
Contact Person Elaine Katen
Email info@tcmconference.org

Date **7–10 October**
Location **Louisville, KY, USA**
Event American Holistic Veterinary Medical Association–Annual Conference
Organizer American Holistic Veterinary Medical Association
Umbrella Organization The American Academy of Veterinary Acupuncture (AAVA)
Language(s) English
Website www.ahvma.org/displaycommon.cfm
Contact Person Dr Carvel G. Tiekert
Email office@ahvma.org

Date **13–15 October**
Location **Balatonfüred, Hungary**
Event Hungarian Medical Acupuncture Society (MAOT)–Annual Congress
Topic TCM: Past–Present–Future
Organizer Hungarian Medical Acupuncture Society
Umbrella Organization Hungarian Medical Acupuncture Society
Language(s) English, Hungarian
Website www.yamamoto.hu/
Contact Person Prof Dr Hegyi Gabriella
Email drhegyi@hu.inter.net

Date **14 October**
Location **USA**
Event Herb Day
Organizer American Botanical Council (ABC); Amercian Herbal Pharmacopoeia (AHP); American Herbal Products Association (AHPA); American Herbalists Guild (AHG); and United Plant Savers (UpS)
Umbrella Organization The Herb Coalition
Language(s) English
Website www.herbday.org/
Contact Person Karen Robin
Email info@herbday.org

Date **15–16 October**
Location **London, UK**
Event Complementary & Natural Healthcare Expo 2006
Organizer Full Moon Communications
Umbrella Organization British Complementary Medicine Association
Language(s) English
Website www.chexpo.com
Email cdown@naturalproducts.co.uk

Date **19–22 October**
Location **Nuremberg, Germany**
Event 2. GGTM/ATF Herbstkurse für Ganzheitliche Tiermedizin
Organizer Gesellschaft für Ganzheitliche Tiermedizin (GGTM) and Akademie für Tierärztliche Fortbildung (ATF)
Umbrella Organization Gesellschaft für Ganzheitliche Tiermedizin (GGTM) and Akademie für Tierärztliche Fortbildung (ATF)
Language(s) German
Website www.ganzheitliche-tiermedizin.de/
Email info@mayer-kongress.de

Date **19–22 October**
Location **New York, NY, USA**
Event 22nd Annual International Symposium on Acupuncture and Electro-Therapeutics
Organizer International College of Acupuncture and Electro-Therapeutics
Umbrella Organization International College of Acupuncture and Electro-Therapeutics
Language(s) English
Website www.icaet.org/symposium.html
Contact Person Yoshiaki Omura, MD, ScD

Date **19–22 October**
Location **Berlin, Germany**
Event Berlin Balance Conference
Organizer Dr Richard The-Fu Tan
Umbrella Organization Praxis Dr Katrin Klose
Language(s) English, German
Website www.dr-katrin-klose.de/
Contact Person Dr Katrin Klose

Date **20–22 October**
Location **Phoenix, AZ, USA**
Event American Association of Oriental Medicine Conference and Exposition 2006
Topic Oriental Medicine – Healing Body, Mind and Spirit
Organizer American Association of Oriental Medicine
Umbrella Organization American Association of Oriental Medicine
Language(s) English
Website www.aaom.org
Email asomseminars@gmai.com

Date **21 October–4 November**
Location **China**
Event China-Reise
Umbrella Organization Schweizerische
  Ärztegesellschaft für Aurikulomedizin
  und Akupunktur
Website www.saegaa.ch
Email saegaa@akupunktur-tcm.ch

Date **23–26 October**
Location **Dublin, Ireland**
Event XIV Cochran Colloquium
Organizer The Cochrane Collaboration
Umbrella Organization The Cochrane
  Collaboration
Language(s) English
Website www.colloquium.info
Contact Person Conference Secretariat
Email colloquium@platinumone.ie

Date **24 October**
Location **Orlando, FL, USA**
Event AOM Day
Topic National Acupuncture and Oriental
  Medicine Day
Organizer Acupuncture and Oriental Medicine
  Day is supported through a unique interna-
  tional partnership of organizations including
  the USA, Canada, Mexico and Pakistan.
  The partnership includes professional asso-
  ciations, research organizations and educa-
  tion institutions.
Umbrella Organization National Certification
  Commission for Acupuncture and Oriental
  Medicine
Language(s) English
Website www.aomday.org
Contact Person Laura Edgar
Email lcedgar@nccaom.org

Date **24 October**
Location **Orlando, FL, USA**
Event AOM Day
Topic Laughing Qigong for Emotional Health,
  History of TCM, Clinic and Treatments, Herbs
Organizer Florida College of Integrative
  Medicine
Umbrella Organization Florida College of
  Integrative Medicine
Language(s) English
Website www.fcim.edu
Contact Person Jon Diament
Email jdiament@fcim.edu

Date **26–29 October**
Location **Boulder, CO, USA**
Event American Herbalists Guild's 17th Annual
  Symposium
Topic Many Ways of Knowing: Evidence in
  Clinical Botanical Medicine
Organizer American Herbalists Guild
Umbrella Organization American Herbalists
  Guild
Language(s) English
Website www.americanherbalistsguild.com
Email ahgoffice@earthlink.net

Date **27 October–2 November**
Location **Baden-Baden, Germany**
Event 40. Medizinische Woche Baden-Baden
Topic Vorsorge statt Nachsorge –
  Prävention mit Komplementärmedizin
Organizer Karl F. Haug Verlag in MVS
  Medizinverlage Stuttgart GmbH & Co. KG
Umbrella Organization Ärztegesellschaft
  für Erfahrungsheilkunde e.V.
Language(s) German
Website www.medwoche.de
Contact Person Caroline Augspurger-Hacker
Email medwoche@medizinverlage.de

Date   **28–29 October**

Location   **Aix-en-Provence, France**

Event   10ème Congrès National de la Fédération Nationale de Médecine Traditionnelle Chinoise (FNMTC)

Organizer   Fédération Nationale de Médecine Traditionnelle Chinoise (FNMTC)

Umbrella Organization   Fédération Nationale de Médecine Traditionnelle Chinoise (FNMTC)

Language(s)   French

Website   www.fnmtc.com

Contact Person   Yves Giarmon

Email   contact@fnmtc.com

Date   **28–29 October**

Location   **Adelaide, Australia**

Event   AMAC 33rd AGM – Scientific Weekend

Topic   Acupuncture's Role In the Healing Process

Organizer   Australian Medical Acupuncture College

Umbrella Organization   Australian Medical Acupuncture College

Language(s)   English

Website   www.acupunctureaustralia.org

Contact Person   Cheryl Moriarty

Email   davmitch@tpg.com.au

Date   **28–29 October**

Location   **Chengdu, Sichuan, China**

Event   50th Anniversary of Chengdu University of TCM

Topic   Celebration and Congress

Organizer   Prof Fan Xinjian, President of Chengdu University of TCM

Umbrella Organization   Chengdu University of TCM

Language(s)   Chinese, English

Website   www.cdutcm.edu.cn

Contact Person   Victor Yao Hongwu, Director of Foreign Affairs Office

Email   Stone30cn@yahoo.com.cn

Date   **2–5 November**

Location   **San Diego, CA, USA**

Event   18th Annual Pacific Symposium 2006

Organizer   Pacific College of Oriental Medicine

Umbrella Organization   Pacific College of Oriental Medicine

Language(s)   English

Website   www.pacificcollege.edu/symposium/index.html

Contact Person   Jack Miller

Email   symposium@PacificCollege.edu

Date   **10–12 November**

Location   **Los Angeles, CA, USA**

Event   The International Complementary and Natural Healthcare Conference and Expo (CAM Expo West)

Topic   Featuring the 9th World Congress on Qigong and Traditional Chinese Medicine 2006

Umbrella Organization   Organic Trade Association

Language(s)   English

Website   www.camexpowest.com

Email   info@camexpo.com

Date   **11–12 November**

Location   **Paris, France**

Event   Troisième Symposium Endocrinologie et MTC

Organizer   Fédération Pan-Européenne des Spécialistes de Médecine Traditionnelle Chinoise (PEFCTCM)

Umbrella Organization   Fédération Pan-Européenne des Spécialistes de Médecine Traditionnelle Chinoise (PEFCTCM)

Language(s)   French

Website   www.pefctcm.org

Email   pefctcm@wanadoo.fr

Date **15–18 November**
Location **Horn-Bad Meinberg, Germany**
Event 15. Bad Meinberger Woche
Organizer Internationale Medizinische
  Gesellschaft für Neuraltherapie nach Huneke –
  Regulationstherapie e.V.
Umbrella Organization Internationale
  Medizinische Gesellschaft für Neuraltherapie
  nach Huneke – Regulationstherapie e.V.
Language(s) German
Website www.neuraltherapie-huneke.de/
Email mail@ignh.de

Date **17–19 November**
Location **Brighton, UK**
Event European Legislation
  and Complementary Medicine
  (Second Symposium of the ETCMA)
Topic Hopes and Fears for the Future
Organizer European Traditional Chinese
  Medicine Association (ETCMA)
Umbrella Organization European Traditional
  Chinese Medicine Association (ETCMA)
Language(s) English
Website www.etcma.org
Contact Person Joan Maynard
Email joan@ouziebust.wanadoo.co.uk

Date **17–19 November**
Location **São Paulo, Brazil**
Event I Congresso Médico de Acupuntura do
  Instituto Van Nghi do Brasil
Organizer Instituto Van Nghi do Brasil
Umbrella Organization Instituto Van Nghi do
  Brasil
Language(s) French, Portuguese
Website www.acupunturaivn.com.br
Email contato@acupunturaivn.com.br

Date **23–25 November**
Location **Hong Kong, China**
Event 2006 World Congress on Chinese
  Medicine
Organizer School of Chinese Medicine, Hong
  Kong Baptist University
Umbrella Organization School of Chinese
  Medicine, Hong Kong Baptist University
Language(s) English, Putonghua (Chinese)
Website www.mvdmc.com/cm2006/index.htm
Contact Person Congress Secretariat
Email cm2006@mvdmc.com

Date **24–27 November**
Location **Aurangabad, India**
Event International Congress of Medical &
  Cosmetic Acupuncture – Acupressure
Topic Scientific & Clinical Research in Medical &
  Cosmetic Acupuncture – Acupressure
Organizer Indian Academy of Acupuncture
  Science
Umbrella Organization Indian Academy
  of Acupuncture Science
Language(s) English, German
Website www.acupunctureindia.org/conf.html
Contact Person Prof Sir Dr P. B. Lohiya
Email lohiyaacus@satyam.net.in

Date **1–4 December**
Location **San Francisco, CA, USA**
Event Microcurrent & Color Light Therapy
  Acupuncture for Advanced Pain Manage-
  ment & Energetic Balancing
Organizer East-West Seminars
Umbrella Organization East-West Seminars
Language(s) English
Website www.east-westseminars.com
Contact Person Katt Warfield
Email seminars@neta.com

2007

Date **8–10 February**
Location **New York, NY, USA**
Event The International Complementary and
Natural Healthcare Conference and Expo
(CAM Expo East)
Umbrella Organization Organic Trade
Association
Language(s) English
Website www.camexpoeast.com/
Email info@camexpo.com

Date **9–11 February**
Location **Cologne, Germany**
Event YNSA Seminar with Toshikatsu Yama-
moto MD, PhD, Founder, YNSA
Topic Yamamoto New Scalp Acupuncture
Organizer International Association and
Network for Yamamoto New Scalp Acu-
puncture e.V.
Umbrella Organization ICMART
Language(s) German
Website www.ynsa.de
Contact Person Susan Schreiber
Email info@ian-med.de

Date **18–22 February**
Location **Las Vegas, NV, USA**
Event 79th Annual Western Veterinary
Conference
Topic Putting Progress into Practice
Organizer Western Veterinary Conference
Umbrella Organization Western Veterinary
Conference
Language(s) English
Website www.wvc.org/
Contact Person Carolyn Verduzco
Email carolyn@wvc.org

Date **1–6 March**
Location **Freudenstadt, Germany**
Event 112. ZÄN-Kongress
Organizer Zentralverband der Ärzte für
Naturheilverfahren und Regulationsmedizin
Umbrella Organization Zentralverband
der Ärzte für Naturheilverfahren und
Regulationsmedizin
Language(s) German
Website www.zaen.org
Email info@zaen.org

Date **10–11 March**
Location **Paris, France**
Event Congrès de la Confédération Française de
Médecine Traditionnelle Chinoise (CFMTC)
Organizer Confédération Française de
Médecine Traditionnelle Chinoise (CFMTC)
Umbrella Organization FNMTC, UFPMTC,
SIATTEC, PEFCTCM
Language(s) French
Website www.cfmtc.org
Contact Person Yves Giamon
Email presidence@cfmtc.org

Date **24–25 March**
Location **Wyboston, Bedfordshire, UK**
Event Acupuncture Association
of Chartered Physiotherapists (AACP) –
Annual Conference
Organizer Acupuncture Association
of Chartered Physiotherapists (AACP)
Umbrella Organization Acupuncture Associa-
tion of Chartered Physiotherapists (AACP)
Language(s) English
Website www.aacp.uk.com/
Contact Person Kim Rowe
Email kimrowe4@fsmail.net

Date **13–15 April**
Location **Nuremberg, Germany**
Event 7. Internationaler Kongress für
Ganzheitliche Tiermedizin
Topic Schmerztherapie beim Kleintier
Organizer Gesellschaft für Ganzheitliche Tier-
medizin (GGTM) and Akademie für Tierärzt-
liche Fortbildung (ATF)
Umbrella Organization Gesellschaft für Ganz-
heitliche Tiermedizin (GGTM) and Akademie
für Tierärztliche Fortbildung (ATF)
Language(s) German, English
Website www.ganzheitliche-tiermedizin.de
Contact Person Markus Mayer
Email info@mayer-kongress.de

Date **21–22 April**
Location **London, UK**
Event 1st International Conference:
  Traditional East Asian Medicines in the West
Topic Demonstrating Efficacy, Safeguarding
  Authenticity: The Challenge of Integrating
  Traditional East Asian Medicines into Western
  Health Care
Organizer Dr Volker Scheid and Mark Bovey
Umbrella Organization School of Integrated
  Medicine, University of Westminster
  in conjuction with the Acupuncture
  Research Council
Language(s) English
Contact Person Volker Scheid
Email scheidv@wmin.ac.uk

Date **27–28 April**
Location **Prague, Czech Republic**
Event Electroacupuncture nach Voll (EAV)
  Conference
Organizer Czech Medical Acupuncture Society
Umbrella Organization J. E. Purkyně Czech
  Medical Association
Language(s) Czech, German
Website www.akupunktura.cz
Contact Person Dr Stránecký
Email stranecky@volny.cz

Date **27–29 April**
Location **Baltimore, MD, USA**
Event American Academy of Medical
  Acupuncture (AAMA) Symposium
Topic Medical Acupuncture
Organizer American Academy of Medical
  Acupuncture (AAMA)
Umbrella Organization American Academy
  of Medical Acupuncture (AAMA)
Language(s) English
Website www.medicalacupuncture.org
Contact Person C. James Dowden
Email cjdowden@pacbell.net

Date **28 April**
Event **World T'ai Chi & Qigong Day**
Organizer World T'ai Chi & Qigong Day
Umbrella Organization World T'ai Chi &
  Qigong Day
Website www.worldtaichiday.org
Contact Person Bill Douglas
Email wtcqd2000@aol.com

Date **8–13 May**
Location **New Orleans, LA, USA**
Event Council of Colleges of Acupuncture and
  Oriental Medicine (CCAOM)
Topic None-General Semi-Annual Meeting
Organizer Council of Colleges of Acupuncture
  and Oriental medicine (CCAOM)
Umbrella Organization Acupuncture and
  Oriental Medicine Alliance (AOMA)
Language(s) English
Website www.ccaom.org;
  www.aomalliance.org
Contact Person CCAOM: David M. Sale,
  Executive Director; AOMAlliance: Michael
  McCoy, Executive Director
Email CCAOM: Executivedirector@ccaom.org
  AOMAlliance: Director@aomalliance.org

Date **11–13 May**
Location **Munich, Germany**
Event International Congress on
  Complementary Medicine Research
Organizer Centre for Complementary Medicine
  Research, Technical University Munich in
  cooperation with The International Society of
  Complementary Medicine Research (ISCMR)
Umbrella Organization Centre for Comple-
  mentary Medicine Research, Technical
  University Munich in cooperation with The
  International Society of Complementary
  Medicine Research (ISCMR)
Language(s) English, German
Website www.cmr-muc2007.de
Email info@CMR-Muc2007.de

Date **16–20 May**
Location **Rothenburg, Germany**
Event 38th TCM Conference
Topic Psyche and Soma/Transmission East–West
Organizer Arbeitsgemeinschaft für Klassische Akupunktur und Traditionelle Chinesische Medizin e.V. (AGTCM)
Umbrella Organization Arbeitsgemeinschaft für Klassische Akupunktur und Traditionelle Chinesische Medizin e.V. (AGTCM)
Language(s) English, German
Website www.tcm-kongress.de
Contact Person Ms. Kuras
Email kongress@tcm-kongress.de

Date **18–19 May**
Location **Roanoke, VA, USA**
Event National Acupuncture Detoxification Association–18th Annual Conference
Topic Acupuncture Detoxification: A New Gateway to Recovery
Organizer National Acupuncture Detoxification Association
Umbrella Organization National Acupuncture Detoxification Association
Language(s) English
Website www.acudetox.com
Contact Person Jay Renaud
Email NADAOffice@Acudetox.com

Date **18–20 May**
Location **Brisbane, QLD, Australia**
Event Australasian Acupuncture & Chinese Medicine–Annual Conference
Topic Clinical Practice, Research, Theory & Philosophy, Policy, Regulation, Education, Standards, Safety
Organizer Australasian Acupuncture and Chinese Medicine Association Ltd. (AACMA)
Umbrella Organization Australasian Acupuncture and Chinese Medicine Association Ltd. (AACMA)
Language(s) English
Website www.acupuncture.org.au
Contact Person Jazz Tyrill
Email publications@acupuncture.org.au

Date **1–3 June**
Location **Barcelona, Spain**
Event ICMART 2007 International Symposium of Medical Acupuncture and Related Techniques
Topic Acupuncture: Art, Evidence, and Challenges
Organizer ICMART & Medical Acupuncturist Section, Medical College Barcelona
Umbrella Organization ICMART & Medical Acupuncturist Section, Medical College Barcelona
Language(s) English, Spanish
Website www.icmart2007.com/
Contact Person Technical Secretariat
Email icmart2007@activacongresos.com

Date **2–6 June**
Location **Vancouver, Canada**
Event World Physical Therapy Congress
Topic Moving Physical Therapy Forward
Organizer Canadian Physiotherapy Association
Umbrella Organization World Confederation for Physical Therapy
Language(s) English
Website www.wcpt.org
Email congress@wcpt.org

Date **9–11 June**
Location **Atlanta, GA, USA**
Event World Tea Expo
Topic Tea, Tisanes, Gifts & Gourmet
Organizer World Tea Expo
Umbrella Organization World Tea Expo
Language(s) English
Website www.worldteaexpo.com
Email info@worldexpo.com

Date **14–18 June**
Location **Washington, DC, USA**
Event 144th Annual American Veterinary Medical Association Conference
Organizer American Veterinary Medical Association
Umbrella Organization American Veterinary Medical Association
Language(s) English
Website www.avma.org
Email avmainfo@avma.orgoo

Date **16–20 August**
Location **Hong Kong, China**
Event   Hong Kong International Medical & Health Care Fair; International Conference & Exhibition of the Modernization of Chinese Medicine & Health Products
Organizer   Hong Kong Trade Development Council
Language(s)   Cantonese
Website   www.icmcm.com; www.hkmed-healthfair.com
Email   exhibitions@tdc.org.hk

Date **6–9 September**
Location **Slettestrand, Fjerritslev, Denmark**
Event   1st Scandinavian TCM Congress
Topic   Sexuality & Health. Gynecology, Andrology, and TCM Philosophy
Organizer   TCM Lectures
Language(s)   English
Website   www.tcm-kongres.dk
Contact Person   Marian R. Nielsen Joos, Congress Manager
Email   info@tcm-lectures.com

Date **27–30 September**
Location **Las Vegas, NV, USA**
Event   American Academy of Pain Management–18th Annual Clinical Meeting
Organizer   American Academy of Pain Management
Umbrella Organization   American Academy of Pain Management
Language(s)   English
Website   www.aapainmanage.org/conference/ConferenceNext.php
Contact Person   Jolene Montoya
Email   jolene@aapainmanage.org

Date **27 September–2 October**
Location **Freudenstadt, Germany**
Event   113. ZÄN-Kongress
Organizer   Zentralverband der Ärzte für Naturheilverfahren und Regulationsmedizin
Umbrella Organization   Zentralverband der Ärzte für Naturheilverfahren und Regulationsmedizin
Language(s)   German
Website   www.zaen.org
Email   info@zaen.org

Date **4–7 October**
Location **New York, NY, USA**
Event   Traditional Chinese Medicine World Foundation–Annual Conference
Topic   Building Bridges of Integration for Traditional Chinese Medicine–True Health, True Healing
Organizer   Traditional Chinese Medicine World Foundation
Umbrella Organization   Traditional Chinese Medicine World Foundation
Language(s)   English
Website   www.tcmconference.org
Contact Person   Elaine Katen
Email   ekaten@tcmconference.org

Date **21–25 October**
Location **São Paulo, Brazil**
Event   15th Cochrane Colloquium
Organizer   The Cochrane Collaboration
Umbrella Organization   The Cochrane Collaboration
Language(s)   English
Website   www.colloquium.info/
Contact Person   Conference Secretariat
Email   colloquium@platinumone.ie

Date **24 October**
Location **Orlando, FL, USA**
Event   AOM Day
Topic   Laughing Qigong for Emotional Health, History of TCM, Clinic and Treatments, Herbs
Organizer   Florida College of Integrative Medicine
Umbrella Organization   Florida College of Integrative Medicine
Language(s)   English
Website   www.fcim.edu
Contact Person   Jon Diament
Email   jdiament@fcim.edu

Date **27–28 October**

Location **Aix-en-Provence, France**

Event   11e Congrès National de la Fédération Nationale de Médecine Traditionnelle Chinoise (FNMTC)

Organizer   Fédération Nationale de Médecine Traditionnelle Chinoise (FNMTC)

Umbrella Organization   Fédération Nationale de Médecine Traditionnelle Chinoise (FNMTC)

Language(s)   French

Website   www.fnmtc.fr

Contact Person   Yves Giarmon, President

Email   contact@fnmtc.fr

Date   **27 October–1 November**

Location   **Baden-Baden**

Event   41. Medizinische Woche Baden-Baden

Topic   Complementary Medicine

Organizer   Karl F. Haug Verlag in MVS Medizin-verlage Stuttgart GmbH & Co. KG

Umbrella Organization   Ärztegesellschaft für Erfahrungsheilkunde e.V.

Language (s)   German

Website   www.medwoche.de

Contact Person   Caroline Augspurger-Hacker

Email   medwoche@medizinverlage.de

Date   **9–11 November**

Location   **Baltimore, MD, USA**

Event   Society for Acupuncture Research – Annual Conference 2007

Topic   Acupuncture Research 1997–2007: A Decade After the NIH Consensus Conference: Progress, Challenges, and Future Directions

Organizer   Society for Acupuncture Research

Umbrella Organization   Society for Acupuncture Research

Language(s)   English

Website   www.acupunctureresearch.org/

Email   info@acupunctureresearch.org

Date   **21–25 November**

Location   **Hong Kong, China**

Event   4th International Conference on Daoism

Topic   Daoism in Action

Organizer   Department of Asian Studies, Institute of Sinology, Ludwig-Maximilians-University Munich; Medical Association for Qigong Yangsheng, Bonn; Societas Medicinae Sinensis (International Society for Chinese Medicine), Munich

Umbrella Organization   Medical Association for Qigong Yangsheng, e.V.

Language(s)   English

Website   www.daoism-conference.de/ Conf2007.html

Email   info@daoism-conference.de

JANUARY

Monday

1

Tuesday

2

Wednesday

3

Thursday

4

Friday

5

Saturday

6

Sunday

7

cal·en·dar (kăl'əndər)

n.
1. Any of various systems of reckoning time in which the beginning, length, and divisions of a year are defined.
2. A table showing the months, weeks, and days in at least one specific year.
3. A schedule of events.
4. An ordered list of matters to be considered: *a calendar of court cases; the bills on a legislative calendar.*
5. *Chiefly British* A catalog of a university.

The American Heritage® Dictionary of the English Language, Fourth Edition. S.v. "calendar." Retrieved 7 August 2006, from http://www.thefreedictionary.com/calendar

Monday

8

Tuesday

9

Wednesday

10

Thursday

11

Friday

12

Saturday

13

Sunday

14

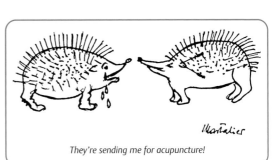

© Mastalier

They're sending me for acupuncture!

JANUARY

Monday
15

Tuesday
16

Wednesday
17

Thursday
18

Friday
19

Saturday
20

Sunday
21

JANUARY

Monday

22

Tuesday

23

Wednesday

24

Thursday

25

Friday

26

Saturday

27

Sunday

28

FEBRUARY

Monday

29

Tuesday

30

Wednesday

31

Thursday

1

Friday

2

Saturday

3

Sunday

4

**Learning is a treasure that will
follow its owner everywhere.**

Chinese proverb

Monday

5

Tuesday

6

Wednesday

7

Thursday

8

The International Complementary and Natural Healthcare Conference and Expo, New York, NY, USA (8–10 February)

Friday

9

YNSA (Yamamoto New Scalp Acupuncture) Seminar with Toshikatsu Yamamoto MD, PhD, Founder of YNSA, Cologne, Germany (9–11 February)

Saturday

10

Sunday

11

FEBRUARY

Monday

12

Tuesday

13

Wednesday

14

Thursday

15

Friday

16

Saturday

17

Sunday

18

A book holds a house of gold.

Chinese proverb

Monday

19

Tuesday

20

Wednesday

21

Thursday

22

Friday

23

Saturday

24

Sunday

25

MARCH

Monday

26

Tuesday

27

Wednesday

28

Thursday

1

112. ZÄN-Kongress, Freudenstadt, Germany (1–6 March)

Friday

2

Saturday

3

Sunday

4

Frequently Used Conversions

Metric to US Customary

If you have:	Multiply by:		To get:
Length			
millimeters	0.04	(0.03937)	inches
centimeters	0.4	(0.3937)	inches
meters	39	(39.37)	inches
meters	3.3	(3.280840)	feet
meters	1.1	(1.093613)	yards
kilometers	0.6	(0.621371)	miles
Area			
sq. cm	0.16	(0.15500)	sq. inches
sq. meters	10.8	(10.76391)	sq. feet
sq. meters	1.2	(1.195990)	sq. yards
hectares	2.5	(2.471044)	acres
sq. kilometers	0.39	(0.386102)	sq. miles
Weight			
grams	0.035	(0.03527396)	ounces
grams	0.002	(0.00220462)	pounds
kilograms	2.2	(2.204623)	pounds
metric tons	0.98	(0.9842065)	tons
Liquid measures			
liters	33.8	(33.81402)	ounces
liters	4.2	(4.226752)	cups
liters	2.1	(2.113376)	pints
liters	1.1	(1.056688)	quarts
liters	0.26	(0.264172)	gallons

Monday

5

Tuesday

6

Wednesday

7

Thursday

8

Friday

9

Saturday

10

Congrès de la Confédération Française de Médecine Traditionnelle Chinoise (CFMTC), Paris, France (10–11 March)

Sunday

11

MARCH

Monday
12

Tuesday
13

Wednesday
14

Thursday
15

Friday
16

Saturday
17

Sunday
18

Daylight saving time (DST) is the name which is used for the time during which clocks are set one hour or more ahead of standard time to provide more daylight at the end of the working day during late spring, summer, and early fall.

However, daylight saving time is the term which is mainly used in North America. Some regions (Europe, Russia, South America) rather use the name "summer time" (in their respective language; German: "Sommerzeit," French: "l'heure d'été"). This could lead to confusion in the meaning of abbreviatons related to time. ST could stand for "summer time" +1 hour (Europe, Russia, South America) and for "standard time" (North America).

Daylight saving time used to begin in the USA on the first Sunday in April and end on the last Sunday in October. In 2007 it will begin on 11 March and end on 4 November. In most countries in Western Europe and in the countries belonging to the EU (European Union), "summer time" begins on the last Sunday of March and ends on the last Sunday of October.

Monday

19

Tuesday

20

Wednesday

21

Thursday

22

Friday

23

Saturday

24

Acupuncture Association of Chartered Physiotherapists (AACP)—Annual Conference, Wyboston, Bedfordshire, UK (24–25 March)

Sunday

25

APRIL

Monday

26

Tuesday

27

Wednesday

28

Thursday

29

Friday

30

Saturday

31

Sunday

1

Frequently Used Conversions

Boldface indicates exact values

US Customary to Metric

If you have:	Multiply by:		To get:
Length			
inches	**25.4**		millimeters
inches	**2.54**		centimeters
inches	**0.0254**		meters
feet	0.3	**(0.3048)**	meters
yards	0.9	**(0.9144)**	meters
miles	1.6	**(1.609344)**	kilometers
Area			
sq. inches	6.5	**(6.4516)**	sq. cm.
sq. feet	0.09	(0.09290341)	sq. meters
sq. yards	0.84	(0.83612736)	sq. meters
acres	0.4	(0.4046873)	hectares
sq. miles	2.6	(2.58998811)	sq. kilometers
Weight			
ounces	28	**(28.349523125)**	grams
pounds	454	**(453.59237)**	grams
pounds	0.45	**(0.45359237)**	kilograms
tons	1	**(1.0160469088)**	metric tons
Liquid measures			
ounces	0.03	(0.02957353)	liters
cups	0.24	(0.23658824)	liters
pints	0.47	(0.473176473)	liters
quarts	0.95	(0.946352946)	liters
gallons	3.79	(3.785411784)	liters

APRIL

Monday

2

Tuesday

3

Wednesday

4

Thursday

5

Friday

6

Saturday

7

Sunday

8

Monday

9

Tuesday

10

Wednesday

11

Thursday

12

Friday

13

7. Internationaler Kongress für Ganzheitliche Tiermedizin, Nuremberg, Germany (13–15 April)

Saturday

14

Sunday

15

**To avoid sickness eat less;
to prolong life worry less.**

Chu Hui Weng

Monday

16

Tuesday

17

Wednesday

18

Thursday

19

Friday

20

Saturday

21

1st International Conference: Traditional East Asian Medicines in the West, London, UK (21–22 April)

Sunday

22

Monday

23

Tuesday

24

Wednesday

25

Thursday

26

Friday

27

Electroacupuncture according to Voll (EAV) Conference, Prague, Czech Republic (27–28 April)

Saturday

28

World T'ai Chi & Qigong Day (28 April)

Sunday

29

American Academy of Medical Acupuncture (AAMA) Symposium, Baltimore, MD, USA (27–29 April)

Monday

30

Tuesday

1

Wednesday

2

Thursday

3

Friday

4

Saturday

5

Sunday

6

MAY

Monday

7

Tuesday

8

Wednesday

9

Thursday

10

Friday

11

Saturday

12

Sunday

13

Monday

14

Tuesday

15

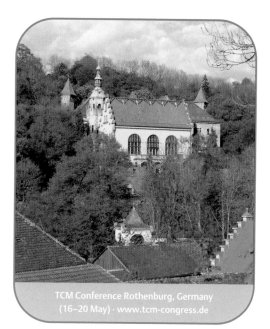

TCM Conference Rothenburg, Germany
(16–20 May) · www.tcm-congress.de

Wednesday

16

38th TCM Conference, Rothenburg, Germany (16–20 May)

Thursday

17

Friday

18

Australian Acupuncture & Chinese Medicine Annual Conference, Brisbane, QLD, Australia (18–20 May)

Saturday

19

National Acupuncture Detoxification Association–18th Annual Conference, Roanoke, VA, USA (18–19 May)

Sunday

20

MAY

Monday
21

Tuesday
22

Wednesday
23

Thursday
24

Friday
25

Saturday
26

Sunday
27

Monday

28

Tuesday

29

Wednesday

30

Thursday

31

Friday

1

ICMART International Symposium of Medical Acupuncture and Related Techniques 2007, Barcelona, Spain (1–3 June)

Saturday

2

Sunday

3

JUNE

Monday

4

Tuesday

5

Wednesday

6

Thursday

7

Friday

8

Saturday

9

Sunday

10

JUNE

Monday

11

Tuesday

12

Wednesday

13

Thursday

14

Friday

15

Saturday

16

Sunday

17

JUNE

Monday

18

Tuesday

19

Wednesday

20

Thursday

21

Friday

22

Saturday

23

A bird does not sing because it has an answer. It sings because it has a song.

Chinese proverb

Sunday

24

Monday

25

Tuesday

26

Wednesday

27

Thursday

28

Friday

29

Saturday

30

Sunday

1

JULY

Monday

2

Tuesday

3

Wednesday

4

Thursday

5

Friday

6

Saturday

7

Sunday

8

JULY

Monday

9

Tuesday

10

Wednesday

11

Thursday

12

Friday

13

Saturday

14

Sunday

15

JULY

Monday

16

Tuesday

17

Wednesday

18

Thursday

19

Friday

20

Saturday

21

Sunday

22

Names of Days

ENGLISH	CHINESE	PINYIN
Sunday	星期日	*xīng qí rì*
Monday	星期一	*xīng qí yī*
Tuesday	星期二	*xīng qí èr*
Wednesday	星期三	*xīng qí sān*
Thursday	星期四	*xīng qí sì*
Friday	星期五	*xīng qí wǔ*
Saturday	星期六	*xīng qí liù*

FRENCH	GERMAN	HEBREW
dimanche	Sonntag	yom rishon
lundi	Montag	yom sheni
mardi	Dienstag	yom shlishi
mercredi	Mittwoch	yom ravii
jeudi	Donnerstag	yom hamishi
vendredi	Freitag	yom shishi
samedi	Samstag	shabbat

JULY

Monday

23

Tuesday

24

Wednesday

25

Thursday

26

Friday

27

Saturday

28

Sunday

29

Names of Days

ENGLISH	ICELANDIC	ITALIAN
Sunday	sunnudagur	domenica
Monday	mánudagur	lunedi
Tuesday	þriðjudagur	martedi
Wednesday	miðvikudagur	mercoledi
Thursday	fimmtudagur	giovedi
Friday	föstudagur	venerdi
Saturday	laugardagur	sabato

JAPANESE	RUSSIAN	SPANISH
nichiyoubi	voskresenye	domingo
getsuyoubi	ponedelnik	lunes
kayoubi	vtornik	martes
suiyoubi	sreda	miércoles
mokuyoubi	chetverg	jueves
kinyoubi	pyatnitsa	viernes
doyoubi	subbota	sábado

Monday

30

Tuesday

31

Wednesday

1

Thursday

2

Friday

3

Saturday

4

Sunday

5

AUGUST

Monday
6

Tuesday
7

Wednesday
8

Thursday
9

Friday
10

Saturday
11

Sunday
12

Ginkgo
Ginkgo Biloba

Forgetting where you put the key
Or what you ate for snack?
The issue is your memory
You'd like to get that back
Here's an ancient Chinese tree
The leaves affect the brain
An extract for the elderly
More facts they will retain
Improve cerebral circulation
A neuropathic gift
Enhance a sexual situation
When the penis needs a lift
And if your feet are cold
The circulation is too slow
Ginkgo Biloba, it is told
Improves the blood to flow
If your ears are ringing
You've tinnitus or vertigo
You're getting very frustrated …
This calls for some Ginkgo!
The benefits may take some time
So take it in full swing
Remember to take your Ginkgo
You might remember everything!

Sylvia Seroussi Chatroux, MD, Ashland, OR, USA
(*Botanica Poetica—Herbs in Verse*:
www.poeticapress.com)

Monday

13

Tuesday

14

Wednesday

15

Thursday

16

Hong Kong International Medical & Health Care Fair; International Conference & Exhibition of the Modernization of Chinese Medicine & Health Products, Hong Kong, China (16–20 August)

Friday

17

Saturday

18

Sunday

19

Monday

20

Tuesday

21

Wednesday

22

Thursday

23

Friday

24

Saturday

25

Sunday

26

SEPTEMBER

Monday

27

Tuesday

28

Wednesday

29

Thursday

30

Friday

31

Saturday

1

Sunday

2

Monday

3

Tuesday

4

Wednesday

5

1st Scandinavian TCM Congress in Denmark
(6–9 September) · www.tcm-kongres.dk

Thursday

6

1st Scandinavian TCM Congress, Slettestrand, Fjerritslev, Denmark (6–9 September)

Friday

7

Saturday

8

Sunday

9

SEPTEMBER

Monday

10

Tuesday

11

Wednesday

12

Thursday

13

Friday

14

Saturday

15

Sunday

16

SEPTEMBER

Monday

17

Tuesday

18

Wednesday

19

Thursday

20

Friday

21

Saturday

22

Sunday

23

The greatest wealth is health.

Virgil

SEPTEMBER

Monday

24

Tuesday

25

Wednesday

26

Thursday

27

American Academy of Pain Management—18th Annual Clinic Meeting, Las Vegas, NV, USA (27–30 September)

Friday

28

113. ZÄN-Kongress, Freudenstadt, Germany (27 September–2 October)

Saturday

29

Sunday

30

Monday

1

Tuesday

2

Wednesday

3

Thursday

4

Traditional Chinese Medicine World Foundation–Annual Conference, New York, NY, USA (4–7 October)

Friday

5

Saturday

6

Sunday

7

OCTOBER

Monday

8

Tuesday

9

Wednesday

10

Thursday

11

Friday

12

Saturday

13

Sunday

14

OCTOBER

Monday
15

Tuesday
16

Wednesday
17

Thursday
18

Friday
19

Saturday
20

Sunday
21

Medicine for the soul

Inscription over the door of the Library at Thebes

OCTOBER

Monday

22

Tuesday

23

Wednesday

24

AOM Day, Orlando, FL, USA (24 October)

Thursday

25

Friday

26

Saturday

27

41. Medizinische Woche, Baden-Baden, Germany (27 October–1 November)

Sunday

28

11e Congrès National de la Fédération Nationale de Médecine Traditionelle Chinoise (FNMTC), Aix-en-Provence, France (27–28 October)

Monday

29

Tuesday

30

Wednesday

31

Thursday

1

Friday

2

Saturday

3

Sunday

4

NOVEMBER

Monday

5

Tuesday

6

Wednesday

7

Thursday

8

Friday

9

Society for Acupuncture Research—Annual Conference, Baltimore, MD, USA (9–11 November)

Saturday

10

Sunday

11

Monday

12

Tuesday

13

Wednesday

14

Thursday

15

Friday

16

Saturday

17

Sunday

18

NOVEMBER

Monday

19

Tuesday

20

Wednesday

21

4th International Conference on Daoism, Hong Kong, China (21–25 November)

Thursday

22

Friday

23

Saturday

24

Sunday

25

Monday

26

Tuesday

27

Wednesday

28

Thursday

29

Friday

30

Saturday

1

Sunday

2

DECEMBER

Monday
3

Tuesday
4

Wednesday
5

Thursday
6

Friday
7

Saturday
8

Sunday
9

DECEMBER

Monday

10

Tuesday

11

Wednesday

12

Thursday

13

Friday

14

Saturday

15

Sunday

16

Temperature Conversions

Celsius °C	Fahrenheit °F
−17.8	**0**
−12.2	10
−10	14
−6.7	20
−1.1	30
0	**32**
4.4	40
10	50
15.6	60
20	68
21.1	70
23.9	75
25	77
26.7	80
29.4	85
30	86
32.2	90
35	95
37	98.6
37.8	**100**
40	104
43	110
49	120
50	122
54	130
60	140
66	150
70	158
80	176
90	194
93	200
100	**212**

DECEMBER

Monday

17

Tuesday

18

Wednesday

19

Thursday

20

Friday

21

Saturday

22

Sunday

23

DECEMBER

Monday

24

Tuesday

25

Wednesday

26

Thursday

27

Friday

28

Saturday

29

Sunday

30

DECEMBER

Monday

31

Tuesday

1

Wednesday

2

Thursday

3

Friday

4

Saturday

5

Sunday

6

ICMART Congress 2006—The 3B Acupuncture Awards

Stefan M. Baudis, Hamburg, Germany

"Once a year, outstanding scientific achievements within acupuncture are celebrated with the 3B Acupuncture Awards," said the Belgian Secretary-General, Baron François Beyens, of the International Council of Medical Acupuncture and Related Techniques (ICMART), concerning this new form of prize-giving within the world of acupuncture. The prizes were donated by the Hamburg-based company 3B Scientific GmbH, which has been representing and promoting high-quality acupuncture for a number of years. It was thought that the best platform to initiate a prize-giving of this sort that would be consistent over a number of years was the 2006 ICMART Congress in Washington.

An independent jury, made up of Palle Rosted (UK) and Marshall Seeger (USA), was tasked to select a winner from a total of 50 entrants in the category of free papers. Florian Pfab from Munich, a 28-year-old medical professional, was the lucky winner of this year's 3B Acupuncture Awards. The jury recognized the particularly innovative research of the German scientist. The title of his work was "Preventive Effect of Acupuncture with Experimentally Induced Itching—A Randomized, Placebo-Controlled Study," relating to the preventive effect of acupuncture on skin reaction and emotional perception of histamine-induced itch.

Florian Pfab was greatly helped in the study he submitted by the German Medical Association of Acupuncture (DÄGfA). He was congratulated, together with Evemarie Wolkenstein and Katharina Rubi-Klein from Austria who won the second prize, and Patrick Sautreuil from France, who won the third prize. The Austrian acupuncturists were praised for their study on the influence of acupuncture as an adjuvant pain therapy for endometriosis ("Acupuncture as Pain Treatment in Patients with Endometriosis").

Sautreuil was able to prove in a case study the positive influence of acupuncture during the pain treatment of amputated patients ("Amputation, Pain Caused by Neuromas and Acupuncture").

The prizewinners received their awards with both surprise and joy, as the results were announced only at the conclusion of the ICMART Congress. Once the 300 delegates had applauded, the distinguished Baron François Beyens (ICMART Secretary-General) and Bryan Frank (ICMART President 2004–2006) announced the winners and gave out the prizes.

The prize-giving for the best scientific poster presentation had already taken place one day previously. In this category, the jury of the Chairman Robert Gross (USA) was tasked to select a winner out of 42 entrants.

The first prize went to the University of São Paulo. Fernanda G. Martins accepted the

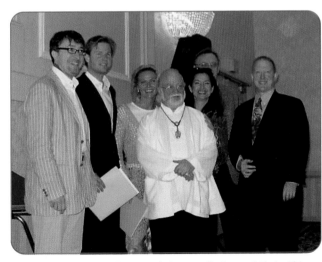

Fig. 1 From left to right: Stefan M. Baudis (3B Scientific, Germany); Florian Pfab (Germany); Katharina Rubi-Klein (Austria); Francois Beyens (ICMART Secretary-General, Belgium); Evemarie Wolkenstein (Austria); Patrick Satreuil (France); Bryan Frank (ICMART President 2004–2006, USA).

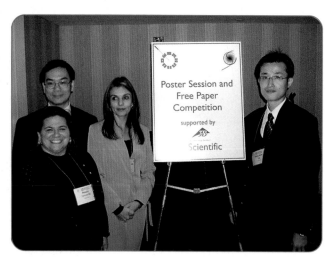

Fig. 2   From left to right: Rosalie Tassone; Yuan Chi-Lin (USA); Fernanda G. Martins (Brazil); Youn Byoung Chae (Korea).

prize on behalf of her research team for their work entitled "Treatment of Moderate Obstructive Sleep Apnea Syndrome with Acupuncture." The Brazilian researchers were able to prove the positive effect of acupuncture in the occurrence of heavy sleep disturbances in a controlled study.

The second prize went to a research group at the Harvard University in Boston, which focused on the acupuncture treatment of children in an intensive care unit. The title of the work by Yuan-Chi Lin and Rosalie Tassone was "Acupuncture Therapy Reduces Emergence Agitation and Pain in Children After Bilateral Myringotomy and Tympanostomy Tube Insertion: A Randomized Controlled Trial."

The third prize went to Youn Byoung Chae and his co-workers in Seoul. The title of the work was "The Effect of Acupuncture on Carrageenan-Induced Inflammation: Evidence from Protein Array Analysis of Cytokine Levels."

The donated prize of the 3B Acupuncture Awards was worth $4500 in total.

The founder of this prize-giving, Hamburg-based 3B Scientific GmbH, is the market leader in medical teaching materials and the exclusive importer for SEIRIN acupuncture needles in Europe.

The next 3B Acupuncture Awards competition will take place at the ICMART Congress in Barcelona in 2007.

Contact Details

Stefan M. Baudis
3B Scientific GmbH
Rudorffweg 8
21031 Hamburg, Germany
www.3b-akupunktur.de
www.3bscientific.com

Traditional Chinese Almanac Information

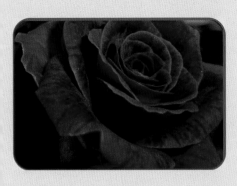

uhuan Zhang

Introduction

As one of the oldest agricultural communities in human civilization, the Chinese people long ago developed a highly sophisticated time system related to the rhythms of nature, to aid agricultural activity. The effect of this time system was to influence human activity and interaction with their physical environment in order to bring about harmony with the Greater World. It also had the effect of influencing other human activities, both at the social level and in matters of personal health. Certain rituals and cultural events at particular times of the year were conceived to enable the person to make the link between the individual and the environment. This time system was never just a system for measuring time; it is a system, or rather a structure, upon which an understanding of the universe and the individual's participation in it, can be built.

Traditional Chinese Medicine (TCM) is rooted in a rich, classical, multifaceted tradition that speaks to the essence of what we call Chinese culture. Over the millennia it has also made use of other systems, cultures, and structures to produce a uniquely comprehensive, composite body of knowledge. The paradigm in its contemporary form gives us a glimpse of the many aspects of Chinese culture and life.

The ancient Chinese came to realize the importance of living one's life in harmony with time and with nature, moving to the rhythms of the changes in the seasons, in temperature, in humidity. This time system is one of the fundamental principles of Chinese medicine, measuring the many cycles of both the microcosm and the macrocosm, thus creating a connection between human beings and their environment. In TCM, the view of how our body corresponds to the changes in the environment lays the ground for its principles and strategies of diagnosis and treatment. In the seminal work Huang Di Nei Jing *(The Yellow Emperor's Classic of Medicine) the idea that "Heaven and Man are one" iterates one of the key philosophical medical concepts in Chinese Medicine. A considerable body of work has since been done specifically on this topic; from general guidelines on how to live one's life, including emotional and physical adjustments, to detailed daily habits. The Chinese highly respect and value this system and view it as the way to maintain good health and ensure longevity.*

The time system in TCM not only serves as part of a general philosophical framework but is also deeply embedded in its diagnostic and treatment methodologies. It can give rise to prohibitions or restrictions as regards the use of herbs and acupuncture and can lead to recommendations regarding whether or not to take specific herbs according to the different times of the year. The same is true for the timing of acupuncture treatments. The study of these time cycles is important in understanding both the path and the flow of qi and blood in the body. Chinese doctors therefore predict the opening and closing of certain acupuncture points on our body at certain times of the day and year, enabling appropriate treatment strategies to be devised to gain optimal results. This method of acupuncture treatment according to time is sometimes now referred to as chrono-acupuncture.

Chinese people through the ages have put this system into practice in their daily lives. The Chinese signs of the zodiac, birth characters, and farming are based on the Chinese time system. It still plays a central role in the Chinese philosophy on life. Understanding this system helps us to deepen our understanding of Chinese culture and Chinese medicine. This section of the Almanac provides a general introduction to some aspects of Chinese culture and philosophy, as well as to the importance of understanding the Chinese calendar as a "roadmap" for change. The "Chinese Almanac Forecast" article can help to highlight for the reader how to navigate the change. Another article outlines the basis of the Chinese calendar, providing information on the standard terminologies and theories in the Chinese time system.

It gives readers a cultural sense of how the Chinese view time in relation to their physical environment. It also provides a simple historical exploration of the Chinese calendar, as well as a comparison of the Chinese and Western calendars. The articles on health preservation according to the seasons, the 24 solar divisional points, and dietary principles contain practical advice and useful strategies that readers can apply in their lives. This section of the Almanac not only contains theoretical discussions, but also information on how to incorporate that theory in everyday life. We hope that readers will find the quotations from ancient sages on how to preserve one's health and prolong one's life according to time, as well as basic instructions on what to do and what not to do, helpful.

What Will You Find In This Section?

This section contains diverse articles, some on the external environment and some on the body, which provide a comprehensive picture of what a Chinese traditional almanac might be like and how it is used in Chinese culture. From advice on how to live one's daily life to medical care, each article provides information on a different aspect of a Chinese traditional almanac.

The "Chinese Almanac Forecast" article gives a detailed month-by-month forecast with advice for the year 2007. As in Western culture the tradition of almanac forecasting has been a central part of the Chinese way of life. Almanacs not only refer to agricultural activities, but also to social and personal matters. The short article "The Chinese Calendar" gives a concise description of what a Chinese calendar is. This article not only gives a short description of the background to the configuration of the Chinese calendar and its method of calculation, it also gives a good explanation of the terminology used in the Chinese calendar system. There is also a brief discussion of comparing and contrasting the terminology used in the Chinese lunar calendar system and the Western solar calendar system. Overall, this article is a good introduction for someone who is unfamiliar with the concept of the Chinese calendar.

The author of the article "Seasonal Health Advice from Ancient Chinese Sources," has selected a chapter from one of the most important traditional Chinese books on diet in Chinese history: The Orthodox Essence of Drink and Food, [1279–1368 CE]. This work is renowned as the basic Chinese book on diet, focusing on overall seasonal advice on both physical and mental activities. It also gives suggestions on what habits one should adopt in the different seasons. There are four sections classified according to the four seasons and each section begins by analyzing the nature or character of each season followed by the advice on food, drink, and daily activities. The article "The 24 Seasonal Division Points and Their Implications for the Preservation of Life" gives detailed advice on how to go about one's daily life in the different seasonal and solar divisional segments. The article quotes extensively from the section in the Huang Di Nei Jing (The Yellow Emperor's Classic of Medicine) on the season and health. It provides a more comprehensive picture of how one should make changes in one's life according to changes in the environment.

The final article entitled "Theoretical Discussion of Health Preservation Using Nutritional Therapy in Traditional Chinese Medicine" merges the TCM theories with basic dietary advice. It provides general principles that people should follow in applying those dietary guidelines. Nutritional therapy guided by TCM theory in health preservation has a long history. This article systematically discusses how nutritional therapy is guided by TCM theory in terms of the origin of food and medicine, differentiation according to *flavor and nature and pattern differentiation, as well as prohibitions in its application. It thus provides helpful advice on maintaining and on improving quality of life guided by TCM theory, culture, and philosophy.*

Yuhuan Zhang, San Francisco, CA, USA

Bibliography

1. Veith I. *Huang Ti Nei Ching Su Wen*. Berkeley: University of California Press; 2002.
2. Zhang Yuhuan, Rose K. *A Brief History of Qi*. Massachusetts: Paradigm Publication; 2001.
3. Zhang Yuhuan, Rose K. *Who Can Ride the Dragon?* Massachusetts: Paradigm Publication; 1995.

Chinese Almanac Forecast

Lillian Garnier Bridges, Kirkland, Washington, USA

Year of the Pig—2007

This is the last year of the 12-year animal cycle. The pig is a water sign and this particular year is fire. Therefore, there is fire sitting on top of water. These are opposite elements in the five-element cycle, however this combination does not signify much conflict since the water puts out the fire. Therefore, this should be a relatively peaceful year. Steady business growth can be expected, especially in well-established companies, but rash schemes of all kinds should be avoided. This is a year for focusing on the home and the family.

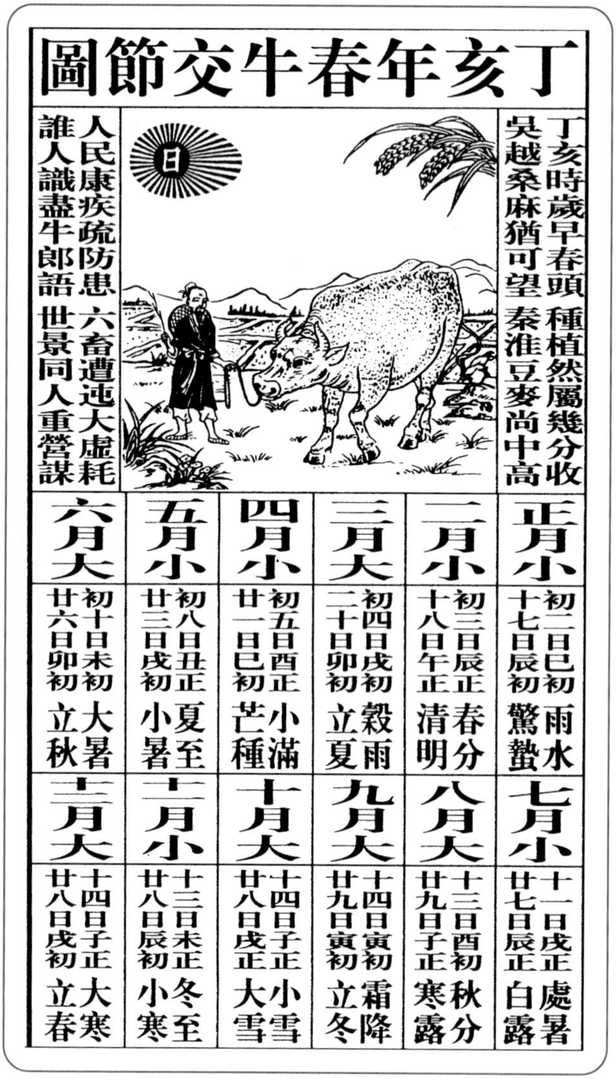

The pig is the sign of completion. Pigs are considered special by the Chinese because nearly every part can be eaten or used to make things; also they were the favored animal of farmers because they were easy to raise and lived on scraps and leftovers. Therefore, the energy of recycling, reupholstering, remodeling, fixing and repairing, cooking and making things by hand are highlighted personally and in business. Projects left unfinished can be easily completed within this year and, if not, may take a long time to get done.

Pig energy is concerned with the rewards of home at the end of the day and retirement at the end of a career. We will likely see some public figures and famous celebrities retire. Additionally, there will be more marriages, pregnancies, and births. It is a good sign for the home and family and socializing. Pig years are also good for home building and design, repairs, and domestic arts like decorating and cooking.

This is an excellent year for all of the nurturing and caretaking professions—including medicine, psychology, counseling, and teaching—and also for real estate involving home sales. It is also a good year for food products and the manufacturing of decorative items, for volunteer work and for getting along with neighbors and especially friends. The primary urge of the pig year is to rest, relax, and enjoy life with family and friends. Socializing is

Fig. 1 Dates for the 24 solar divisional points in the Chinese lunar calendar.

highlighted. Home and family are the most important energies. Pig years are good years for marriage, fertility and pregnancy, adoption, and buying a home.

It is not really a good year for business expansion or for speculation, but instead for letting things continue the way they have been. Change is not the best energy at this time; the focus is much more on the status quo. It should be a more peaceful year around the world, as most countries will worry more about their own problems than their problems with others. There is a good chance of military withdrawal from other countries and it is also an outstanding year for peaceful negotiations and the signing of treaties.

Individual Animal Forecasts

Rat—water element: 1912, 1924, 1936, 1948, 1960, 1972, 1984, 1996, 2008

This is an up and down year for the rat. You must finish all projects that you start and work more by yourself than usual. Finances are variable so watch your investments carefully. Your love life should be good and it will be a good year socially.

Ox—earth element: 1913, 1925, 1937, 1949, 1961, 1973, 1985, 1997, 2009

This should be a happy year overall for the ox. Your social position and finances will improve and promotion is likely. Travel is indicated and you will end the year feeling more successful.

Tiger—wood element: 1914, 1926, 1938, 1950, 1962, 1974, 1986, 1998, 2010

Tigers are lucky overall this year but watch out for potential legal problems. Business and investments should do well. Love life is happy but there may be some unexpected problems within the family.

Rabbit—wood element: 1915, 1927, 1939, 1951, 1963, 1975, 1987, 1999, 2011

This is a very happy year for rabbits, especially romantically. This is a good year to get engaged, married, or to have children. Financially only moderate gains can be expected

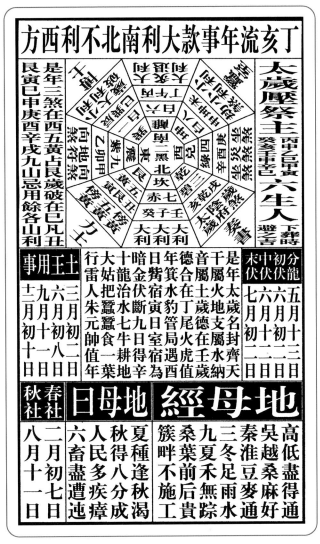

Fig. 2 *South and North are the grand lucky directions and West is the unlucky direction.*

this year, but this is a very creative year for rabbits.

Dragon—earth element: 1916, 1928, 1940, 1952, 1964, 1976, 1988, 2000, 2012

This is a difficult year for dragons. There will be a lot of socializing but there is also the potential for many fights. Romance is also somewhat conflicted. This is not a year for any big moves or for speculation. Dragons need to remain calm.

Snake—fire element: 1917, 1929, 1941, 1953, 1965, 1977, 1989, 2001, 2013

This is a difficult year for snakes regarding family, but romance is good. Snakes feel very artistic this year and need to nourish their creativity, but business and finances can be rocky and lawsuits should be avoided. Stay close to home and lay low.

Horse—fire element: 1918, 1930, 1942, 1954, 1966, 1978, 1990, 2002, 2014

This is a comfortable year with little to be concerned about. Horses can move forward with plans, and both business and social life look good. Home repairs are likely and may cost some money but family life is happy.

Sheep—earth element: 1919, 1931, 1943, 1955, 1967, 1979, 1991, 2003, 2015

This is a great year for sheep overall. It is a happy year for family; there may be children born and marriages occurring as the family increases in size. Traveling is good, especially for short distances. Business shows improvement.

Monkey—metal element: 1920, 1932, 1944, 1956, 1968, 1980, 1992, 2004, 2016

Monkeys need to be careful this year. They have lots of good ideas but need to be careful when implementing them. This is, however, a good year for business growth and finances.

Rooster—metal element: 1921, 1933, 1945, 1957, 1969, 1981, 1993, 2005, 2017

This is a more exciting year for roosters. It is a good year for family relationships but there may be some problems with home repairs. Some rewards in business can be expected but since it is a social and romantic year business may be put on the back burner.

Dog—earth element: 1922, 1934, 1946, 1958, 1970, 1982, 1994, 2006, 2018

Dogs are companions to pigs so this will be a happy year with a focus on a good home life. However, there may be some problems with health. It is a slow, easy year for business but there is luck in money.

Pig—water element: 1923, 1935, 1947, 1959, 1971, 1983, 1995, 2007, 2019

This is a peaceful year for pigs and is a year of rest. However, pigs feel confident and successful and see the rewards of the previous years' hard work. Home and family life is happy and pigs see a wish or dream fulfilled.

Contact Details

Lillian Garnier Bridges
Lotus Institute
Kirkland, WA, USA
www.lotusinstitute.com

The Chinese Calendar

Yuhuan Zhang, San Francisco, California, USA

Before trying to understand what the Chinese calendar is, we should spend a little time considering what a calendar is. It is a term we live so closely with in our daily life, but just like other familiar concepts and objects in our everyday environment, we have stopped trying to understand their definition. However, it is important for us to pause for a moment before we start to tap into a cultural concept that belongs to another cultural setting. Let us first try to understand what our culture tells us. The *Merriam-Webster Dictionary* defines the term "calendar" as follows:

"A system for fixing the beginning, length, and divisions of the civil year and arranging days and longer divisions of time (as weeks and months) in a definite order."

In plain language, a calendar is a system for measuring time, from hours and minutes, to months and days, and to years and centuries. The terms "hour," "day," "month," "year," and "century" are the units of time in the calendar system. But what is "measuring time"? It is well known that time is measured by observing the movements of the sun, moon, and stars. In almost all major cultures people have used this method since prehistoric times.

So, what determines a "day"? We all know that the earth rotates about its axis, causing the apparent movement of the sun from the east to the west across the sky. Therefore, one "day" is defined as one cycle of movement of the sun. The concept is plainly embedded in the Chinese character 日 *ri* (sun), which is used to denote both the sun and the day.

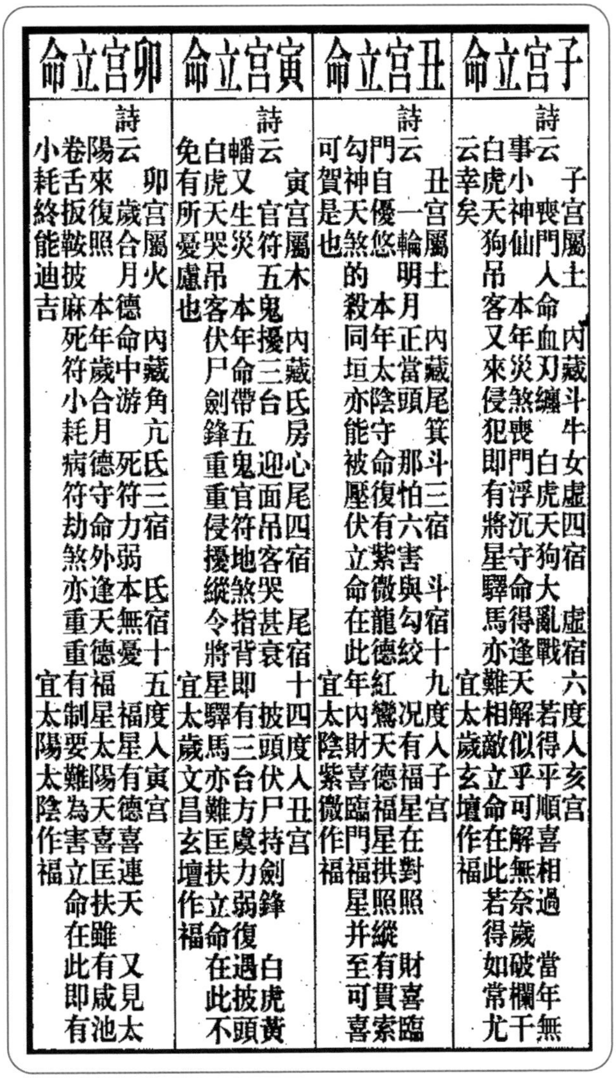

Fig. **1** *The first four earthly branches in correspondence with celestial bodies and their implications in human affairs.*

命立宮未	命立宮午	命立宮巳	命立宮辰
詩	詩	詩	詩
在月華云	德刃暗云	弄天開云	神劍天云
此德大　未	行太明　午	瓦厄抱　巳	破鋒解　辰
平拱白命宮	善歲劍白宮	之同麟紅宮	財伏不歲宮
安照明逢屬	可劍　虎屬	喜垣兒鷥屬	尤尸明破屬
納劫　天太	為鋒本守太	可六　行水	其災　入金
福煞本德陰	安伏年命陽	為害本運	幸煞本命
矣勾年又	康尸將將	預劫年入內	矣浮年遇內
絞天福內	為星星內	賀殺龍紫藏	沉歲耗藏
咸德星藏	害守　藏	勾德微星	相破星翌
池福　參	雖命對井	神紫　張	侵欄　軫
晦星披井	有內面鬼	欲微太翌	即干月角
氣守麻二	天有連柳	來紅陽三	有月煞三
的命卷宿	解天天星	侵鷥臨宿	驛煞欄宿
殺扳舌	正雄哭四	犯守照	馬守千
受鞍無井	照披災宿	亦命萬翌	天命也角
制卷尅宿	但頭情	退外事宿	解外無宿
于舌應廿	助白　星	處有宜六	終逢情六
宜本已　四	宜力虎華宿	宜無太　度	宜恐天　度
太宮經太度	太不侵蓋三	太權陽還入	太難狗太入
陽凶無陽入	歲大擾三度	陽立天有辰	歲化吊歲卯
太神妨月午	玄立外台入	太命喜太宮	文立客劍宮
陰安又德宮	壇命又相巳	陰在太陰	昌命喪鋒
作敢得喜	作在官護宮	紫此陰傍	作在門當
福出太合	福此符拱	微桃朝處	福此飛頭
而陽照	吉五	作天拱拱	積廉落
為天	凶鬼遂	福之雛	善大
害喜月	交地使	慶有桃	消殺疲
立太色	集煞劍	弄亡天	災太馬
命陰光	修血鋒	璋神花	勞歲連

Fig. 2 The second four earthly branches in correspondence with celestial bodies and their implications in human affairs.

What about the concept of the "week"? This concept is less important in the Chinese calendar. However, just like the ancient Egyptians, the Chinese had a 10-day week. It was the ancient Assyrians who invented the seven-day week. As to the names of the days of the week we use today, these are based on the system that assigns the five planets visible to our naked eye, the sun, and the moon to the seven days of the week. Arranged in their supposed order of decreasing distance from the Earth, they are: Saturn, Jupiter, Mars, the Sun, Venus, Mercury, and the Moon. The relevant Chinese material appears in a book called the *Bai Hu Tong* by Ban Gu (32–92 CE). It lists the 五行 *wu xing*, the Five Phases, in a unique order. The Five Phases concept lies at the very foundation of Chinese metaphysics. It is used to explain other things both subjectively and objectively. It is clear that the Five Phases are metaphysical constituents of reality, while their foundation lays in cosmic *yin* and cosmic *yang*. More importantly, it is their inherent motion and cyclic passage that enables them to "phase" into each other in definite sequence or sequences. The best known ordinary sequences are the cycle of production and the cycle of destruction. This is best found in Chinese medical theory. Chinese philosophy draws elaborate correspondences between sets of five: There are the five notes of the musical scale, the five planets, the five colors, the five flavors, and so forth. In Chinese astronomy, the names of the five planets have the same names as the five metaphysical "elements"—the five terms mentioned above: metal, wood, water, fire, and earth.

What about "month"? We must turn to the moon for this concept. The observation of the periodical waxing and waning of the moon defines a "month" as the time it takes for the moon to go through one full periodic cycle. In reality, the cycle takes about 29.5 days. Thus, we round the period of one month up or down to be either 29 or 30 days. Just like the concept of "day" in Chinese, the concept of "month" is embedded in the Chinese character 月 *yue*, which is used to denote both the moon and the month.

The next unit of time measurement is the "year." We must now go back to our observation of the sun again. Careful observation and calculation reveals that the sun shifts from very high overhead to a much lower point at noon. This shift in the sun's height also corresponds proportionally to the change in the length of the day, namely from longer to shorter as the sun shifts from high overhead to a lower point. Another major corresponding change that takes place following this shift is the change in the weather. The weather changes from hot to cold, giving rise to the four seasons of winter, spring, summer, and fall. The Chinese character to denote this concept is 年 *nian*, that is, "year." What about the length of a year? In 104 BCE the length of a year was calculated as 365.2502 days. However, the great mathematician and astronomer Zhu Chong-Zhi recalculated this number in 480 CE and arrived at 365.2428 days, only 52 seconds more than the modern figure of 365.2422 days. As this small discrepancy shows, the Chinese devised the system for measuring time that more accurately reflects reality. The Chinese did not stop at this, though. Indeed, in order to justify the discrepancy of

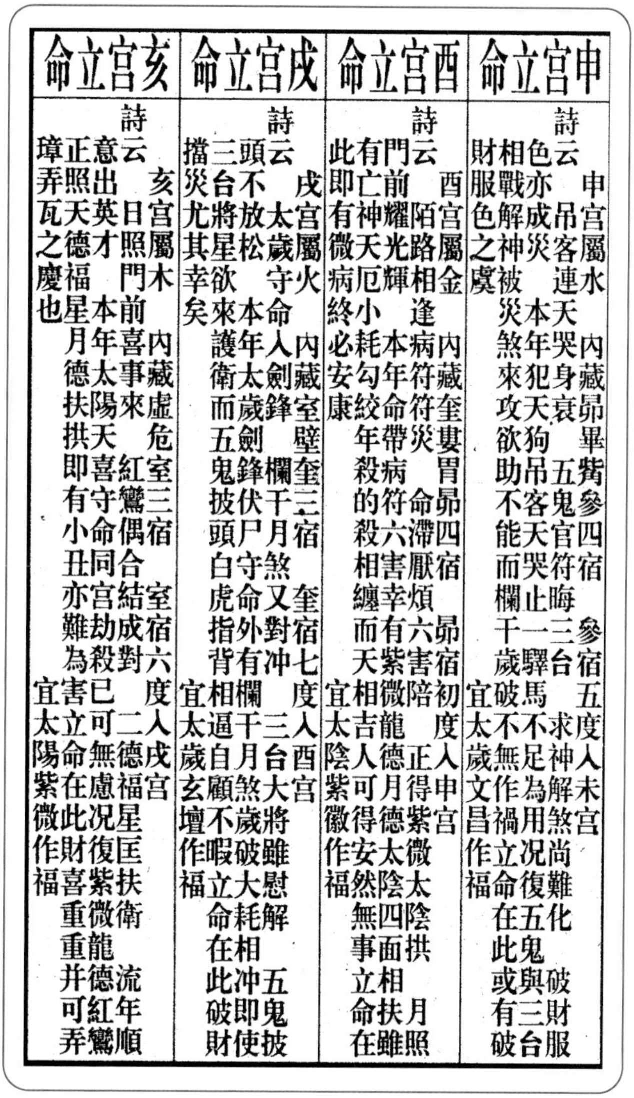

Fig. 3 The third four earthly branches in correspondence with celestial bodies and their implications in human affairs.

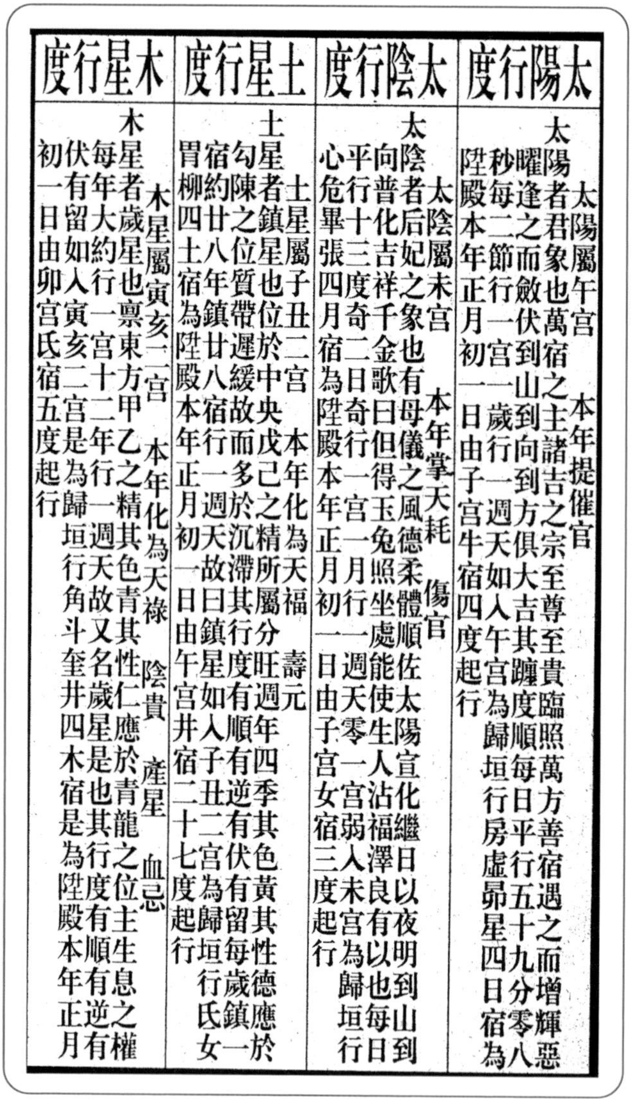

度行星木	度行星土	度行陰太	度行陽太
木	土	太	太

木初伏每星 一有年者木 日留大歲星 由如約星屬 卯入行也寅 宮寅一稟亥 氐亥宮東一 宿二十方宮 五宮二甲 度是年乙木 起為行之本 行歸一精化 垣週其為 行天色天 角故青祿 斗又其 奎名歲陰 井星仁貴 四星應 木是於產 宿也青星 是其龍 為行之血 陛度位忌 殿有主 本順生 年有息 正逆之 月有權

土胃宿勾星 柳約陳者土 四廿之鎮星 土八位星屬 宿年質也子 為鎮帶位丑 陛廿遲於二 殿八緩中宮 本宿故央 年行而戊本 正一多己年 月週於之化 初天沉精為 一故滯所天 日日其屬福 由鎮行分 午星度旺壽 宮如有週元 并入順年 宿子有四 二丑逆季 十二有其 七宮伏色 度為有黃 起歸留其 行垣每性 行歲德 氐鎮應 女一於

太心平向陰 危行普者太 畢十化后陰 張三吉妃屬 四度祥之未 月奇千象宮 宿二金也 為日歌有 陛奇日母本 殿行但儀年 本一得之掌 年宮玉風天 正一兔德耗 月月照柔 初行坐體傷 一一處順官 日週能佐 由天使太 子零生陽 宮一人宣 女宮沾化 宿弱福繼 三人澤日 度未良以 起宮有夜 行為以明 歸也到 垣每山 行日到

太陛秒曜陽 殿每逢者太 本二之君陽 年節而象屬 正行斂也午 月一伏萬宮 初宮到宿 一山之 日歲到主 由行向諸 子一到吉 宮週方之宗 牛天俱至 宿如大尊 四入吉至 度午其貴 起宮躊臨 行為度照 歸順萬 垣每方善 行日平宿 房虛行遇 昴五之 星十而 四九增 日分零輝 宿為八惡

Fig. **4** *Cycling of celestial bodies in the Chinese calendar and their astronomical implications in human affairs in the coming year.*

0.24 days, the system of rounding off was devised to deal with this off-set day. The traditional Chinese method is the "lunar calendar," which forms the basis for all traditional Chinese festivals. So, traditionally, it fixes the schedules for social events such as markets, court sessions, temple affairs, and all private agreements to meet to do business.

History of the Chinese Lunar Calendar

In general, a lunar calendar (wherein a month corresponds to the cycle of phases of the moon), makes sense in a society where there is little artificial lighting and the presence or absence of a bright moon makes a big difference to nocturnal activity. By contrast, a solar calendar, with the year anchored to the solstices and equinoxes, more realistically reflects our experience of the seasons, and helps us to discuss longer-term historical phenomena (such as death).

By the middle of the second millennium BCE, Chinese observers had concluded that the solar year was pretty nearly 365.2502 days long.

Each cycle of the moon is very close to 29.5 days long. To accommodate the half day, some Chinese months are 29 days long and some 30 days long. However, as in all calendars, it has to fit the length of the solar year:

1 year = 365 days
12 lunar months = 29.5 × 12 = 354 days
(11 days short per year)

In other words, there are (365.25 : 29.5 =) 12.3813559322 … lunar months per year. It would not be very felicitous if this were used to make a calendar that fits the movement of both celestial bodies. Since each solar year is about a third of a lunar month longer than 12 lunar months, the error can be reduced by adding an extra month to every fourth year, a leap year, in order to make up the 365.24 days.

3 years = 365.25 × 3 days = 1095.75 days
37 months = 29.5 × 37 = 1091.5 days
Difference = 4.25 days in three years,
1.4167 days per year

That is still a relatively large error. The problem was partially solved, probably by about the Spring and Autumn Period (770–476 BCE), by using a cycle of 19 years, in seven of which intercalary months were inserted:

19 years = 365.25 days = 6939.75 days
(6935 if one ignores the quarter days)
19 years × 12 months = 228 months,
plus 7 intercalary months = 235 months
235 months × 29.5 days = 6932.5 days

However, this still involved an error of 7.25 days in 19 years, or over a third of a day per year.

Conclusion

As discussed above, the Chinese have devised a very different system to calculate time. Knowledge of this system could not only help us to understand more about how Chinese

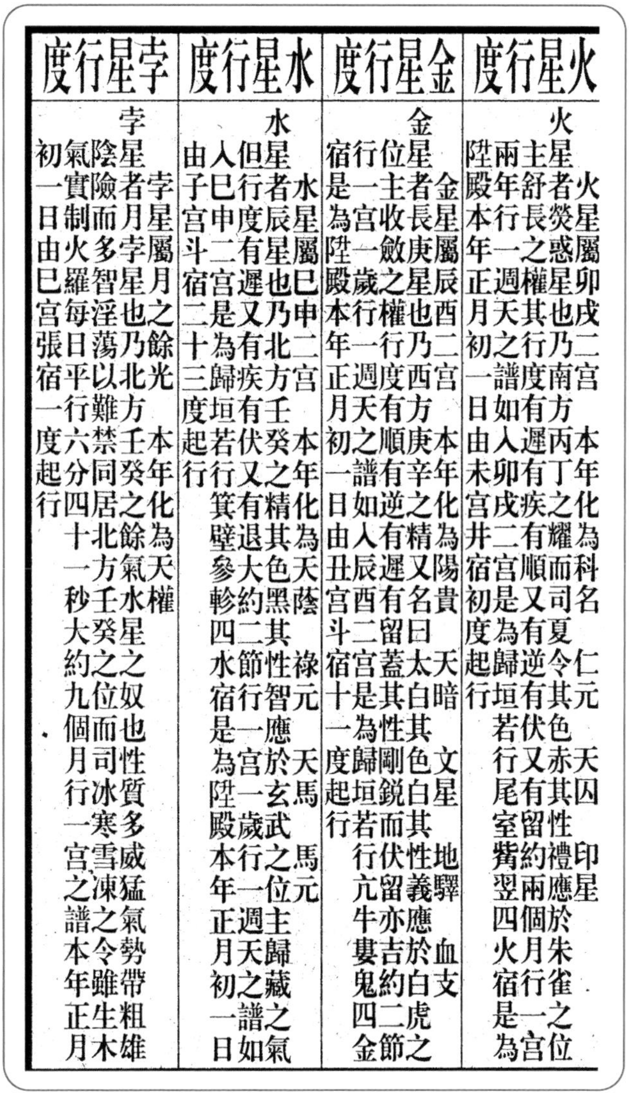

度行星孛	度行星水	度行星金	度行星火
孛 初氣陰星 一實險者孛 日制而月星 由火多孛屬 巳羅智星月 宮每淫也之 張日蕩乃餘 宿平以北光 一行難方 度六禁壬本 起分同癸年 行四居之化 十北餘為 一方氣天 秒壬水權 大癸星 約之之 九位奴 個而也 月司性 行冰質 一寒多 宮雪威 之凍猛 譜之氣 本令勢 年雖帶 正生粗 月木雄	水 由入但星 子巳行者水 宮中度辰星 斗二有星屬 宿宮遲也巳 二是又乃申 十為有北二 三歸疾方宮 度垣有壬 起若伏癸本 行行又之年 箕有精化 壁退其為 參大色天 軫約黑陰 四二其 水節性祿 宿行智元 是一應 為宮於天 陞一玄馬 殿歲武 本行之馬 年一位元 正週主 月天歸 初之藏 一譜之 日如氣	金 宿行位星 是一主者金 為宮收長星 陞一斂庚屬 殿歲之星辰 本行權也酉 年一行乃二 正週度西宮 月天有方 初之順庚本 一譜有辛年 日如逆之化 由入有精為 丑辰遲又陽 宮酉有名貴 斗二留日 宿宮蓋太天 十是其白暗 一為性其 度歸剛色文 起垣銳白星 行若而其 行伏性地 亢留義驛 牛亦應 婁吉於血 鬼約白支 四二虎 金節之	火 陞兩主星 殿年舒者火 本行長熒星 年一之惑屬 正週權星卯 月天其也戌 初之行乃二 一譜度南宮 日如有方 由入遲丙本 未卯有丁年 宮戌疾之化 井二有耀為 宿宮順而科 初是又司名 度為有夏 起歸逆令仁 行垣有其元 若伏色 行又赤天 尾有其囚 室留性 觜約禮印 翌兩應星 四個於 火月朱 宿行雀 是一之 為宮位

Fig. 5 *Cycling of celestial bodies in the Chinese calendar and their astronomical implications in human affairs in the coming year.*

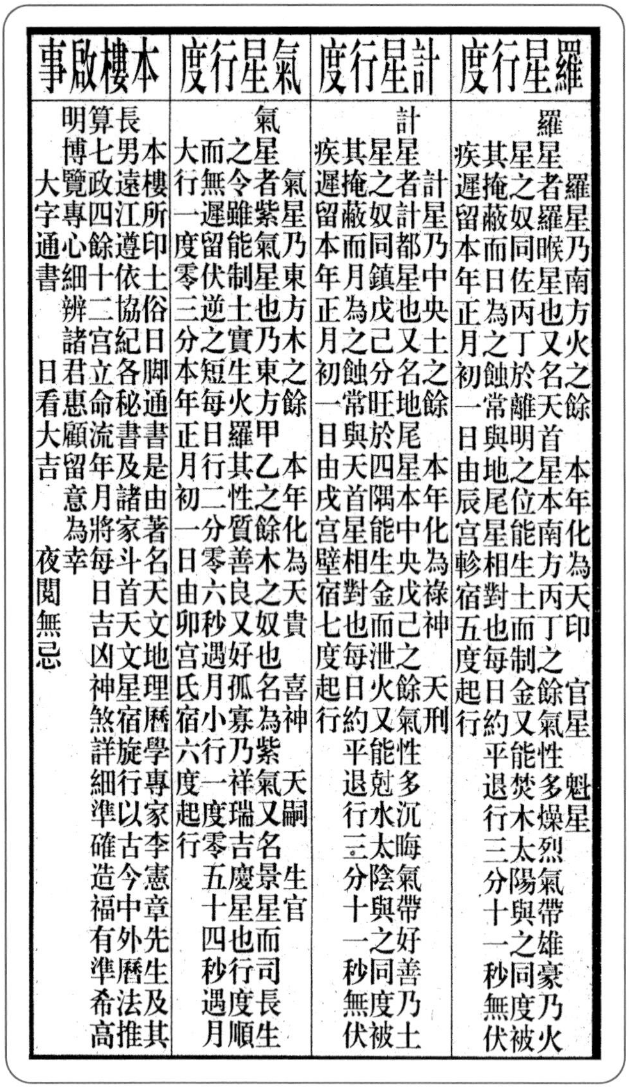

本樓啟事　氣星行度　計星行度　羅星行度

本遠樓長算明
男政七博算覽
所江四專字心
印遵依十餘通
土俗協二細書
紀日宮宮協辨
腳各立君諸宮
通秘命惠日看
書書流顧大吉
是及留意月留
著家諸將為意
名斗每幸夜閣
天首日無忌
文天吉
地文凶
理星神
曆宿煞
學旋詳
專行細
家以準
李古確
憲今造
章中福
先外有
生曆準
及法希
其推高

氣
星之而大
星紫雖遲行
乃氣能令無
東星鎮伏留度
方木乃星三零
餘之實本逆
甲羅日正年火每短本分
乙其行月初二性之餘質一善木
之年化為木善之良又卯秒遇好也
氏月孤寡宿小寡六行度一祥瑞吉
名為紫氣天又嗣吉名行零五慶十
星官四也而秒行司遇度長月順生

計
星星其疾
計者掩遲
乃奴藏留
中星都同而本
央鎮月星為正
土戊為己之月
名分蝕初地餘
尾於與日常一
本星四天由餘
化能星宮戊首
為祿戊金對相壁宿
神己之泄火日每度起
喜紫為名孤宿
多沉水行魁戰退能平
氣陰太三晦太三
好之一帶與十
善同秒好之一
土被伏乃度無

羅
星星其疾
羅者掩遲
星奴藏留
南星佐日同而本
方丙為丁之月
火又丁之月
名於蝕初首天離一餘
尾辰地之由首明與日
化能星宮南對相生轍宿
神丙土對五也而印丁制之
星官餘金起日
豪之一雄之一帶與十
善同秒好之一
火被伏乃度無

Fig. **6** *Cycling of celestial bodies in the Chinese calendar and their astronomical implications in human affairs in the coming year.*

people perceive themselves in the midst of the universe and their relationship to the external universe, but also about the metaphors they employ in the medical realm. Time, as one of the indicators of our state of being in this infinitely changing universe, allows us to gain a better knowledge of ourselves, and thus of how to change accordingly. The philosophy of wholeness and impermanence that gives rise to this time system also gives rise to the fundamental principles in Traditional Chinese Medicine. As stated by one of greatest Chinese medical doctors of the Tang dynasty, Sun Simiao: "… a great doctor must not only study the medical theory, but to understand the astrology and geology is vital in differentiating a good doctor from the mediocre …"

Chinese Calendar Terminology

Great Year = 12 years
Cycle = 5 Great Years = 60 years
Epoch = 60 Cycles = 60 × 60 years = 3600 years

We are currently in the second Epoch.

Western Calendar Terminology

Decade = 10 years
Century = 100 years
Millennium = 1000 years
2006 is in the third millennium, 21st century, first decade, and sixth year.

Seasonal Health Advice from Ancient Chinese Sources

Yuhuan Zhang, San Francisco, California, USA

Ever since the beginning of Chinese civilization, the Chinese have paid great respect and close attention to what they eat and drink, as well as to their physical living conditions. According to Chinese belief, we are what we eat and we are part of the greater universe. Therefore, our health is affected by external factors such as seasonal changes, monthly lunar changes, etc. The types of food we should eat and clothes we should wear are thus prescribed. In most cases, this advice is categorized according to the seasons, sometimes according to the 24 solar divisional points in the Chinese calendar. This advice is not only common culture, it is also highly regarded in Chinese medical texts. For instance, we can find extensive descriptions of seasonal advice not only in the Chinese medical texts such as *Huang Di Nei Jing* (The Yellow Emperor's Classic of Medicine), but also in Chinese traditional dietary books such as *The Orthodox Essence of Drink and Food*, 饮膳正要, from the *Yuan* dynasty (1279–1368 CE); similar advice is to be found in numerous Chinese Daoist sutras.

Below are excerpts from *The Orthodox Essence of Drink and Food*. It is renowned as the basic Chinese dietary book and not only describes the properties of food ingredients, but also gives extensive descriptions of how to use those foods appropriately according to the seasons.

Spring

The three months of spring constitute the season of engendering. The space between heaven and earth is filled with robust life force. Everything in nature is thriving. At this time, one should go to bed early and rise early. After rising in the morning, one should let

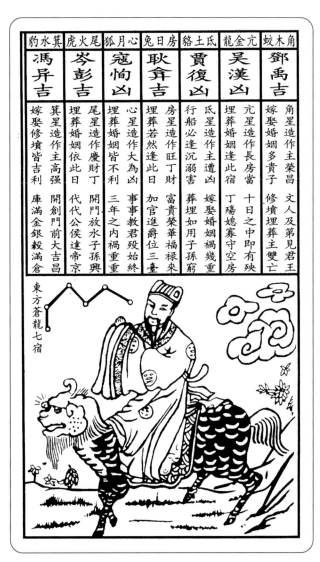

Fig. 1 Seven celestial bodies in eastern direction and their implications in human activities, such as marriage, house building, and moving.

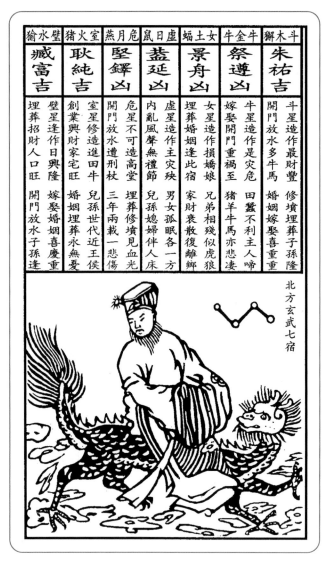

Fig. 2 Seven celestial bodies in northern direction and their implications in human activities, such as marriage, house building, and moving.

in the season and make internal changes accordingly. Any other ways would be injurious to one's health and, most immediately, to one's liver *qi*, which would result in cold-natured disease in the summer and decrease the body's constitution in the summer.

Spring weather is generally warm; it is beneficial to eat more millet and related foods, because millet is cool in nature. One should not only be mindful of the warmth in nature. Food that is warm in nature is forbidden. It is not advisable to wear too much clothing.

Summer

The three summer months constitute the season of exuberant growth. At this time, the heavenly *qi* descends from above and the earthly *qi* ascends from below. The two *qi* meet in the middle and mingle. Most vegetation is in bloom and bears fruit at this time. Thus, one should adjust one's life accordingly by going to bed late but rising early. One should not fret about the heat in the weather. One should not let one's emotions swing in haste. One should not retain anger. One should try to remain joyful and peaceful, try to keep one's spirit focused and abundant. This is just like all things that are in exuberant and firm growth. One should let one's skin breathe and keep the mind at ease. This is the way of life in summer. Any other ways would injure the heart *qi*. Damage to heart *qi* would result in swamp fever (or malaria), which decreases one's adaptability to the harvesting *qi* in the fall; in severe cases, it would cause illness in the winter.

Summer is the season of heat; it is beneficial to eat more beans and related foods, because they are cold in nature and have the function of clearing summer heat. It is not advisable to use warm and hot herbs. Foods that are warm in nature are prohibited. One should not overeat. One should not dwell in a damp place and not wear wet clothing.

one's hair hang loose and take a stroll in the courtyard or simply walk in the open air in loose robes. Throughout the day, one should try to shape one's mind and will according to the nature of spring. One should be active both physically and mentally; one should not let one's mind and spirit sit and stagnate, as this is contradictory to the engendering nature of spring. The way to life is to follow the change

Autumn

The three months of autumn constitute the season of harvesting. During this season, the sky is high and the air is crisp; weeds and woods are bleak and silent; the weather cools down from the summer heat. One should now go to sleep early and rise early. One should adopt the daily schedule of a rooster. One should try to keep one's mind in a peaceful, pure, and quiet state. Only by constraining one's spirit and *qi* and remaining in a state of peace and quietness can one soften and yield the solemn and punishing nature of fall and purify the lung *qi*. This is the "nourishing and constraining" way of fall. If the life nourishing way of fall is disobeyed, this will injure lung *qi*, which results in diarrhea and undigested food in the stool in the winter, which in turn decreases one's adaptive ability to the hidden and storage *qi* of winter.

In autumn the weather is dry; it is beneficial to eat more sesame and related foods, because of their moist and nourishing nature, which soothes the dryness of autumn. Foods that are cold in nature should not be eaten. It is advisable to wear sufficient clothing.

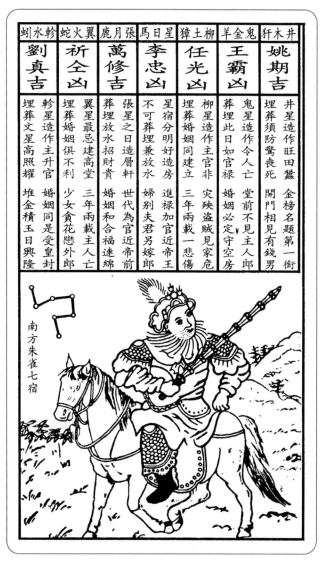

Fig. 3 Seven celestial bodies in southern direction and their implications in human activities, such as marriage, house building, and moving.

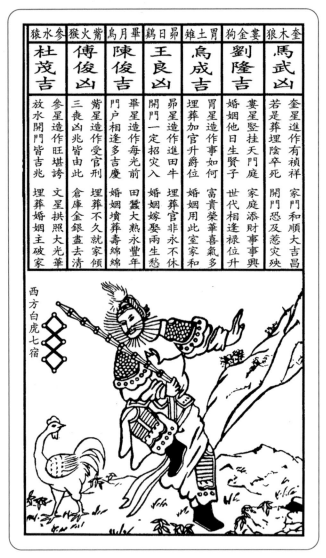

猿水參	猴火觜	烏月畢	鷄日昴	雉土胃	狗金婁	狼木奎
杜茂吉	傅俊凶	陳俊吉	王良凶	烏成吉	劉隆吉	馬武凶
放水開門皆吉兆	參星造作旺堪誇	觜星凶兆皆由此	畢星造作每光前	昴星造作進田牛	胃星造作事如何	婁星竪挂天門庭	若是葬埋陰卒死	奎星進作有禎祥
埋葬婚姻主破家	文星拱照大光華	三喪凶兆皆受官刑	門户相逢多吉慶	開門一定招災入	田蠶大熟永豐年	埋葬加官升爵位	富貴榮華喜氣多	婚姻他日生賢子	世代相逢禄位升	家庭添財事事興	開門恐惹災殃	家門和順大吉昌
		倉庫金銀盡去清	埋葬不久就家傾	婚姻嫁娶兩生愁	婚姻葬壽綿綿	埋葬官非永不休	婚姻用此室家和	

西方白虎七宿

Fig. 4 Seven celestial bodies in western direction and their implications in human activities, such as marriage, house building, and moving.

Winter

The three winter months constitute the season of hibernation and storage. Water turns into ice because of the cold. The Earth is cracked because of the cold. The engendering nature of things in the world is now obstructed and the transition to the hibernating stage is made. At this time, man should go to bed early and rise late. It is best to rise after the sun has risen high into the sky. One should keep one's state of mind and one's will crouching and in hiding, as if these are tangible things one has in one's possession. One should avoid the cold. One should use heating, but not allow the skin and pores to open to the point of sweating, as this will damage yang *qi*. These are the ways of the winter, of "nourishment and storage." If the nourishing way of winter is disobeyed, one can expect wilting reversal illness the following spring, which decreases one's ability to adapt to the engendering *qi* of spring.

The weather in winter is cold; it is beneficial to eat broomcorn millet and related foods in order to use their hot nature to cure coldness. Food that is very hot in temperature should not be eaten. It is not advisable to dress in clothes that have been dried over a fire.

The 24 Seasonal Division Points and Their Implications for the Preservation of Life

Yuhuan Zhang, San Francisco, California, USA

Chinese farmers have long depended on the 24 seasonal division points in the Chinese calendar to provide them with horticultural advice. Even more so, Chinese Daoists and Chinese medical doctors and ancient professional life preservers all depended on this subdivision of the Chinese calendar to give them indications of time and changes in the atmosphere, so they could make appropriate changes to their own existence accordingly. This idea of change in accordance with the environment fits the general treatment principle of diseases and lifestyle in general and was prescribed in the *Huang Di Nei Jing* (The Yellow Emperor's Classic of Medicine). In contrast to the changes according to the seasons, the 24 solar terms represent seasonal division points that segment each year into 24 parts. These detail habits including diet, exercise, dress codes, daily schedules, and even sexual habits and acts, which should all be adapted accordingly. The purpose is a long and healthy life. As the great physician and Daoist of the Tang dynasty, Sun Si Miao, said in his *Qian Jin Fang* (Chapter 27):

Intercourse should be avoided on the dates associated with S3 and S4. One should also avoid the waning and waxing dates of the month, or when there is excessive wind, excessive rain, excessive fog, excessive cold, excessive heat, thunder and lightening, extreme darkness during the day, eclipses, and earthquakes. If one has intercourse with a woman, it can damage one's spirit. It is not a lucky thing to do. The damage this can bring a man is a hundred times greater; it could also cause the female partner ill. If one intends to conceive under such atmospheric circumstances, the child will be crazy, mentally retarded, blind, mute, deaf, crippled, chronically ill, with a short life expectancy, barbaric, uneducable.

In the same chapter, Dr Sun even gives specific dates in each month that are the best for intercourse. This shows that the ancient Chinese lived precisely according to space and time.

In order to understand this philosophy of life, we need to understand what the so-called 24 seasonal division points are. The Chinese believe that the 24 seasonal division points are determined by segmenting the changes in the sun's position at eclipses as well as the consequent changes in the atmosphere on earth into 24 segments. Each segment covers a period of about 15 days, i.e., there are two seasonal division points in each month. Those seasonal division points in the first half of the month are called 节气 *jie qi*, seasonal *qi*; those seasonal division points in the second half of the month are called 中气 *zhong qi*, middle *qi*. The word "*qi*" here refers to weather and the atmosphere. The following is taken from the *Huang Di Nei Jing* (The Yellow Emperor's Classic of Medicine), Book 9: Treatise on the Six Regulations Governing the Manifestations of the Viscera:

… Five days are called a "period of five days," three of those five-day periods are called "one of the 24 solar periods of the year"; six of these solar periods are called "one season"; four seasons are called "one year"; and each of these periods is subject to a different control.

Below is the chart listing the names and order of the 24 seasonal division points

Within those seasonal division points, the 立春 *li chun*, Beginning of Spring, 春分 *chun fen*, Vernal Equinox, 立夏 *li xia*, Beginning of Summer, 夏至 *xia zhi*, Summer Solstice, 立秋 *li qiu*, Beginning of Autumn, 秋分 *qiu fen*, Autumnal Equinox, 立冬 *li dong*, Beginning of Winter, and 冬至 *dong zhi*, Winter Solstice, indicate the partition of the four seasons of the year. The two "equinoxes" and two

THIEME Almanac 2007 **325**

The 24 Seasonal Division Points

	Order and Name of Seasonal Division Point	Sun's Position at Ecliptic	Date on Gregorian Calendar
Spring	1. Beginning of Spring (*lì chūn*)	315°	February, 4th or 5th
	2. Rain Water (*yǔ shuǐ*)	330°	February, 19th or 20th
	3. Waking of Insects (*jing zhé*)	345°	March, 5th or 6th
	4. Vernal Equinox (*chūn fēn*)	0°	March, 20th or 21st
	5. Pure Brightness (*qīng ming*)	15°	April, 5th or 6th
	6. Grain Rain (*gǔ yǔ*)	30°	April, 20th or 21st
Summer	7. Beginning of Summer (*lì xià*)	45°	May, 5th or 6th
	8. Grain Budding (*xiǎo mǎn*)	60°	May, 21st or 22nd
	9. Grain in Ear (*máng zhǒng*)	75°	June, 6th or 7th
	10. Summer Solstice (*xià zhi*)	90°	June, 21st or 22nd
	11. Slight Heat (*xiǎo shǔ*)	105°	July, 7th or 8th
	12. Great Heat (*dà shǔ*)	120°	July, 23rd or 24th
Autumn	13. Beginning of Autumn (*lì qiū*)	135°	August, 7th or 8th
	14. Limit of Heat (*chù shǔ*)	150°	August, 23rd or 24th
	15. White Dew (*bái lù*)	165°	September, 7th or 8th
	16. Autumnal Equinox (*qīu fēn*)	180°	September, 23rd or 24th
	17. Cold Dew (*hán lù*)	195°	October, 8th or 9th
	18. Frost's Descent (*shuāng jiàng*)	210°	October, 23rd or 24th
Winter	19. Beginning of Winter (*lì dōng*)	225°	November, 7th or 8th
	20. Slight Snow (*xiǎo xuě*)	240°	November, 22nd or 23rd
	21. Great Snow (*dà xuě*)	255°	December, 7th or 8th
	22. Winter Solstice (*dōng zhì*)	270°	December, 22nd or 23rd
	23. Slight Cold (*xiǎo hán*)	285°	January, 5th or 6th
	24. Great Cold (*dà hán*)	300°	January, 20th or 21st

"solstices" mark the turning point of the seasons; the four "beginnings" mark the beginning of each season.

The 小暑 *xiao shu*, Slight Heat, 大暑 *da shu*, Great Heat, 处暑 *chu shu*, Limit of Heat, 小寒 *xiao han*, Slight Cold, and 大寒 *da han*, Great Cold, each mark the hottest and coldest time of the year.

The 白露 *bai lu*, White Dew, 寒露 *han lu*, Cold Dew, and 霜降 *shuang jiang*, Frost's Descent, each reflect the process and the degrees of decreasing temperature. The 雨水 *yu shui*, Rain Water, 谷雨 *gu yu*, Grain Rain, 小雪 *xiao xue*, Slight Snow, and 大雪 *da xue*, Great Snow, each reflect the level of rain or snow.

Lastly, the 惊蛰 *jing zhe*, Waking of Insects, 清明 *qing ming*, Pure Brightness, 小满 *xiao man*, Grain Budding, and 芒种 *mang zhong*, Grain in Ear, each reflect horticultural and seasonal phenomena.

As listed above, we can see that each of these 24 seasonal division points is based on the agricultural phenomenon of a particular time in the year. The naming of those divisional points reflects the characteristics of each period.

The Chinese have long realized the relation between our health and the external world. It is by connecting bodily functions to the outside physical world that we are able to exist and maintain our health. Therefore, it is natural for philosophers and Chinese medical doctors to perceive and conceptualize phenomena. It is pivotal in understanding the correlation and functioning of our internal being and the outer world.

In the *Huang Di Nei Jing* (The Yellow Emperor's Classic of Medicine), Qi Bo, the Yellow Emperor's divine doctor and teacher also emphasizes the correlation between bodily functions and the changes in the seasons and the importance of understanding this as the gateway to good health:

The interaction of the five elements brings harmony and everything is in order. At the end of one year the sun has completed its course and everything starts anew with the first season, which is the beginning of Spring. This system is comparable to a ring which has neither beginning nor end. The periods of five days each also share this arrangement. Therefore I must say: those who are ignorant about the increase of the year, and about that which is produced through the flourishing, deteriorating, emptying, and filling powers of the four seasons cannot produce good work.

The point is emphasized by the Yellow Emperor when he asks:

'*The interaction of the five elements is like a ring—it has no beginning; is this an excessive or inadequate description?'*

Qi Bo answered: 'The five atmospheric influences change their spheres of activity; they counteract one another and there is constancy in their transformation from abundance to emptiness.'

The Emperor asked: 'How can one achieve a tranquil atmosphere?'

Qi Bo answered: 'By avoiding transgression of the laws of nature.'

The Emperor asked: 'If this perfection cannot be achieved— what then?'

Qi Bo answered: 'This perfection is contained in the invariable rules of conduct.'

The Emperor asked: 'What is the meaning of counteraction?'

Qi Bo answered: 'Spring counteracts the Long Summer; the Long Summer counteracts Winter; Winter counteracts Autumn; Autumn counteracts Spring. This is called the effect of the counteraction of all the five elements and their respective seasons. Each element uses its life-giving principles to influence the destiny of its particular viscera.'

The Emperor asked: 'How can one use this knowledge of their counteraction?'

Qi Bo answered: 'By seeking the highest (good). Everything is restored at the beginning of Spring. If people have not yet arrived at the highest (good) but nevertheless reach out for it, their action is called 'excessive.' Then there is carelessness everywhere, which cannot be counteracted, and that which must be overcome is multiplied. General behavior becomes immoral and licentious, and people no longer segregate those whose inner life is depraved and heterodox, and those in office cannot enforce restrictions and prohibitions.

'*Those who strive for the highest (good), yet cannot attain it, are called unequal to the task. Then that which has already been gained is squandered in foolish and reckless conduct. This produces suffering of diseases because of carelessness, which cannot be overcome. At these critical times those who seek the highest (good) turn to the highest life-giving principles of the respective season.*

'*Even though one attends respectfully to the periods of five days, to the seasons and their atmospheric influences, it is still possible to make mistakes in regard to the full year and to act against the system of the five-day periods and the five elements. Then one can no longer segregate oneself from those whose inner life is depraved and heterodox; and those in office can no longer enforce restrictions and prohibitions.'*

The Emperor asked: 'Is there no hereditary influence?'

Qi Bo answered: 'The atmospheric influence of the blue sky is constant, but this climate cannot be inherited and it is called 'extraordinary and unusual.' Because it is extraordinary it changes (while Heaven remains constant and invariable).'

The Emperor asked: 'How can it be extraordinary and yet change?'

Qi Bo answered: 'The change affects the body and thus brings disease. If this disease can be overcome it remains invisible and trifling; if it cannot be overcome it will become more important than its cause and very severe; and if evil influences are added death will ensue. Thus if one acts wrongly in regard to the seasons his action may remain secret and hidden, but if one follow the laws of the seasons he will be considered great.'

The Emperor said: 'Excellent indeed! I have also heard that the atmospheric influences unite and take shape, and because of this change one can define them in precise terms. The revolution of Heaven and Earth and the transformation brought about by Yin and Yang have their effect upon everything in creation. Can we also obtain knowledge about the extent of this influence?'

Qi Bo said: 'How brilliant a question! Heaven is boundless and cannot be measured.

二十四节气卦象阴阳损益图

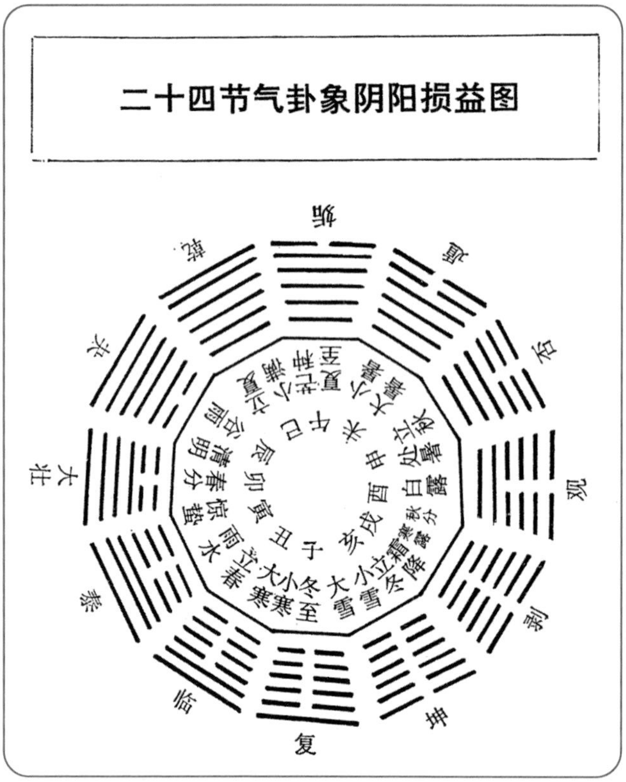

Fig. 1 Increasing of yin and yang in the 24 solar periods.

The Earth is large and without limit. In order to find out how large one must ask Ling Shen and beg him for information on the extent of those regions.

'Grass and herbs bring forth the five colors; nothing that can be seen excels the variation of those five colors. Grass and herbs also produce the five flavors; nothing excels the deliciousness of those five flavors. Human desires are not alike, therefore everyone has at his disposal all of them.

'Man receives the five atmospheric influences as food from Heaven and the five flavors as food from Earth.

'The five atmospheric influences enter the nostrils and are stored by the heart and the lungs and then they are allowed to rise. The five colors restore brightness and light. The (musical) sounds are manifestations of talent and ability. The five flavors enter the mouth and are stored by the stomach. The flavors which are stored nourish the five atmospheric influences, and when these influences are well-blended they produce saliva. Together all those influences help to perfect the mind, which then begins to function spontaneously.'

The Emperor asked: 'How can you explain the outer appearances of the viscera?'

Qi Bo answered: 'The heart is the root of life and causes the versatility of the spiritual faculties. The heart influences the face and fills the pulse with blood. Within Yang, the principle of light and life, the heart acts as the Great Yang which permeates the climate of Summer.

'The lungs are the origin of breath and the dwelling of the animal spirits or inferior soul. The lungs influence the body hair and have their effect upon the skin. Within Yang, the lungs act as the Great Yin which permeates the climate in Fall.

'The kidneys (testicles) call to life that which is dormant and sealed up; they are the natural organ for storing away, and they are the place where the secretions are lodged. The kidneys influence the hair on the head and have an effect upon the bones. Within Yin the kidneys act as the Lesser Yin which permeates the climate of Winter.

'The liver causes utmost weariness and is the dwelling place of the soul, or spiritual part of man that ascends to Heaven. The liver influences the nails and is effective upon the muscles; its brings forth animal desires and vigor. The taste connected with the liver is sour and the color connected with the liver is green. Within Yang the liver acts as the Lesser Yang which permeates the air in Spring.

'In the stomach, the lower intestines, the small intestines, the three foci, the groin, and the bladder, one can find the basic principle for the public granaries and the encampment of the regiment. These organs are called 'vessels,' and have the power to transform the dregs and the sediment, and cause the flavors to revolve so that they enter the vessels and leave them. These organs are effective upon the flesh and the muscles. The flavor connected with these organs is sweet and the color is yellow. They belong to the organs of Yin which permeates the climate of the earth.

'In general one can say that the eleven viscera either receive from the gallbladder or expel into it.

'When people have one pulse full and abundant, the disease is in the region of the Lesser Yang. When two pulses are full and abundant, the disease is in the region of the Great Yang; when three pulses are full and abundant, the disease is located in the region of the 'sunlight.' When four pulses are full and abundant, the disease has come to an end and the powers above act as regulators of Yang.

'When the 'inch' (寸 cun) pulse at the wrist beats once fully and abundantly, the disease is located in the region of the Absolute Yin. When the 'inch' pulse at the wrist beats twice fully and abundantly, the disease is located in the region of the Lesser Yin. When the 'inch' pulse at the wrist beats three times fully and abundantly, the disease is located in the region of the Great Yin. When the 'inch' pulse beats four times fully and abundantly, the disease has come to an end and the powers above close Yin.

'When all the 'inch' pulses at the wrist are concurrent and flourishing, the four pulses join and come to an end, and the powers above of closing and regulate the pulse. Through this system of closing and regulating the pulse there can never be a surplus, when the essence of Heaven and Earth has come to an end (has been exhausted), death follows.'

The text below gives general health advice, dietary, and *qi gong* exercises for each season and 24 seasonal division points gathered from various ancient texts and modern resources.

Spring

The three months of Spring are called the period of the beginning and development (of life). The breaths (qi) of Heaven and Earth are prepared to give birth; thus everything is developing and flourishing.

After a night of sleep people should get up early (in the morning); they should walk briskly around the yard; they should loosen their hair and slow down their (body) movements; by these means they can (fulfill) their wish to live healthfully.

During this period (one's body) should be encouraged and not be killed; one should give (to it) freely and not take away (from it); one should reward (it) and not punish (it).

All this is in harmony with the breath of Spring and all this is the method for the protection of one's life.

Those who disobey the laws of Spring will be punished with an injury of the liver. For them the following Summer will bring chills and (bad) changes; thus they will have little to support their development (in Summer).

…

Those who do not conform with the breath of Spring will not bring to life the region of the Lesser Yang. The atmosphere of their heart will become empty.[1]

The six seasonal division points in this season are:
1. Beginning of Spring, 立春 *li chun*
2. Rain Water, 雨水 *yu shui*
3. Waking of Insects, 惊蛰 *jing zhe*
4. Vernal Equinox, 春分 *chun fen*
5. Pure Brightness, 清明 *qing ming*
6. Grain Rain, 谷雨 *gu yu*

Summer

The three months of Summer are called the period of luxurious growth. The breaths of Heaven and Earth intermingle and are beneficial. Everything is in bloom and begins to bear fruit.

After a night of sleep people should get up early (in the morning). They should not be weary during daytime and they should not allow their mind to become angry.

They should enable the best parts (of their body and spirit) to develop; they should enable their breath to communicate with the outside world; and they should act as though they loved everything outside.

All this is in harmony with the atmosphere of Summer and all this is the method for the protection of one's development.

Those who disobey the laws of Summer will be punished with an injury of the heart. For them Fall will bring intermittent fevers; thus they will have little to support them for harvest (in Fall); and hence, at Winter solstice they will suffer from grave disease.

...

Those who do not conform with the atmosphere of Summer will not develop their Great Yang. The atmosphere of their heart will become empty.[1]

The six seasonal division points in this season are:

7. Beginning of Summer, 立夏; *li xia*
8. Grain Budding, 小满 *xiao man*
9. Grain in Ear, 芒种 *mang zhong*
10. Summer Solstice, 夏至 *xia zhi*
11. Slight Heat, 小暑 *xiao shu*
12. Great Heat, 大暑 *da shu*

Autumn

The three months of Autumn are called the period of tranquility of one's conduct. The atmosphere of Heaven is quick and the atmosphere of the Earth is clear.

People should retire early at night and rise early (in the morning) with (the crowing of) the rooster. They should have their minds at peace in order to lessen the punishment of Fall. Soul and spirit should be gathered together in order to make the breath of Autumn tranquil; and to keep their lungs pure they should not give vent to their desires.

All this is in harmony with the atmosphere of Autumn and all this is the method for the protection of one's harvest.

Those who disobey the laws of Autumn will be punished with an injury of the lungs. For them Winter will bring indigestion and diarrhea; thus they will have little to support their storing (of Winter).

...

Those who do not conform with the atmosphere of Autumn will not harvest their Great Yin. The atmosphere of their lungs will be blocked from the lower burning space.[1]

The six seasonal division points in this season are:

13. Beginning of Autumn, 立秋 *li qiu*
14. Limit of Heat, 处暑 *chu shu*
15. White Dew, 白露 *bai lu*
16. Autumnal Equinox, 秋分 *qiu fen*
17. Cold Dew, 寒露 *han lu*
18. Frost's Descent, 霜降 *shuang jiang*

Winter

The three months of Winter are called the period of closing and storing. Water freezes and the Earth cracks open. One should not disturb one's Yang.

People should retire early at night and rise late in the morning and they should wait for the rising of the sun. They should suppress and conceal their wishes, as though they had no internal purpose, as though they should seek warmth; they should not perspire upon the skin, should let themselves be deprived of breath of the cold.

All this is in harmony with the atmosphere of Winter and all this is the method for the protection of one's storing.

Those who disobey (the laws of Winter) will suffer an injury of the kidneys (testicles); for them Spring will bring impotence, and they will produce little.

...

Those who do not conform with the atmosphere of Winter will not store their Lesser Yin. The atmosphere of their testes (kidneys) will be isolated and decreased.[1]

The six seasonal division points in this season are:

19. Beginning of Winter, 立冬 *li dong*
20. Slight Snow, 小雪 *xiao xue*
21. Great Snow, 大雪 *da xue*
22. Winter Solstice, 冬至 *dong zhi*
23. Slight Cold, 小寒 *xiao han*
24. Great Cold, 大寒 *da han*

---

1   Excerpt from the *Huang Di Nei Jing* (The Yellow Emperor's Classic of Medicine), Book 2: Great Treatise on the Harmony of the Atmosphere of the Four Seasons with the (Human) Spirit.

Heavenly Stems and Earthly Branches

Heavenly Stems and Earthly Branches
Tiān Gān Dì Zhī

Heavenly Stems	Corresponding Phase	Corresponding Star
First Heavenly Stem (jiǎ, 甲)	Wood	Jupiter
Second Heavenly Stem (yǐ, 乙)		
Third Heavenly Stem (bīng, 丙)	Fire	Mars
Fourth Heavenly Stem (dīng, 丁)		
Fifth Heavenly Stem (wù, 戊)	Earth	Saturn
Sixth Heavenly Stem (jǐ, 己)		
Seventh Heavenly Stem (gēng, 庚)	Metal	Venus
Eighth Heavenly Stem (xīn, 辛)		
Ninth Heavenly Stem (rén, 壬)	Water	Mercury
Tenth Heavenly Stem (guǐ, 癸)		

Earthly Branches	Chinese Zodiac	Corresponding Hours
First Earthly Branch (zǐ, 子)	Rat	23:00–01:00
Second Earthly Branch (chōu, 丑)	Ox	01:00–03:00
Third Earthly Branch (yín, 寅)	Tiger	03:00–05:00
Fourth Earthly Branch (mǎo, 卯)	Rabbit	05:00–07:00
Fifth Earthly Branch (chén, 辰)	Dragon	07:00–09:00
Sixth Earthly Branch (sí, 巳)	Snake	09:00–11:00
Seventh Earthly Branch (wǔ, 午)	Horse	11:00–13:00
Eighth Earthly Branch (wèi, 未)	Sheep	13:00–15:00
Ninth Earthly Branch (shēn, 申)	Monkey	15:00–17:00
Tenth Earthly Branch (yǒu, 酉)	Rooster	17:00–19:00
Eleventh Earthly Branch (xū, 戌)	Dog	19:00–21:00
Twelfth Earthly Branch (hài, 亥)	Pig	21:00–23:00

The 24 Solar Division Point Recipes

Yuhuan Zhang, San Francisco, California, USA

Flowery Knotweed with Liver Slices

Main Ingredients
8 oz fresh flowery knotweed juice
1 oz dried black wood ear
1 cup leafy greens
8 oz pork liver

Ingredients—Quantities According To Taste
Light chicken broth
Cooking wine
Vinegar
Cornstarch
Soy sauce
Vegetable oil
Sesame oil
Green onion
Fresh ginger
Fresh garlic

Method
1 Boil the flowery knotweed in a pot of water and condense the juice to about 8 oz. Place in a utensil on the side. Clean the pork liver and slice it into thin pieces. Clean the green onion, ginger, and garlic. Shred the ginger and slice the garlic into thin pieces; wash the leafy greens and lay out to dry.
2 Pour half of the flowery knotweed extract into a bowl and add the liver slices, cornstarch, and a pinch of salt to marinate.
3 Add soy sauce, cornstarch, and light chicken broth, cooking wine and vinegar to the rest of the flowery knotweed extract; mix well.
4 Heat the oil in a wok at a high temperature, add the liver along with its marinade; stir it quickly then take it out and place on a plate.
5 Add a little more oil to the wok. When the oil is heated, pour in the ginger and garlic slices, stir a little until they start to release an aromatic fragrance, then add the green leaves; stir quickly.
6 Pour in the rest of the flowery knotweed extract mix. When it has boiled, add the green onion slices. Stir only a few times before removing it from the heat and pour the sauce onto the already cooked liver slices.

Function
Supplements liver and kidney *yang*, beneficial to essence and blood, darkens the hair, and brightens the eyesight. (Flowery knotweed does not only secure the liver, but it can also reduce cholesterol levels and blood pressure. Black wood ear has the function of freeing the blood vessels; it is good for general health.)

Precautions
- It is not advisable to eat pork liver along with tofu products because it could induce intractable diseases.
- This dish should not be eaten in combination with fish.

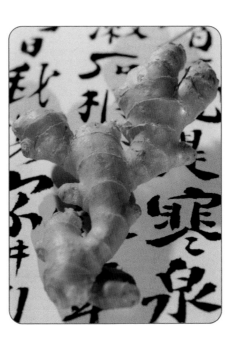

Fresh Prawns with Chinese Leek

Main Ingredients
4 oz fresh prawns
8 oz chinese leek
1 egg

Ingredients—Quantities According to Taste
Cornstarch
Soy sauce
Vegetable oil
Sesame oil

Method
1 Rinse the fresh prawns under cold water to clean, lay them on a clean paper towel to dry; wash the Chinese leek, then section it into 1 in lengths.
2 Put about 2 tbsp of cornstarch into a bowl and break the egg into the same bowl. Beat well.
3 Add a dash of sesame oil and the fresh prawns, mix well.
4 Heat up a little vegetable oil in a wok, pour the prawn/egg mixture into the hot oil and stir.
5 When the starch begins to glaze on the prawns, add the sectioned Chinese leek.
6 When the Chinese leek is well cooked but still tender, add another dash of sesame oil, quickly stir a few more times, transfer to a plate.

Function
Supplements kidney *yang*, secures kidney *qi*, promotes lactation. This dish is also beneficial for constipation because the Chinese leek is rich in fiber, which induces peristalsis. Warms the center and supplements *qi*, tonifies es-

sence and replenishes marrow, clears heat and eliminates vexation.

Pearl Triple Freshness Soup

Main Ingredients
2 oz chicken breast (de-skinned and minced)
1 large tomato
2 oz fresh soybeans
2 tbsp cornstarch
2 tbsp milk
1 egg white

Ingredients—Quantities According to Taste
White cooking wine
Chicken broth or water
Salt
Sesame oil

Method
1 Rinse the tomato with boiling water to de-skin it then cut it into small cubes.
2 Clean the fresh soybeans with cold water; reserve them in a bowl for later use.
3 Crack open the egg, extract only the egg white.
4 Moisten the 1 tbsp of cornstarch with 2 tbsp of milk and egg white.
5 Pour the mixture from step 4 into the bowl of minced chicken breast, beat well.
6 Put a pot of water (or light chicken broth) onto heat. Add a pinch of salt if the taste is too mild, and a third of a cup of white cooking wine. Add soybeans after the broth has boiled.
7 Turn the heat down after it boils again, but let the pot continue steaming without stirring the ingredients. Add meatballs of minced chicken rounded into shape with a spoon.
8 Turn the heat up to bring the pot to the boil again. Add the rest of the cornstarch moistened with water to thicken the juice in the pot. Add a dash of sesame seed oil once it boils again.

Function
Warms the center and supplements *qi*, tonifies essence and replenishes marrow, clears heat and eliminates vexation.

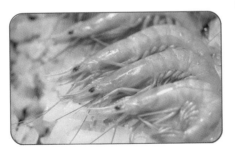

Theoretical Discussion of Health Preservation Using Nutritional Therapy in Traditional Chinese Medicine

Chen Xuexi, PhD, OMD, Chengdu, Sichuan Province, China
Chen Zhan, OMD and Ao Hui, OMD, Jinan, Shandong Province, China

Abstract: Nutritional therapy in health preservation based on the theory of Traditional Chinese Medicine (TCM) has a long history. This article discusses how nutritional therapy is guided by TCM theory in terms of the origin of food and medicine, differentiation of flavor and nature and pattern differentiation, as well as prohibitions in its application. It thus provides helpful advice on health preservation guided by TCM theory and on improving quality of life.

Keywords: Traditional Chinese Medicine (TCM); nutritional therapy; health preservation; theoretical discussion

In more than two thousand years of TCM history in China, people have accumulated and documented abundant experience of nutritional therapy. The *Book of Plain Questions* in *The Yellow Emperor's Classic of Medicine* put forward the following lines of argumentation: "The five cereals are staple food; the five fruits are auxiliary food; the five meats are beneficial, and the five vegetables should be taken in abundance." Zhang Zhang Zhongjing in the Han dynasty says in his book *Synopsis of Prescription of the Golden Chamber*: "Some foods are helpful in the treatment of diseases and some are harmful to the body. So, if they are helpful, they will do good to the body and if they are harmful, they may cause diseases." This book also collected some nutritional therapies and advice on what foods and drinks to avoid. Many influential books on nutritional therapy were published in subsequent centuries, such as the article about nutritional therapy in *Valuable Prescriptions Worth A Thousand Gold Pieces for Emergencies* by Sun Simiao written during the Tang dynasty, *Treatise on Dietetic Therapy* written by Meng Shen during the Tang dynasty, *Principles of Correct Diet* written by Hu Sihui during the Yuan dynasty, *Suggestions on Health Preservation* written by Gao Lian during the Ming dynasty, and *Differentiation of Dietetic Therapy* written by Zhang Mu during the Qing dynasty. The theories and methods of nutritional therapy in TCM have provided us with an abundant and priceless legacy with which to develop nutritional therapy for all kinds of diseases.

The Same Source for Food and Medicine

Just like in medicine, people have many kinds of animals and plants to choose from as regards the food, the need for survival, and reproduction. Choosing useful foods and avoiding harmful foods is the first stage in nutritional therapy. The *Longitude of Rites* records that: "The Suiren drilled wood to get fire. They cooked food, which helped people to get rid of abdominal diseases." The transition from uncooked foods to cooked foods is the original nutritional therapy. It is said that Yi Yin, a great doctor in the Shang dynasty, used ginger and bay leaves as a condiment in cooking. However, these herbs were much more than just flavoring, they were considered as medicine. Through cooking, Yi Yin created a decoction of medicinal ingredients for treating diseases. The *Book of Rite of Zhou: Heavenly Official* also records that there was an official position in court for a medical doctor. Because of his unique method of combining food and medicine, Yi Yin was appointed head of nutritional therapy at the Zhou court. He was called "food doctor." According to his theory, physicians should try to cure diseases by using the five flavors, five cereals, and five kinds of Chinese herbs. Here, medicine is equal to common food. Yi Yin emphasized the positive correlation between diet and the treatment of illnesses. The close link between medicine and food is one of the origins of Chinese medical treatment. Other doctors have since done more work in this field, which has helped to enrich and develop this theory.

As Chinese medical theory developed further, it included nutritional therapy as part of the treatment method as well as the foundation of human well-being. This was the beginning of Chinese nutritional therapy.

The Difference
between Nature and Flavor

In Chinese medicine, herbs are categorized according to their property—called the four natures—and five flavors prescribed by the theory of Chinese medicine. The same theory applies to foods as well, i.e., there are cold, hot, warm, and cool foods, and five flavors—sour, bitter, sweet, acrid, and salty. By utilizing the properties of natural herbs, Chinese doctors could adjust *qi* and blood circulation, balance *yin* and *yang* in the body, and strengthen vital *qi* and eliminate evil *qi* in order to help the body to recover and to achieve a state of *yin* and *yang* in relative equilibrium. Unlike medicinal herbs, which have four clearly differentiated natures, food may be divided into three main kinds according to the influence they have on the body: warm and hot foods, cold and cool foods, and neutral foods. Foods that relieve or eliminate cold syndrome warm the interior and reverse vacuity to rid the body of symptoms of contractions and crymodynia in the abdominal cavity. Examples are ginger, mutton, and brown sugar, which belong to the warm and hot food category. Foods that relieve or eliminate heat syndrome expel heat and promote the production of fluid to relieve thirst. Examples are watermelon and pear, which belong to the cold and cool category. Foods that do not clear cold or warm influences in the body belong to the neutral category. Examples are haricot beans and lotus.

The five flavors are closely related to the treatment of diseases, because foods of different flavors have different effects. For example, the acrid flavor has the effect of inducing dia-phorrsis and promoting the flow of *qi* and blood circulation. This is advantageous in activating *qi* to eliminate stasis and purge accumulated heat, relieving exterior and dispelling cold, promoting blood circulation, and stopping pain. The sweet flavor has the effect of tonifying, harmonizing, and relieving spasms. It is advantageous in tonifying vacuity, normalizing the function of the stomach and spleen, as well as nourishing body fluids. The sour flavor is astringent, which is good for increasing or alleviating excessive loss of the vital essences and body fluid. The bitter flavor eliminates evils and dries dampness. It thus has the effect of purging heat accumulation, eliminating evils from the lungs, and clearing away heat–fire and eliminating dampness. The salty flavor softens hard masses and purges evils. It thus has the effect of resolving hard lumps and diarrhea. Therefore, only by combining natures with flavor can doctors create appropriate formulae.

The *Plain Questions* thus states that the five cereals are staple food, the five fruits are auxiliary food, the five meats are benificial, and the five vegetables should be taken in abundance. So, in order to tonify essence and *qi*, people must take food with complementary flavors and natures according to their individual body type. Even though different foods have different natures, flavors, and functions, they function differently in tonifying vacuity or eliminating repletion, they have the same principal function, which is the same as medicinal herbs, namely supporting vital *qi*, expelling evils, and regulating the balance of *yin* and *yang*. The process may be slow, but this method is especially suitable for tumor patients with deficient vital *qi* and persistent residuals of evil.

In addition, when serving meals prepared according to nutritional therapy, it is very important to complement foods of different natures and flavors. For example, the sweet flavor has the effect of tonifying and soothing spasms, but it has the disadvantage of stagnating the functions of the spleen and stomach. So foods that promote the flow of *qi* and have an acrid flavor, such as ginger, shallot, leek, pepper, and vegetables, should be combined in order to promote the transformation and transportation of spleen and stomach. Fish (sweet water) and seafood (fish and shellfish from the ocean) are mostly cold or cool in nature. They should be used in combination with food that has an acrid flavor, warm nature, and a dispersing function. Examples are wine, ginger, shallot, and pepper. The sour flavor has an astringent effect and should not be overeaten by patients with an accumulation and obstruction of dampness–heat and sputum. The bitter flavor has the effect of eliminating evils and drying dampness. So patients who are deficient of *yang qi* should avoid this category of foods. The salty flavor has the effect of softening hard masses and purging evils. Overeating foods of this flavor can disturb the blood. In practice, these principles should be applied flexibly.

Diet Based on Pattern Differentiation

In TCM the basic principle of diet prescription is pattern differentiation. Doctors must first consider the patient's overall constitutional factors, such as the patient's basic constitution, age, hobbies, and living and working environment. Then they must analyze and synthesize this information according to the principles of TCM. Once a patient's condition has been determined, that is the correct illness has been diagnosed, the doctor should provide the patient with a menu of suitable foods. For example, cold and vacuity condition is treated with warm foods. Heat and repletion condition is treated with cold foods. Overall vacuity is treated with foods of a tonifying nature.

Nutritional therapy has the following objectives: Firstly, it should provide the patient with the necessary nourishment to ensure the body has enough strength to fight off evil and so that whatever has been damaged can recover. For instance, tumor patients generally have deficient vital *qi*, thus most of them need tonification. The *Yellow Emperor's Classic of Medicine* states that people of a weak physique require a *qi* tonifying therapy, while those with essence vacuity need to protect *jing* with a regular diet of healthy and highly

nutritious foods. When applying the *qi* tonifying therapy, people usually eat plant-based foods; while tonifying the physic, people usually eat animal-based foods. What is more, patients' *yin* vacuity or *yang* vacuity should also be considered. Accordingly the patients are given cooling–tonifying (tonifying *yin* blood) foods or warming–tonifying (tonifying *yang qi*) foods.

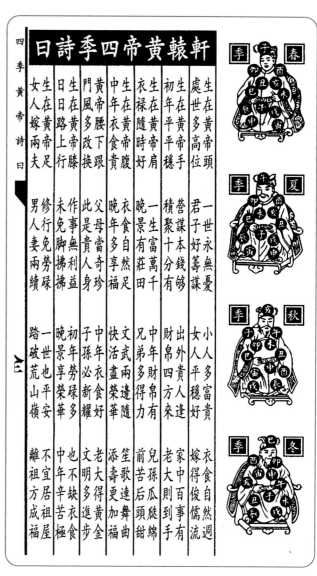

Fig. 1 Seasonal advices attributing to the legend Huangdi.

Secondly, one should select foods that invigorate and transform the spleen and stomach in order to keep the spleen in an excellent condition. Both the adverse effects of harsh tumor treatment and the patients' low emotional state could harm the functionality of the spleen and stomach. Close attention should be paid to the functionality of the spleen and stomach, because these two are regarded as the root of later heaven, the root and the transformation of *qi* and blood. They govern the decomposition, conversion, and transformation of food. Food with a high fat content should be avoided so that the function of the spleen does not stagnate. Acrid and dry foods should also be avoided because these types of food can impair *yin* and waste *qi*. At the same time, patients should also pay attention to the warmth and coldness of their living environment, and take meals at regular times. Doctors should pay attention to patients' nutritional habits and suggest foods with appetizing colors, smells, flavors, and shapes in order to stimulate their appetite and the functioning of the spleen and stomach.

Food Prohibitions

In tumor patients, attention should also be paid to possible drug interactions that may aggravate the disease.

1. Diet Should Correspond to the Nature and Flavor of Drugs

For example, when taking drugs of a hot nature, food should also be hot in nature. Likewise, when taking drugs of a neutral or cool nature, food should also have the same nature. In this way, the effect of the medicine can be amplified rather than reduced. By combining medications with appropriate foods, the combination can reinforce the curative effect. By contrast, if the patient has been taking medication and food that are contradictory in nature and flavor, the combination can reduce or diminish the curative effect. In some extreme cases, such a combination could lead to adverse effects.

2. Diet Should Correspond to the Function of *Zang Fu*

Along with their general effect, each of the five flavors is associated with one of the five phases. This explains the flavor's effect on the specific bowels and viscera (*zang fu*) of a corresponding phase. Different foods have different effects on a particular *zang fu*, which is related to the TCM theory of tonifying *zang* with the corresponding *fu*. This is also one of the basic fundamental principles of nutritional therapy in TCM. For example, it is documented that in the past the Chinese ate sheep or deer thyroid to treat thyroid dysfunction. Furthermore, there is also a nutritional therapy based on *zang fu* pattern differentiation and the five phase relationships. For example, the *Ling Shu* documents a nutritional prescription according to which people use sweet rice, jujube, and sunflower to relieve liver spasm. This can eliminate the potential of neither overwhelming nor restricting the function of the spleen.

3. Prohibitions in Combining Diet and Medications

The incompatibility of foods and medications could result in inefficacy and may even cause adverse effects. Therefore, when taking certain medications, certain foods must be avoided. For example, when taking 地黄 rehmannia (Chinese foxglove), 首乌 multiflower knotweed root, and 土茯苓 smilax glabra rhizome (sarsasparilla), or some preparation containing iron, patients should avoid tea; when taking *gen sheng*, rehmannia, and multiflower knotweed root, patients should avoid radish; when taking turtle shell, patients should avoid amaranth; when taking orange peduncle and ebony, patients should avoid pork. The *Compendium of Food and Herbs* lists dozens of prohibitions that must be followed when taking medications. For example: "Whenever taking drugs, patients should neither eat fatty pork nor dog meat, nor should they overeat foods that have a purging effect, such as garlic, coriander, and ginger." All these prohibitions are worthy of our attention; they should also be researched and put into practice.

4. Diet According to the Three Treatment Factors

The principle of the three treatment factors states that treatment should be based on different patients, different location, and different time. This is one of the fundamental principles of TCM treatment. This treatment principle should also be applied to nutritional therapy. The diet prescribed to a particular patient also needs to be individualized, that is, different places, different time, different patient, and different diet. As regards the basic constitution of patients, common sense tells us that it is better for obese people to avoid fatty foods and to eat more insipid foods and that it is better for slim people to avoid acrid and spicy foods and to eat light and mild foods. The *New Book of Longevity and Health Preservation* states that: "Foods for the elderly should be warm and hot; sticky, hard, and cold food should be avoided." As to the correspondence of location, the *Yellow Emperor's Classic of Medicine* states: "In the north (…) people usually live in the open air and eat more dairy food," i.e., because of the geographical location in the North of China, people should have more dairy in their diet in order to tonify vital *qi* to fight the severe environmental conditions. As regards the correspondence of time, the *Prescriptions Worth A Thousand Pieces of Gold* states: "It is suitable for people to eat leek in February and March, while in August and September people should avoid eating ginger." We can infer from these examples the correlation between nutritional therapy and time.

In conclusion, we infer that when prescribing diets based on pattern differentiation, make sure that the food complements the medication, *zang fu*, and also consider the three treatment factors (different treatment according to different patient, different place, and different time). At the same time, attention should be paid to the possible adverse interactions between food and medication, as well as to their beneficial reinforcement. Only then can nutritional therapy be most effective.

Bibliography

1. Shen Lilong. *The Compendium of Food and Herbs* (in Chinese). Liaoning: Jinchang Press; 2003.
2. Sun Simiao. *Qian Jin Fang* [Valuable Prescriptions Worth a Thousand Gold Pieces for Emergencies]. Beijing: Hua Xia Press; 1994.
3. Zou Xuan. *The New Book of Longevity and Health Preservation* (in Chinese). Tianjin: Tianjin Science and Technology Press; 2003.

Contact Details

Chen Xuexi, PhD, OMD
Chengdu University of TCM
Sichuan Province
China

Chen Zhan, OMD
Shandong University of TCM
Shandong Province
China

Ao Hui, OMD
Shandong University of TCM
Shandong Province
China

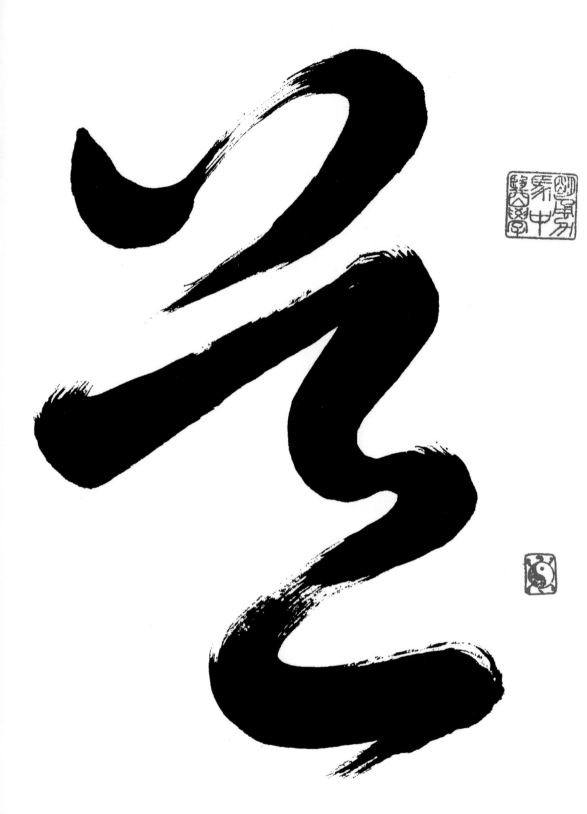

Book Reviews

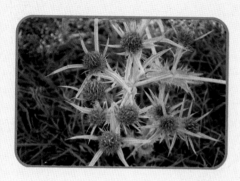

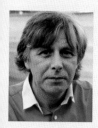

Chris Dhaenens

Introduction

Chinese herbalists and herbalists in general are experiencing troublesome times. Whereas acupuncture is firmly taking root in Western complementary medicine, Chinese herbal medicine seems to have become the icon of herb toxicity, and the classic example of failing quality control. To what extent is this true? And what do Chinese herbalists have to say about the situation? These days, tuition programs in Traditional Chinese Medicine (TCM) herbal medicine courses cover a lot of items that are forbidden, restricted, controversial, or unavailable. Students tend to find this very confusing, and quite understandably wonder why they have to study a delicately integrated system that is both incomplete and impracticable. A traditional Chinese doctor operating in an EU country these days will miss about 30 % to 40 % of the shang han and wen bing formulas, and big chunks of the single substances in the Chinese Pharmacopoeia. This section, among other topics, intends to evaluate if and how our present TCM herbals and handbooks deal with these issues.

Also part of this section is Isaac Cohen's very personal appreciation of Hecker et al's Practice of Acupuncture. Isaac's review is preceded by a critical and honest personal account of his own struggle to reconcile the "alien ways" of Chinese thinking with the ubiquitous modern biomedicine. Under "Other Interesting Publications" you can find a review of Nigel Wiseman and Feng Ye's A Practical Dictionary of Chinese Medicine, the inevitable source for correct and lucid translation of TCM terms and ideas. Next there is a review of Fritz Smith's Alchemy of Touch, the long awaited standard on Zero Balancing, and the section concludes with a brief review of Schnorrenberger's Pocket Atlas of Tongue Diagnosis.

Chris Dhaenens, lic. Filologie, OMD
Melle, Belgium

Chinese Herbal Medicine: Status Quaestionis and Publications

Chris Dhaenens, lic Filologie, OMD, Melle, Belgium

(For François Ramakers. Thanks to Angelika)

"The errors of a great spirit are more instructive than the axioms of a small one"
Ludwig Börne

The Problems Chinese Herbal Medicine is Facing Today

It is true that Chinese herbal medicine has experienced plenty of teething problems in the last few decades. There were (and still are) serious authentication problems in mainland China, and some of the worst cases of herb toxicity in recent history have been associated with Chinese herbal substances. Despite massive improvement in recent years, 100 % adequate quality control has not yet been achieved.

The introduction of Chinese herbal medicine in the West ignited a series of regrettable tendencies for phytotherapy in general. A tidal wave of regulatory fever rushed through EU health administrations, resulting in ludicrous negative lists, futile attempts to separate alimentary from medicinal substances, and a series of unworkable laws and regulations coming into being instead of common sense, empirical knowledge, and education. Throughout Europe, the Chinese materia medica is deprived of a legal framework. If the authorities provide any information, it is always repressive in outlook, and the blueprint for future regulation, the Traditional Herbal Medicinal Products Directive (THMPD), looks particularly gloomy for Chinese phytotherapy. Moreover, the regulatory bodies tend to display an annoying lack of transparency and democracy in their decision-making.

Another striking evolution is the systematic imputation of herbs and herbal medicine by academic pharmacology and the medical establishment in general. Often incited by quack-hunters and other skeptical cenacles of right-mindedness, it is hardly an overstatement to say that a large part of the scientific community suffers from hysterical "phytophobia."

It is very clear to herbalists and suppliers that there cannot be any compromise as far as the quality and safety of herbs is concerned, and there is no one who still believes that a "natural" product is automatically a safe product. However, the level of precautionary measures now in place regarding alleged toxicity (that includes side effects, adverse effects, and interactions) beggars belief. Invariably magnified by press releases "a mile wide and an inch deep," here are some sad examples from different parts of the world.

- Arbitrary, selective, and unscientific evidence to justify the ban on *Kava Kava*.
- A warning about the consumption of red rice, because of the presence of statins.
- The disgraceful story of St John's Wort (*Hypericum perforatum*). Numerous press releases have created a climate of anxiety about this herb, merely because it does what it has always done, namely, to stimulate the liver enzyme system so that toxins and medicine are metabolized faster.
- A (now lifted) ban on lycium berries in Belgium and Holland. Nobody knew why they had been banned.
- *Lycium* species remain banned in Italy though. Furthermore, the Italian authorities recently spread a rapid alert to all EU health authorities warning against the illicit use of Chen Pi (*Citrus aurantium* peel) and Tao Ren (*Prunus persica* pit) in food and food supplements. This would imply that English marmalade and plenty of Italian liquors need to be registered as medicine.
- An official warning from the Canadian authorities against *Magnolia officinalis*, be-

cause adulterants could contain insignificant traces of "turbocurarine." The constituent is actually called tubocurarine, the "turbo" only being the expression of their vigilant zeal.

- A warning against the "alkaloid" trichosanthin in the Chinese Trichosantes gourd. Trichosantes is a vegetable, and trichosanthin is not an alkaloid but a protein, which is completely destroyed by cooking.
- Pennyroyal tea (monograph in the European Pharmacopoeia!) is forbidden as a medicinal substance in Belgium. The reason given for this is that one molecule of pulegone is enough to cause cancer.
- Even more hilarious: The Chinese herb *mu tong* is considered a risk, because in the past an *Aristolochia* species was sometimes used as a source for it. An American FDA inspector suggested that every herb containing the Chinese character "*tong*" in its name should be forbidden, thus introducing the notion of semiotic contamination.

Within the present prohibitive regulatory perspective, another alarming tendency is the straightjacketing of Chinese herbal medicine into a linear, reductionist methodology, essentially designed for mono-components and allopathic medicine. Assessing quality, safety, and efficacy solely by quantitative determination of active markers is in fact almost the opposite of what Chinese herbal medicine is all about. It is clear that measuring brings about knowledge, and for some substances, for example, herbs that are toxic in raw form that need to be detoxified, or herbs for which the active and toxic dose is close to one another, such a quantitative determination is indispensable. However, to make quantitative determination the general principle and sole reference point is not only a waste of time and energy, it also seriously threatens the survival of traditional herbal medicinal systems in their essential form.

The energetics attributed to plants in traditional pharmacopeias reflect the totum (whole) of the plant with its potential synergies, its positive interactions, and its specific form of preparation in the context of a homeo-static and humoral concept of the "body-mind" (*jing shen*). Mainstream pharmacology and toxicology avoid phytochemical complexity and the diffuse pathways of xenobiotics metabolization by a series of scientifically inadmissible reductions: mechanical extrapolation from "in-vitro" results to "in-vivo" results, from animal test results to humans, inconsideration of traditional dosages and specific preparation forms, and so on.

Too rarely, however, are these invariably bad tidings placed in a healthy perspective:

- The vast majority of herb toxicity cases have been attributed to the adulteration of species rather than to the intrinsic toxicity of the plants. Well-known examples are the substitution of *Stephania and Akebia* species by *Aristolochia* species, *Acanthopanax* by *Periploca*, *Scutellaria* by *Teucrium*, and *Illicium verum* by *Illicium religiosum*. Such instances are certainly not confined to Chinese herbs and can be adequately traced before distribution by chromatographic analysis, both in terms of verification and falsification.
- Many studies relating to herb toxicity, interactions, and adverse effects are trivial, deceptively selective, and totally irrelevant for a better understanding of plant molecule pharmacokinetics. Obviously, the determination of what is potentially toxic should not be left to trial and error, and clear cases of toxicity exist. For example, there is the nephrotoxicity of aristolochic acid, the veno-occlusive syndrome caused by some pyrrholizidine alkaloids, the potential toxicity of methylchavicol in infants, and the (unproven but epidemiologically significant) connection between some Chinese plants and hepatotoxicity. The list of clear-cut cases is short, however. Even when taking into account that problems with herbs probably tend to be poorly reported, it is nevertheless the case that, used appropriately, herbal therapy still shows a most favorable safety/efficacy profile, especially when compared to the adverse and idiosyncratic reactions of registered allopathic medicine.

Before accepting toxicity reports and clinical studies on herb toxicity at face value, it is wise to consider the following:

- Because of the complexity of phytochemistry and the poor knowledge relating to the metabolic pathways of plant constituents, the configuration of such a study is very often a self-fulfilling prophecy. In other words, only a reductionist method and choice of axioms allows for a conclusion, and very often a conclusion that is clinically separated from real life.
- Herb toxicity and efficacy reports tend to suffer from the same ailments as pharmaceutical research in general: arbitrary presuppositions, major methodological flaws, inadmissible extrapolations, narrow demographic bases, genetic dispositions being ignored, and the lack of consideration of empirical (traditional) knowledge relating to herbal medicine. Furthermore, examples of clearly biased and fraudulent research exist, and the majority of papers do not survive meta-analysis.
- Toxicity research is somehow poisoned by the myth that it is possible to achieve absolute safety in every instance, and that such safety should be pursued with all means in every case. Not only is this impossible, it is a total misunderstanding of the concerns of both phytotherapy and the whole field of natural medicine. Even practitioners of complementary medicine are seduced by the notion that clinical, cosmetic, and mechanical healing is possible. Experienced Chinese herbalists, while treating *shang han* and *wen bing* epidemic or autoimmune diseases, or endogenous metabolic toxicosis, are very familiar with the healing crises of their patients when they succeed in lifting the ailment to an immunologically more reactive level such as *yang ming* (diuresis) or *tai yang* (diaphoresis). A true healing process is hardly ever achieved without collateral damage, whether we like it or not. Mainstream toxicology studies have been shown to be extremely conservative and dismissive toward these positive aspects of herb toxicity.

All in all, a dictatorship exists in the field of linear safety analytical studies, from which we can only conclude that life is a sexually transmittable fatal disease. In this connection it should be noted that everything that doesn't cause cancer has not been properly analyzed.

The largest ever case of herb toxicity, the ongoing Belgian slimming scandal, should be considered in this instance, as it is a catalog of everything that can go wrong at every level. Misidentified herbs were imported, without elementary quality control, to make a murderous slimming cocktail look like a natural product. Unqualified doctors prescribed the herbs, in an inadmissible form (powder instead of decoction), for a problem totally unrelated to the therapeutic range of the herbs. The subsequent investigations were characterized by highly selective, biased, and partly manipulated information made available to the scientific community and the public.

The paramount question for Chinese herbal medicine is how the vitally necessary issue of quality/safety/efficacy control can be reconciled with the intrinsic creativity and richness of the system. How can we avoid emptying the baby together with the bathwater and TCM herbal medicine being battered into a broken-winged caricature of itself? How can we avoid the introduction of Chinese herb monographs into the European Pharmacopoeia becoming the "mono-graves" of Chinese herbs? Practitioners of Chinese medicine and their professional associations bear a crucial responsibility for the outcome of this issue; it is they who will finally have to determine whether the Chinese materia medica will be a sterile trunk or a living body of knowledge. To ensure the latter they will have to insist on the maximum quality and safety guarantees from their suppliers, but also not give in to absurd or disproportionate restrictions. This is not an easy task, since, as Edgar says at the end of *King Lear*, "the weight of this sad time we must obey." The task requires the love of the art, rather than the unscrupulous pursuit of gain. It requires vision and experience not to yield to the often exorbitant demands of today's patients, who are now no longer at all patient. In fact, an in-

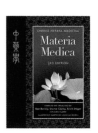

creasing number of patients are im*patient*ly consuming fast health instead of *patient*ly suffering the fate of an existential opportunity. Hence some basic knowledge of pharmacology is required to be able to interpret the energetic and immunological changes caused by allopathic and "life-style" drugs. For it is a sad reality that complementary practices are flooded with desperate hordes of fussy patients seeking natural and painless liberation from their chemically sealed imprisonment in a betrayed body. People deprived of all the joys money cannot buy and usually seeking as much a cure for their solutions as for their problems. The problem tends to manifest as diffuse and borderline pathology, with a higher risk of adverse effects and interactions with allopathic medicine, especially in patients with a pre-existing toxic burden.

To read this "surplus" pathology diagnostically, TCM herbalists can draw amply from their own sources, but they will also need reliable and unbiased information from more recent toxicological research. How do our TCM handbooks and herbal reference books incorporate the relevant information, and how helpful is it for the practitioner?

In the year to come the Chinese materia medica is scheduled to join the UNESCO world patrimonium. The question is: will it be a museum of fine living art, or a mausoleum for obsolete folklore?

Reviews of Recent Publications

For the past 20 years the *Chinese Herbal Medicine Materia Medica* ("The good old Bensky," authored by Dan Bensky, Steven Clavey, Erich Stöger, with Andrew Gamble as the compiler) has been the major reference work for anyone involved in TCM herbal medicine. It is now in its third edition and has grown into a very mature opus. In the new edition the authors wisely decided to focus on traditional facts and botanical authenticity rather than on pharmacological research, since the latter often yields speculative and transitory data.

A major improvement is the in-depth differentiation of all the botanical sources serv-

ing for a specific "*zhong yao*," resulting in a very complete and detailed overview of adulterations, substitutions, fake herbs, non-preferential herbs, valid alternatives, toxic substances, unavailable source materials, alternate names, etc. This material is extremely useful, both for practitioners and for those involved in quality control, not the least because it offers a small but essential picture of the taxonomy of the main problem herbs. This indispensable fieldwork contribution is clearly to the credit of Erich Stöger, co-authoring this edition.

Other subsections also went through a sparkling process of rejuvenation. Drawing amply from their vast clinical experience, the authors list all the important synergies and their mechanisms. The "Commentary" section provides every one of the relevant historical references, and under "Comparisons" the energetic qualities of the herbs are discerningly juxtaposed.

The subsection "Nomenclature and preparation" comments abundantly on the different preparation methods (*pao zhi*). Again, this is very comprehensive and instructive.

Interestingly, the authors decided to leave out the section on pharmacological and toxicological research. This is simply because at this stage the section raises more questions than it provides answers. Given that the actual research in the pharmacodynamics and pharmacokinetics of plant molecules is extremely difficult to interpret in terms of traditional phytotherapy, one can only agree with this excision. Since the relevance and the quality of such research often turns out to be questionable and controversial, the majority of papers on the subject leaves readers with a plethora of volatile and premature conclusions, invariably taken out of context. It is the favorite food for scavenging toxicologists, but it hardly ever stands the test of time and meta-analysis.

This does not mean toxicology is not considered. On the contrary, apart from the traditional subject matter, the book, while not focusing on toxicology, provides information difficult to find in other reference sources. For example, there is a discussion relating to

Rubia cordifolia root (*qian cao gen*) that is undeservedly forbidden in some countries. At the same time, as if to justify their own warning for uncorroborated data, a sad error has survived: it is incorrectly alleged that tropane alkaloids (hyoscyamine and atropine) are present in *Lycium barbarum*. This is a cowboy's tale, that has led to a ban on *gou qi zi* and *di gu pi* in several countries.

What feels so good about this book is that throughout one can sense the TCM pulse throbbing with nuance, balance, and experience. Organically grown over the years, and botanically firmly rooted, it stands out as a titan's labor of love and the major reference source for years to come.

Chinese herbal medicine is still treated in this book as a "path with a heart." An integrating art versus the analytic reduction it is insidiously evolving in. This is a short excerpt of what the authors have to say about toxicology and interactions:

However, to us, it seems that some of the recent discussion is approaching the subject backward, much like talking about how pedestrians get in the way of automobiles. We would suggest instead that the topic be approached in a manner which gives the right of way to the pedestrians of the medical world, that is, herbal medicines.

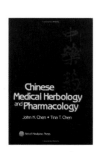

A similar work in magnitude, but with a slightly different approach, is *Chinese Medical Herbology and Pharmacology* by John and Tina Chen. It covers even more single substances than "Bensky," and is more extensive at the level of pharmacology, toxicology, and herb–drug interactions. It also tends to refer more to Western pathology associated with TCM syndromes.

The amount of information brought together here is very impressive. Plenty of data that one previously had to collect from many different sources have now been brought together in this book. It really is the "all in one" guide to TCM herbal medicine, but in an odd way the fact that it is the "all in one" guide is also its Achilles' heel. Despite all the obvious qualities of a systematic approach, together with its comprehensiveness, it never gets beyond the level of a compilation. It is the best compilation of TCM herbs that has ever been achieved, and, according to their preface, the authors are very well aware that the incorporation of all the literature on pharmacology, toxicology, and interactions with allopathic drugs, is a tricky matter. Yet since this book is meant to help prescribing herbalists, questions should be asked that herbalists ask. For example, is it true? Is it relevant? Is it significant? How far can adverse or idiosyncratic reactions be seen to be healthy reactions to chemical saturation?

Professionals prescribing Chinese herbs on a daily basis experience the safety/efficacy profile as being extremely favorable. Knowing that such pharmacological information is at best immature, generally inappropriate, and at worst deceptive, the therapist is burdened with a problem that is either non-existent, unlikely, or inevitable. Since this information is insufficiently placed in perspective, the added value is difficult to justify. This is a little bit strange, as the authors are both ardent advocates of Chinese herbal medicine and qualified in academic pharmacology. They are in the best position to know how weak such information can be and how easily such facts can be diluted in an herbal tea. Nevertheless, this slight quibble about the lack of the personal touch and opinion is about the only difference between four-and-a-half stars and five stars. Along with "Bensky" the book belongs on every herbalist's shelf.

As pointed out above, Dan Bensky et al., in the Preface to the *Materia Medica*, write about the reasons why they didn't include the sections on pharmacology that had existed in the previous edition. They say these sections are essentially the topic of another book, "a book that we'd love to read," they add suggestively. Now, part of such a book has been written—*An introduction to Chinese Herbal Medicine*—and it is simply wonderful.

The author, Mark Wright, is the first Chinese herbalist to write a meaningful story about the "chemistry" between tradition and chemistry. This is a territory for which there is no map, and where Cartesian scientists and Chinese herbalists alike tend to lose their way.

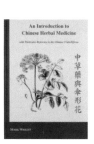

The total absence of a workable paradigm to assess quality, safety, and efficacy issues, and how these should be linked to TCM diagnostics and the physioenergetics of Chinese herbs, is today the major obstacle in regulatory issues worldwide. Health authorities and academic pharmacology invariably flee to the safe havens of their only descriptive language, which is reduction at the molecular level and reduced models of metabolic pathways. All this results in a sterile ultra-conservative no-risk policy, rather than a creative and instructive low-risk policy. This principle, a tortuous interpretation of Ockham's razor*, is totally inadequate to describe the energetics and interactions of herbal substances. Alas, mainstream science, both economically and politically embedded as it is, speaks only one language and uses only one tool. As the old saying goes: "When all you have is a hammer, everything looks like a nail."

On the other hand, quite a few herbalists still think in terms of a romantic notion of nature, and a holism characterized by inadmissible generalizations that might compromise safety. In walking the thin line between science and tradition, Mark Wright has brought about a balanced account of all the trumps and bottlenecks that Chinese herbal medicine holds.

The author explores the historical roots of Chinese medicine, as well as the botany of Chinese plants, with great erudition and painstaking accuracy. The phytochemistry, pharmacokinetics, and pharmacodynamics are covered in depth and, for the first time at this level, are specifically related to the Chinese materia medica. (Here, it would be fair to mention the meritorious *Interactions Between Chinese Herbal Medicinal Products and Orthodox Drugs*, by K. Chan and L. Cheung, Harwood Academic Publishers, 2000. Though more narrow in scope, it is clearly a precursor to this book.)

Equally critical of the tautologies in scientific methodology and the wishful thinking of herbalists, Mark Wright has provided a very solid platform for a neutral, common sense approach to the toxicology of Chinese herbs. Since this is considered to be an "introduction," we can only hope that a man who is so competent can continue to write on the subject using the same fund of knowledge and discerning spirit.

The apotheosis is a selection of monographs for the Umbelliferae family, frequently used in Chinese medicine. If only every monograph were like this, how our treasure house would increase in value! More, please.

Any student genuinely interested in the rationale and risks of his or her discipline should take the trouble to struggle through the tougher sections on phytochemistry and pharmacokinetics. It's worthwhile, and Mark Wright's is one of the few books that might help you to think for yourself, encourage you to use your own experience, and help you to learn from your own mistakes.

This is quite a contrast to Fred Jennes and Bob Flaws' recent publication, *Herb Toxicities and Drug interactions—A Formula Approach*, published by Blue Poppy Press, 2006.

In their introduction, Jennes and Flaws express some sound ideas and opinions on how to avoid adverse effects, possible interactions, and potential toxicity, simply by adhering to the proper practice of Chinese herbal medicine, as well as adhering to the traditional rules on dosages, preparations, and synergies. The authors provide healthy criteria for choosing a supplier and interpreting a certificate of analysis. So far so good. What follows, however, is utterly disappointing: a shallow and poorly documented survey of nephrotoxicity, hepatotoxicity, and fetotoxicity incidence. The authors "copy and paste" their way through 70 classical formulae, endlessly reiterating the possible interactions for every ingredient. Fostering the principle that "copying from one book is plagiary, copying from many books is erudition," this approach merely results in an unprofitable compilation of different sources that are highly divergent in quality and relevance. What, for instance, is the added value of echoing that the presence of potassium can

---

*   Ockham's razor is a principle applied in logic, essentially implying that when there are different solutions for complex problems, the simplest solution should be chosen.

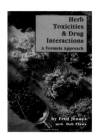

eventually lead to hyperkalemia, when there is no incidence, no risk/benefit profile and no reason at all for the rash extrapolation from a quantitative observation to the qualitative effect of a Chinese soup. Will a herbalist refrain from prescribing a formula containing *dang gui* because of this? Let's hope not. Furthermore, when checking those sources (in this instance, Chan and Cheung), the message is far more subtle and placed in perspective. Also other sources, such as the American Herbal Products Association's (AHPA) *Botanical Safety Handbook*, provide lucid and balanced motives for their safety assessments.

The formulaic approach does not work. Students without a pharmacological background, or, worse, with only a pharmacological background, tend to be scared off unnecessarily when confronted with such gratuitous rendering of opaque, redundant, and derivative data. Worldwide herbs are being banned for trifling reasons. What is the point in nourishing fears with unprocessed food such as this?

One could argue that knowing even a little is better than knowing nothing at all, but frankly, the concept of this publication comes close to a software manual. The more you read, the less you know, and the less you want to know.

Well worth reading is an excellent short article by Trina Ward: "Safety Concerns Involving Chinese Herbal Medicines." It is an eight-page chapter in *The Essential Guide to Herbal Safety*, edited by Simon Mills and Kerry Bone, Elsevier Chuchill Linvingstone, 2005—a publication that is highly recommended as a whole.

Trina Ward covers some of the well-known pain points of Chinese herb toxicity (adulteration, heavy metals, herb–drug interactions, and idiosyncratic reactions) through well-documented cases. Most cases that are dealt with apply to patent remedy pills in mainland China, a long-standing problem. She rightly calls for maximum vigilance and post-launching evaluation and, at the same time, criticizes reputable journals for using incorrect evidence to prove herb toxicity.

For art lovers, there is *An illustrated Chinese Materia Medica*, by Jing Nuan Wu, published by Oxford University Press, 2005. This comprises a collection of small, elementary monographs covering a vast part of the Chinese materia medica. It would be nothing out of the ordinary, if it were not for the superb drawings in the finest tradition of botanical illustration. They are marvelous.

Practice of Acupuncture:
Point Location—Treatment Options—TCM Basics.
Hecker et al. Thieme: Stuttgart–New York; 2005

Isaac Cohen, OMD, LAc, Berkeley, California, USA

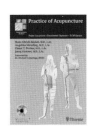

The purpose of medicine is to alleviate suffering, that is, suffering incurred in injury, malfunction, dysfunction, deficiencies and excesses, grief and agony experienced by women, men, children, and all other living creatures. For the most part, medicine evolved from the need to treat and tend to such suffering, as well as from the wish to understand the causes of suffering and its relationships to nature.

Through insight, trial, and error, humanity developed and organized systematic approaches to consider suffering and illnesses, indications, and diseases. Observational organization is essential to educate generations of physicians at both the present time and in the future. Systems allow us shortcuts into knowledge, initially acquired by the efforts of many people striving to explain to themselves what they found. Tenets were developed to produce a language to describe dynamic processes, and measures were formed to permit accuracy and consistency.

Many cultures developed such systems throughout history. These systems retained their essential structure from their beginning. The philosophies, disciplines, and sciences employed as anchors to the approach determine the "taste" of the system, and how it is deployed and learned.

In order to educate and provide tools worth using, medical systems created methods to both learn and teach, as well as to develop their corpus of information. In modern Western medicine, information is now obtained with the help of many scientific disciplines, such as molecular biology, genetics, chemistry, both organic and physical, biochemistry, pharmacology, epidemiology, biostatistics, clinical research, to name but a few. Western medicine also harnesses technologies to sharpen its descriptive and observational abilities, such as—again, to name but a

few—scanning technologies, microscopy, and spectroscopy. An international language has developed to convey the findings, as well as regulatory systems, that control the safe and effective delivery of therapies. Modern biomedicine is now international. The differences in education between poor and developed countries are solely at the level of availability of technologies and costly therapies. Protocols to measure the existence of a peptide or protein in the serum are available through open publications, and are subject to peer scrutiny based on objective measures, not subjective measures that can be repeated regardless of the patient.

In my opinion, Chinese medicine has never arrived at the universality now experienced by Western medicine. Additionally, Chinese medicine, owing to its philosophical roots, never wished to achieve such ubiquity until this century. The reasons are sometimes obvious and sometimes obscure, but nonetheless are a result of what happened to the Chinese empire and civilization in general. For me, coming from the West, the study of Chinese medicine entailed more than studying a method or a technique. It encompassed the study of cultural nuances, behaviors, traditions, mind sets, concepts, and, above all, an "alien" way of thinking. It was a way of thinking for which I had no previous education or training. For me, Chinese medicine provided a systematic approach to the treatment of disease, and a deep and irreplaceable insight into the nature of the human body, together with its complexity of function and organization. It did not, however, provide me with a critical tool to help me test either its capacity or my own skill. I had to listen, internalize, trust, imitate, and then try. After all the years I've practiced, I still don't have conviction in the power of the medicine or in my own skill in practicing it.

The Thieme book *Practice of Acupuncture: Point Location—Treatment Options—TCM Basics*, by Drs Hans-Ulrich Hecker, Angelika Steveling, Elmar T. Peuker, and Joerg Kastner, is refreshingly informative and concise. Reading it, I felt that the authors had tried their best to write about what they knew with great humility. I also thought that they had done this with tremendous skill, producing only the known, accepted, and clinically useful information for the basics of acupuncture education. For the student of acupuncture, knowledge of the channels and the anatomical location of the acupuncture points are of utmost importance. Having the photographs and illustrations next to the anatomical description helps with accurate point location. Point functions are organized in a way that is easy to follow, and the text will not overwhelm any student. Particularly informative is the chapter "Pragmatic Five-Step Concept for Treating Locomotor Pain and Headaches." The concepts are described clearly and relate easily to the illustrations. Including figures in action as illustrations (rather than just invisible "non existent" structures) makes the concept of the channels far more tangible and reasonable. Leaving the more theoretical aspects to the end of the book offsets the usual way we learn Chinese medicine. It takes us straight to the basics, to the core of what an acupuncturist has to learn, that is, to establish an intimate relationship with clients and then to treat them with care.

From the outset, the book emphasizes a discrepancy between the modern theory of acupuncture's mechanism of action and the practice of acupuncture. Also, it states what most texts fail to mention: that acupuncture is a technique that can cause injuries. The authors detail, categorize, and illustrate the safety issues encountered by needling. Although the majority of injuries caused by acupuncture are rare, it is important that we do not discount them, that we know what they are in advance, and know how to avoid them. Then, perhaps, we can possibly start to think of quantifying them. The public deserves to know the precise risk of acupuncture. As an example, none of us can really tell the incidence and severity of pain caused by acupuncture needling. Even if it is a transient and mild pain, the concept of needling nevertheless produces such a high level of anxiety in so many people that they do not wish to even try acupuncture.

In summary, I highly recommend this text to both students and teachers as a basic text for acupuncture. I also recommend it to practitioners who want to have a text that can easily help them to refresh their knowledge of the points and concepts of Chinese medicine. I think this book is a bridge on the way to universalize Chinese medical education. The way it is written leaves no doubt that we need to learn from past knowledge as well as from future tests of our craft.

Contact Details

Isaac Cohen, OMD, LAc
Guest Scientist
Mt. Zion
Carol Frank Buck Breast Care Center
Comprehensive Cancer Center & Center for Reproductive Endocrinology
Department of Obstetrics and Gynecology
University of California
San Francisco, CA, USA

Nigel Wiseman, Feng Ye:
A Practical Dictionary of Chinese Medicine

Hardcover, 945 pages
Published 1998
ISBN: 0-912111-54-2
Including: extensive index ~ glossary
Paradigm Publications, Taos/New Mexico, USA

From the simple and common to the complex and rare, this book contains subtleties, distinctions, and nuances of Chinese medicine never found in beginners' texts. Whether for translational or clinical application, it presents the concepts of Chinese medicine exactly as they would come to the mind of a Chinese physician speaking or writing in their native language.

Arranged as a classical dictionary, definitions are provided in English alphabetical order and include the English term, the source Chinese term, its Pinyin transliteration (including spoken tone), pronounciation, etymology, and one or more definitions as applied in Chinese medicine. Terms used within definitions are cross-referenced and disease and symptom descriptions include the standard therapies applied in the People's Republic of China. Each definition is referenced to one or more Chinese source. In all, it lists the characters, Pinyin, translations, and definitions for

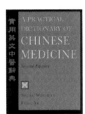

more than 10 000 medical concepts, including treatments for the patterns catalogued, 2000 formulas, 1700 natural drugs, and 1500 acupoints.

The definitions and treatments are drawn from clinically authoritative Chinese medical sources, all of which are cited. The many useful features include a full set of English common and commercial names for medicinal substances, as well as standard Latin scientific names. Western medical correspondences are noted, as is nomenclature put forward by the World Health Organization (WHO). The index is comprehensive and fully cross-referenced; it also includes lesser-used terms and nomenclature so it may be used as a translator's glossary. There is one foreword by Chen Keji, the pioneer of integrated Chinese medicine, and another by Paul Unschuld, the renowned sinologist.

This is a valuable work with a scope that is absolutely breathtaking. It will provide rapid access to an enormous amount of information for the student, researcher, or clinician, and is sure to become the new reference source for academic studies, international exchange, and training in Chinese medicine.

Fritz Smith: Alchemy of Touch

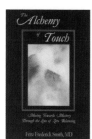

Trade paperback book, 216 pages
Published 2006
ISBN: 0-9673034-6-X
Including: index
Paradigm Publications, Taos/New Mexico, USA

Fritz Smith is the founder of the Zero Balancing method. In his latest book, *Alchemy of Touch,* he uses the "lens" of Zero Balancing to help practitioners move toward mastery in energy-based body work. Rather than a procedural manual, *Alchemy of Touch* is a guide to the universal principles of using touch, both to heal and to enable ourselves and others.

The book begins with a fascinating description of Dr Smith's own spiritual journey and awakening to the power of the spirit and the benefit of touch. In his experiences with Ida Rolf, J.R. Worsley, and initiation by Swami Muktananda, we see the roots of Zero Balancing in the ongoing revelation of his life. By sharing his personal journey in his own words, he establishes a foundation that invites the reader into a deeper exploration of touch and healing.

That deeper exploration takes the form of seven Zero Balancing sessions reported in two coordinated ways, first as the objective description of the session by experienced practitioners and observers, and second as the subjective impressions of the recipient. This unique format aptly illustrates the relationship between the body work and practitioner interaction with the experience of the recipient. We see how a fulcrum, a breath, or a well-timed question or instruction results in a deeper physical, emotional, and spiritual experience.

Each of the seven session chapters is interspersed with Fritz's expert observations about body work. Using Zero Balancing as a focus for experience, Fritz engages topics that broaden and deepen our understanding of the essential interchanges in body work—for example, energetic fields and their relationship to the "body–mind," the integration of energy and structure, how memory is retained in the body, and the various alchemies of body work. Like *yin* and *yang*, these alternating chapters make an integrated whole that advances our understanding of the body and our influences upon it.

Long awaited by Zero Balancing practitioners, and of infinite value to anyone who works with energy and the human body, this work is a most welcome contribution to the literature in the field.

Claus C. Schnorrenberger, Beate Schnorrenberger: Pocket Atlas of Tongue Diagnosis

Softcover, 320 pages with 189 illustrations
Published 2005
ISBN-10: 1-58890-357-5 / 3-13-139831-0
ISBN-13: 978-1-58890-357-0 /
978-3-13-139831-4
Thieme, Stuttgart–New York

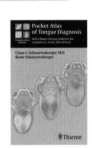

Tongue diagnosis dates back to the Shang dynasty. Together with taking the pulse, it has evolved into a very important tool of Chinese medical diagnosis.

This Color Atlas is concise and to the point. The first half explains individual tongue characteristics and the second half combines these characteristics in real case studies, thus deepening the reader's understanding of tongue diagnosis. The clearly written text is augmented by high-quality, full-color images.

With its compact and user-friendly form, this Color Atlas takes up very little space while at the same time containing a wealth of information of interest to physicians (practitioners) and students of both Chinese and Western scientific medicine.

162 color photographs of Westerners' tongues cleary show the truth of the Chinese proverb "*Bai wén bù rú yi jiàn*" (it is better to see [something] once than to hear [it] a hundred times).

See also "Tongue Diagnosis in Chinese Medicine," p. 88, Clinical Practice.

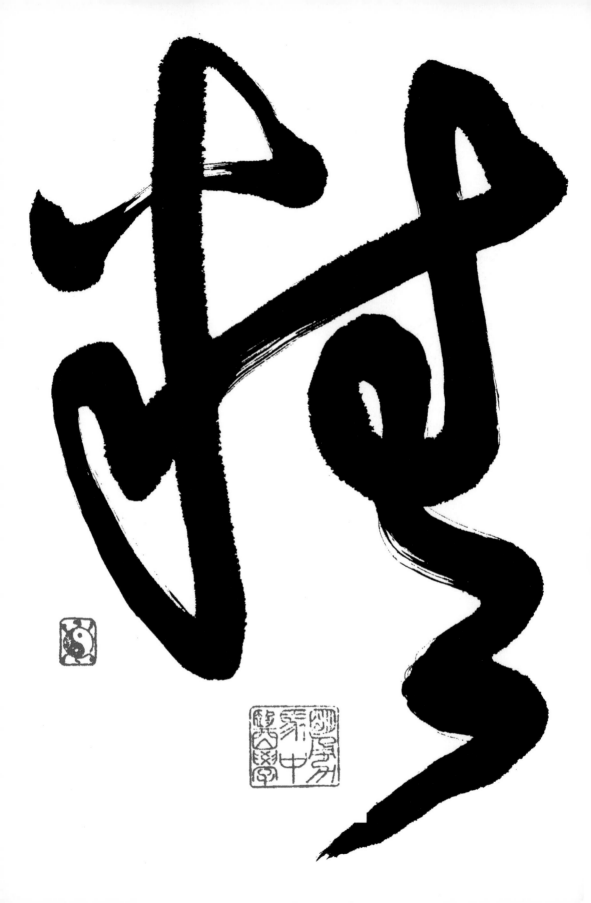

Professional Product and Supplier News

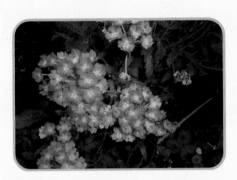

順天堂藥廠股份有限公司
SUN TEN PHARMACEUTICAL CO., LTD.

GMP

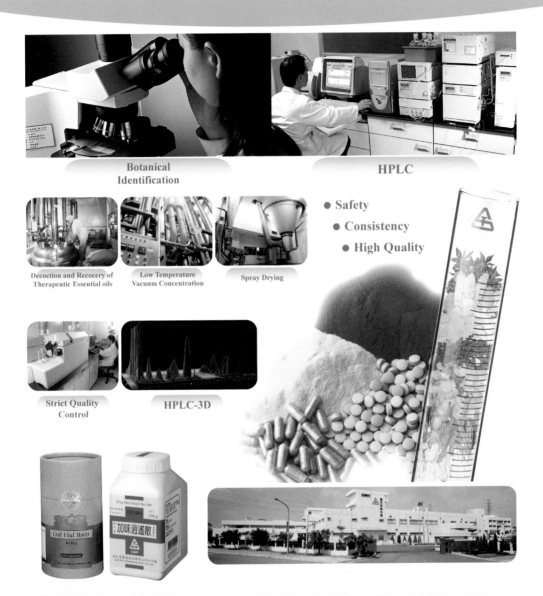

Botanical
Identification

HPLC

- Safety
- Consistency
- High Quality

Decoction and Recocery of
Therapeutic Essential oils

Low Temperature
Vacuum Concentration

Spray Drying

Strict Quality
Control

HPLC-3D

Sun Ten Pharmaceutical Co., Ltd. is a renowned GMP manufacturer of concentrated herbal extracts for 60 years. Sun Ten is dedicated to develop, manufacture, and market the Safe, High Quality, and Efficient natural herbal products for people around the world, because we care about human lives.

Address:3F, No. 11 Roosevelt Rd., Sec. 2, Taipei, Taiwan, R.O.C.
TEL:886-2-2395-7070
FAX:886-2-2321-1926
Website:www.suntenglobal.com

ISO 9001 : 2000
FM52539

3B Scientific and SEIRIN Working Together to Provide Best Quality, Best Value, and Best Service for Excellent Acupuncture Therapy

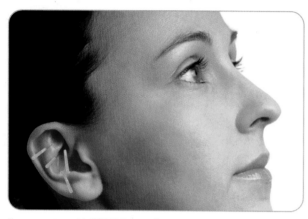

Ear acupuncture with SEIRIN B-Type needles.

The story of the widespread use of acupuncture in Europe started during the early 1980s. Its successful development has been accompanied every step of the way by the SEIRIN brand name.

SEIRIN introduced the first single use needle to the market and has consistently set the highest quality standards for acupuncture needles. The legendary insertion properties of the B-Type and J-Type needles are the reason why SEIRIN is the number one in the acupuncture market.

Additionally, SEIRIN is known for a range of other innovative products such as: the New Pyonex press needle and the SEIRIN Atlas of Acupuncture.

Acupuncture practitioners with an eye for quality believe in the safety and reliability of SEIRIN products. Therapists using SEIRIN needles often follow the Japanese acupuncture methods which are almost painless and stress free. The exceptional material properties and precision manufacturing of the needles make them the perfect product for achieving these goals.

Our partnership began in 2004, when the sole rights for European distribution of SEIRIN products were awarded to 3B Scientific and this has proved to be an excellent complement to the existing 3B Scientific product range.

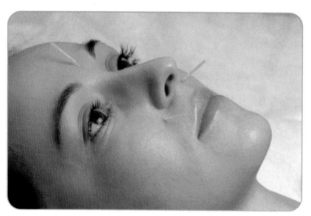

Best quality for excellent acupuncture therapy.

The 3B Scientific Group is the number one manufacturer of anatomical models and a leading supplier of scientific teaching and medical therapy aids. The 3B Scientific brand is well respected in over 100 countries.

Acupuncture models and anatomical charts perfectly complement the SEIRIN product range. The continuing success of 3B Scientific is a result of our commitment to produce and sell high-quality educational, scientific, and medical products at fair prices, such as the new Soft-Laser generation.

3B Scientific is working with many acupuncture societies and training bodies to maintain and increase the standards in acupuncture therapy. We are pleased to sponsor in partnership with ICMART (International Council of Medical Acupuncture and Related Techniques) the 3B Acupuncture Award. It is confered on the best lectures and scientific posters presented at the annual ICMART Congress. See also p. 249 and p. 273, Calendar.

Working with SEIRIN as our partner throughout Europe adds value to the three "b's" in our name, giving 3B Scientific one more reason to say we provide **b**est quality, **b**est value, and **b**est service.

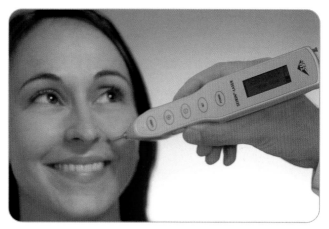
Point accuracy with the new Soft-Laser generation.

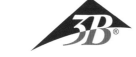
...going one step further

Headquarter: 3B Scientific GmbH
Rudorffweg 8
21031 Hamburg, Germany
www.3b-akupunktur.de
www.3bscientific.com

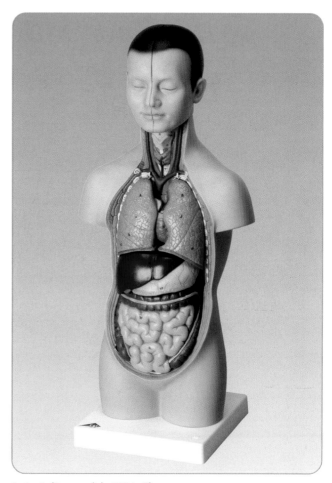
Anatomical torso made by 3B Scientific.

An international Traditional Chinese Medicine (TCM) congress is to take place for the first time in Denmark and will be part of a tradition set up to be followed for many years. The congress will be held from 6th to 9th September 2007 on the west coast of Denmark in a beautiful local seaside hotel.

The theme of this year's congress is "**Sexuality and Health**: Gynecology, Andrology, and the TCM Philosophy." The participants will have the opportunity to experience TCM at its best with international teachers from various countries, such as Norway, Germany, Switzerland, England, Israel, and America.

Lectures, workshops, and a variety of different events will take place all for the purpose of enhancing a higher level of understanding of sexuality and health in the field of TCM. Theoretical as well as practical aspects will be addressed. The overall purpose of the congress is to create a bond between the Scandinavian practitioners and the international TCM community.

The inspirational person behind this initiative is Marian R. Nielsen Joos, the founder of TCM Lectures, who, through her experience of promoting international lectures in Scandinavia, felt the need for an exchange of knowledge and networking.

Anybody from the international community is invited to join and enjoy this unique first International Scandinavian TCM Congress.

Website: www.tcm-kongres.dk

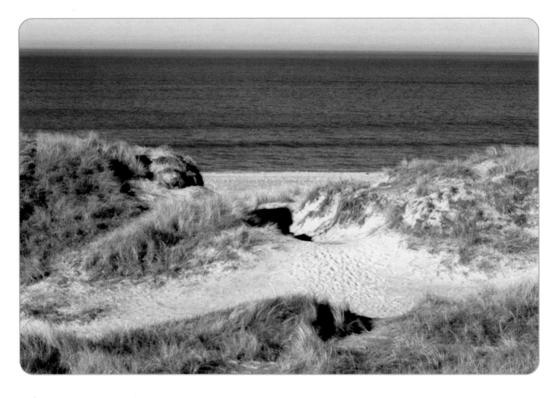

Redwing Book Company has served the complementary medicine professions for 30 years, making available to students, professionals, and institutions a full offering of books and media.

Our imprints, **Paradigm Publications** and **Complementary Medicine Press**, provide the field with translations of classical Chinese medicine, modern TCM texts, and works by sinologists, scholars, and practitioners renowned in their fields.

Paradigm Publications focuses on bringing the knowledge of Chinese medicine, both classical and modern, to the West through means of a thorough and exact terminology.

Complementary Medicine Press brings readers the voices, knowledge base, and skill of eminent teachers and practitioners.

In addition to worldwide ordering capability and full web access to information concerning the 1500 titles we carry, Redwing publishes a full-color printed catalog, *Redwing Reviews,* which allows readers to browse offerings in acupuncture, classical Chinese medicine, Asian healing, energetic arts, manual arts and traditions, energetic bodywork, homeopathy, flower remedies, and naturopathy.

Please view our websites, www.redwingbooks.com and www.paradigm-publications.com.

To regularly receive our printed catalogs, send your name and address via email to us at info@redwingbooks.com, or reach us by fax at 1.505.758.7768, and by voice at 1.505.758.7758.

If you wish to write us, please direct your correspondence to:
Redwing Book Company
202 Bendix St
Taos, NM 87571
USA

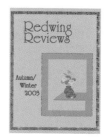

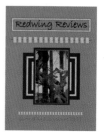

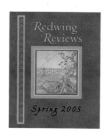

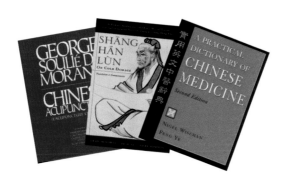

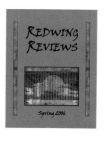

Expand Your Knowledge with These Thieme Titles

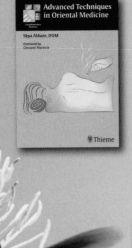

Skya Abbate

Advanced Techniques in Oriental Medicine

This uncommonly useful guidebook presents an overview of all aspects of needling, from the parameters of the needle itself to the importance of treating and anchoring the patient's spirit. Skya Abbate's clear language and detailed descriptions guide you step-by-step through thirteen categories of disease, ranging from anxiety, geriatric and chronic degenerative diseases to those illnesses thought to be untreatable.

Rounding out the text is a practical appendix with a glossary of Chinese medical terminology, sample instructions for patients, as well as an index with more than 2,000 disorders.

© 2006. 183 pages, 34 illustrations, hardcover
The Americas: ISBN 978-1-58890-493-5, US$ 59.95
Rest of World: ISBN 978-3-13-143051-9, € 49.95

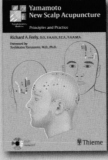

Richard A. Feely

Yamamoto New Scalp Acupuncture

Principles and Practice

Highlights include:

- DVD with easy-to-follow video instruction in point identification and palpatory training
- A laminated chart insert distinguishes YNSA points in color
- More than 70 figures and algorithms supplement descriptions of points and treatments

© 2007. 156 pages, 80 illustrations, hardcover
The Americas: ISBN 978-1-58890-297-9, US$ 69.95
Rest of World: ISBN 978-3-13-141831-9, € 59.95

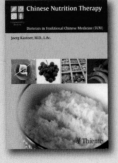

Joerg Kastner

Chinese Nutrition Therapy

Dietetics in Traditional Chinese Medicine (TCM)

This title includes a comprehensive classification of more than 300 readily available foods as well as:

- Descriptions of Chinese Dietetics in practice and discussions of dietary factors, such as seasonal adaptations and differing requirements for children and seniors
- Practical tips on how to adapt Chinese nutritional therapy to Western products and cooking methods
- A handy "A to Z" list of common foods and their healing characteristics.

© 2004. 288 pages, 20 illustrations, softcover
The Americas: ISBN 978-1-58890-107-1, US$ 44.95
Rest of World: ISBN 978-3-13-130961-7, € 39.95

Prices subject to change without notice.

www.thieme.com/cam

Thieme

Suppliers List

Company	Country	Products
3B Scientific GmbH	Germany	Acupuncture and/or Medical Supplies
Active eBase Pty Ltd	Australia	Acupuncture and/or Medical Supplies
Active Herb	USA	Herbal Product Lines
Acu-Market	USA	Acupuncture and/or Medical Supplies
Acumed	USA	Acupuncture and/or Medical Supplies
Acupuncture Medical Arts. LLC.	USA	Acupuncture and/or Medical Supplies
Akupunkturbedarf Karl Blum	Germany	Acupuncture and/or Medical Supplies
American Botanicals	USA	Herbal Product Lines
American Healing Technologies	USA	Herbal Product Lines
American Specialty Health	USA	Acupuncture and/or Medical Supplies
Asiamed Professional, L.P.	USA	Acupuncture and/or Medical Supplies
Austin medical Equipment	USA	Acupuncture and/or Medical Supplies
BI Nutraceuticals	USA	Research & Natural Products
Bio Essence Corporation	USA	Herbal Product Lines
BIOS PHARMACEUTICALS B.V.	Germany	Research & Natural Products
Biotics Research Corporation	USA	Research & Natural Products
Blue Poppy Enterprises	USA	Acupuncture and/or Medical Supplies
Brion Herbs Corporation	USA	Herbal Product Lines
Caesar & Loretz GmbH	Germany	Herbal Product Lines
Carbo Trading	Canada	Acupuncture and/or Medical Supplies
China Herb Company	USA	Herbal Product Lines
China Medical GmbH	Switzerland	Herbal Product Lines
China Natur	Germany	Herbal Product Lines
China Nature N.V.	Belgium	Herbal Product Lines
China Purmed GmbH	Germany	Acupuncture and/or Medical Supplies
Chinese Herbs	USA	Herbal Product Lines
Coastal Medical Supplies, Inc.	USA	Acupuncture and/or Medical Supplies
Complemedis AG	Switzerland	Herbal Product Lines
Cortex Scientific Botanicals	USA	Research & Natural Products
Crane Herb Company	USA	Herbal Product Lines
Cyano Biotech GmbH	Germany	Research & Natural Products
Deutscher Akupunktur Vertrieb GbR	Germany	Acupuncture and/or Medical Supplies
Equilibre	Belgium	Herbal Product Lines
Euroherbs	Netherlands	Herbal Product Lines
Evergreen Herbals	Netherlands	Herbal Product Lines
Evergreen Herbs and Medical Supplies	USA	Herbal Product Lines
Eyefive	USA	Acupuncture and/or Medical Supplies
Far East Summit	USA	Herbal Product Lines
Gaia Herbs	USA	Herbal Product Lines
Ginkgo Software	USA	Software
Go Acupuncture	USA	Acupuncture and/or Medical Supplies
Golden Flower Chinese Herbs	USA	Herbal Product Lines
Golden Sunshine USA	USA	Herbal Product Lines
Guangzhou Zhongyi Pharmaceutical Company Ltd	PRC	Research & Natural Products
Health Body World Supply, Inc.	USA	Acupuncture and/or Medical Supplies
Health Concerns	USA	Herbal Product Lines
Health Point Products	USA	Acupuncture and/or Medical Supplies
Heilpflanzenforschung	Germany	Herbal Product Lines
Helio Mecial Supplies, Inc.	USA	Acupuncture and/or Medical Supplies
Helio Supply Co. Pty Ltd	Australia	Acupuncture and/or Medical Supplies
Herb Product Store	USA	Herbal Product Lines
Herbal International	Australia	Herbal Product Lines
Herbcare Pty. Ltd	Australia	Herbal Product Lines
Hermann Heltschl GmbH	Austria	Acupuncture and/or Medical Supplies
Honso USA	USA	Research & Natural Products

Kamedis Laboratories Ltd	Israel	Research & Natural Products
K'An Herb Company	USA	Herbal Product Lines
Kenshin Trading Corporation	USA	Acupuncture and/or Medical Supplies
King Tim International	Australia	Herbal Product Lines
KPC	USA	Herbal Product Lines
Kronen Apotheke Wuppertal	Germany	Herbal Product Lines
Kunming Shenghuo Pharmaceutical Co., Ltd	PRC	Research & Natural Products
LASERneedle	Switzerland	Acupuncture and/or Medical Supplies
Leader Trading Pty Ltd	Australia	Herbal Product Lines
Lhasa OMS, Inc.	USA	Acupuncture and/or Medical Supplies
LIAN Chinaherb	Switzerland	Herbal Product Lines
Lotusherbs	USA	Herbal Product Lines
Marknew Products	USA	Acupuncture and/or Medical Supplies
Martin Bauer GmbH & Co. KG	Germany	Herbal Product Lines
MayWay Chinese Herbs and Herbal Products	USA	Herbal Product Lines
MB North America	USA	Herbal Product Lines
Medic Herb UK Ltd	UK	Herbal Product Lines
Medichin	Belgium	Acupuncture and/or Medical Supplies
Nalbolaget	Sweden	Acupuncture and/or Medical Supplies
Nereus Pharmaceuticals, Inc.	USA	Research & Natural Products
Nuherbs Co.	USA	Herbal Product Lines
OHCO Oriental Herb Company	USA	Herbal Product Lines
Oxford Medical Supplies, Ltd.	UK	Acupuncture and/or Medical Supplies
P.P.C. (Galway) Ltd.	Ireland	Acupuncture and/or Medical Supplies
Pantheon Research	USA	Acupuncture and/or Medical Supplies
PharmaChin GmbH	Germany	Acupuncture and/or Medical Supplies
PhytoComm	Germany	Herbal Product Lines
Plant Bioactives Research Institute	USA	Research & Natural Products
Prime Herbs Corporation	USA	Herbal Product Lines
Quality Chinese Herbs	USA	Herbal Product Lines
Renaissance Herbs, Inc.	USA	Herbal Product Lines
Royal Dynasty Tea	USA	Herbal Product Lines
Schwa-Medico GmbH	Germany	Acupuncture and/or Medical Supplies
Sedatelec	France	Acupuncture and/or Medical Supplies
SEIRIN Corporation	Japan	Acupuncture and/or Medical Supplies
Shanghai Herbs Group Ltd	UK	Acupuncture and/or Medical Supplies
Shulan UK Ltd	UK	Acupuncture and/or Medical Supplies
SINECURA	Belgium	Herbal Product Lines
Sun Ten Herb	TW	Herbal Product Lines
Superdragon TCM UK Ltd	UK	Acupuncture and/or Medical Supplies
Taodao	Germany	Acupuncture and/or Medical Supplies
Taomedic Software Int. Ltd	Isarel	Software
TCMWindows	USA	Software
The Green Medicine Company	USA	Herbal Product Lines
The Herbalist	USA	Herbal Product Lines
The Supply Center	USA	Acupuncture and/or Medical Supplies
Thorne Research	USA	Research & Natural Products
TIDhealth	USA	Herbal Product Lines
Unigen Pharmaceuticals	USA	Research & Natural Products

Disclaimer

Thieme Publishers does not take any responsibility regarding the quality of the products provided from the companies listed above.

Please note the product column is only a *rough guide* to the types of products that may be found or produced by listed companies.

To have your company listed in the *Thieme Almanac 2008* or to place an advert, please send an email to request more information to almanac@thieme.com.